Epidemiology

An Introduction

To Emily, Margaret, and Samantha

PREFACE TO SECOND EDITION

Some observers appear to believe that epidemiology is no more than the application of statistical methods to the problems of disease occurrence and causation. But epidemiology is much more than applied statistics. It is a scientific discipline with roots in biology, logic, and the philosophy of science. For epidemiologists, statistical methods serve as an important tool but not a foundation. My aim in this book is to present a simple overview of the concepts that are the underpinnings of epidemiology, so that a coherent picture of epidemiologic thinking emerges for the student. The emphasis is not on statistics, formulas, or computation but on epidemiologic principles and concepts.

For some, epidemiology is too simple to warrant serious attention, and for others it is too convoluted to understand. I hope to persuade the reader that neither view is correct. The first chapter illustrates that epidemiology is more than just applying "common sense," unless one has uncommonly good common sense. Although it is unusual to begin an epidemiology text with a presentation of confounding, I believe that the problem of confounding exemplifies why we need to understand epidemiologic principles lest we fall victim to fallacious inferences. At the other extreme, those who believe that epidemiology is too complicated might think differently if they had a unifying set of ideas that extended across the many separate topics within epidemiology. My goal in this book has been to provide that unifying set of ideas.

The second chapter, new to this second edition, adds a historical perspective for the reader who is new to epidemiology, in the form of capsule profiles of pioneers in epidemiology and public health. The chapter illustrates the deep historical roots of epidemiology, highlighting important contributions from trailblazers such as Avicenna, Graunt, Nightingale, and Lane-Claypon. Chapter 3 lays a conceptual foundation by elucidating a general model of causation and discussing the process of causal inference. All too often, these concepts are skipped over in scientific education. Nevertheless, for epidemiologists they are bedrock concerns that belong in any introduction to the field. Chapter 4 continues with a description of the basic epidemiologic measures, and Chapter 5 covers the main study types. An important thread for the student is the emphasis on measurement and how to reduce or describe measurement error. Chapter 6, also new to the second edition, presents a capsule summary of the key ideas in infectious disease epidemiology.

The next two chapters deal with measurement error. Systematic error, or bias, is treated first, in Chapter 7, and random error in Chapter 8. Chapter 9 introduces the basic analytic methods for estimating epidemiologic effects; these methods are extended in Chapter 10 to stratified data. Chapters 11 and 12 address the more advanced topics of interaction and regression modeling. These are subjects to be explored in detail in more advanced courses, but their presentation here in elementary terms lays the groundwork for advanced study. It also draws a boundary between the epidemiologic approach to these topics and nonepidemiologic approaches that can take the analysis in the wrong direction. The final chapter deals with clinical epidemiology, a branch of epidemiology that continues to grow in scope and importance.

Epidemiologic concepts are evolving, as any comparison of this volume with earlier texts will reveal. To complement the book, the publisher has graciously agreed to host a Website that will support reader participation in discussing, extending, and revising points presented in the book. The Website will post contributed answers to the questions raised at the end of each chapter in the text. Interested readers can find this site at www.oup.com/us/epi/.

Along the way I have received invaluable feedback from many students and colleagues. I am especially grateful to Kristin Anderson, Georgette Baghdady, Dan Brooks, Robert Green, Sander Greenland, Tizzy Hatch, Bettie Nelson, Ya-Fen Purvis, Igor Schillevoort, Bahi Takkouche, and Noel Weiss. Cristina Cann provided unflagging and generous encouragement; now that she is no longer here to continue advising me, she is sorely missed. Katarina Bälter deserves special mention for her careful reading of the manuscript and patient, helpful criticisms. Finally, I am indebted to my colleague Janet Lang, who gently prodded me at the right time and was an inspiration throughout.

Kenneth J. Rothman
Newton, Massachusetts
July, 2011

CONTENTS

Epidemiology

An Introduction

Introduction to
Epidemiologic Thinking

This book presents the basic concepts and methods of epidemiology, which is the core science of public health. Epidemiology has been defined as "the study of the distribution and determinants of disease frequency,"[1] or even more simply as "the study of the occurrence of illness."[2]

The principles of epidemiologic research appear deceptively simple. This appearance seduces some people into believing that anyone can master epidemiology just by applying some common sense. In a way that view is correct, but it is nevertheless an oversimplification. The problem is that the kind of common sense that is required may be elusive without training in epidemiologic concepts and methods. As a means of introducing epidemiologic thinking, I shall illustrate this point with some examples of the fundamental epidemiologic concept known as *confounding*. Confounding is described in greater detail in Chapter 7. Here I aim only to demonstrate the kind of problem that epidemiology deals with routinely. I will also point out some basic fallacies, the kind that can be found in the newspapers on a regular basis and that occur commonly among those who are not well versed in epidemiologic thinking.

Common sense tells us that residents of Sweden, where the standard of living is generally high, should have lower death rates than residents of Panama, where poverty and more limited health care take their toll. Surprisingly, however, a greater proportion of Swedish residents than Panamanian residents die each year. This fact belies common sense. The explanation lies in the age distribution of the populations of Sweden and Panama. Figure 1–1 shows the population pyramids of the two countries. A *population pyramid* displays the age distribution of a population graphically. The population pyramid for Panama tapers dramatically from younger to older age groups, reflecting the fact that most Panamanians are in the younger age categories. In contrast, the population pyramid of Sweden is more rectangular, with roughly the same number of people in each of the age categories up to about age 60 years and some tapering above that age. As these graphs

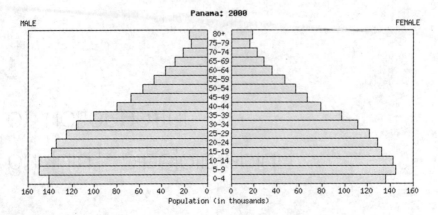

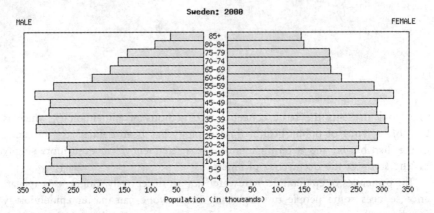

Figure 1–1   Age distribution of the populations of Panama and Sweden (population pyramids).
SOURCE: U.S. Census Bureau, International Data Base.

make clear, Swedes tend to be older than Panamanians. For people of the same age in the two countries, the death rate among Swedes is indeed lower than that of Panamanians, but in both places older people die at a greater rate than younger people. Because Sweden has a population that is on the average older than that of Panama, a greater proportion of all Swedes die in a given year, despite the lower death rates within age categories in Sweden compared with Panama.

This situation illustrates what epidemiologists call *confounding*. In this example, age differences between the countries are confounding the differences in death rates. Confounding occurs commonly in epidemiologic comparisons. Consider the following mortality data, summarized from a study that looked at smoking habits of residents of Whickham, England, in the period 1972–1974 and then tracked the survival over the next 20 years of those who were interviewed.[3-5] Among 1314 women in the survey, almost half were smokers. Oddly, proportionately fewer of the smokers died during the ensuing 20 years than nonsmokers. The data are reproduced in Table 1–1.

Only 24% of the women who were smokers at the time of the initial survey died during the 20-year follow-up period. In contrast, 31% of those who were

Table 1-1 RISK OF DEATH IN A 20-YEAR PERIOD
AMONG WOMEN IN WHICKHAM, ENGLAND,
ACCORDING TO SMOKING STATUS AT THE
BEGINNING OF THE PERIOD*

	Smoking		
Vital Status	Yes	No	Total
Dead	139	230	369
Alive	443	502	945
Total	582	732	1314
Risk (Dead/Total)	0.24	0.31	0.28

*Data from Vanderpump et al.[5]

nonsmokers died during the follow-up period. Does this difference indicate that women who were smokers fared better than women who were not smokers? Not necessarily. One difficulty that many researchers quickly spot is that the smoking information was obtained only once, at the start of the follow-up period. Smoking habits for some women will have changed during the follow-up. Could those changes explain the results that appear to confer an advantage on the smokers? It is theoretically possible that all or many of the smokers quit soon after the survey and that many of the nonsmokers started smoking. Although this scenario is possible, it is implausible; without evidence for these changes in smoking behavior, this implausible scenario is not a reasonable criticism of the study findings. A more realistic explanation for the unusual finding becomes clear if we examine the data within age categories, as shown in Table 1-2. (The risks for each age group are calculated by dividing the number who died in each smoking group by the total number of those dead or alive.)

Table 1-1 combines all of the age categories listed in Table 1-2 into a single table, which is called the *crude* data. It is obtained by adding together, or collapsing, the data for each age category in Table 1-2. The more detailed display of the same data in Table 1-2 is called an *age-specific* display, or a display *stratified* by age. The age-specific data show that in the youngest and oldest age categories there was little difference between smokers and nonsmokers in risk of death. Few died among those in the youngest age categories, regardless of whether they were smokers or not, whereas among the oldest women, almost everyone died during the 20 years of follow-up. For women in the middle age categories, however, there was a consistently greater risk of death among smokers than nonsmokers, a pattern contrary to the impression gained from the crude data in Table 1-1.

Why did the nonsmokers have a higher risk of death in the study population as a whole? The reason is evident in Table 1-2: A much greater proportion of the nonsmoking women were in the highest age categories, the categories that contributed a proportionately greater number of deaths. The difference in age distribution between smokers and nonsmokers reflects the fact that, for most people, lifelong smoking habits are determined early in life. During the decades preceding the study in Whickham, there was a trend for increasing proportions of young women to become smokers. The oldest women in the Whickham study grew up during a period when few women became smokers, and they tended to remain nonsmokers for the duration of their lives. As time went by, a greater proportion

Table 1–2 RISK OF DEATH IN A 20-YEAR PERIOD AMONG
WOMEN IN WHICKHAM, ENGLAND, ACCORDING TO SMOKING
STATUS AT THE BEGINNING OF THE PERIOD, BY AGE

| Age | Vital Status | Smoking | | Total |
		Yes	No	
18–24	Dead	2	1	3
	Alive	53	61	114
	Risk	0.04	0.02	0.03
25–34	Dead	3	5	8
	Alive	121	152	273
	Risk	0.02	0.03	0.03
35–44	Dead	14	7	21
	Alive	95	114	209
	Risk	0.13	0.06	0.09
45–54	Dead	27	12	39
	Alive	103	66	169
	Risk	0.21	0.15	0.19
55–64	Dead	51	40	91
	Alive	64	81	145
	Risk	0.44	0.33	0.39
65–74	Dead	29	101	130
	Alive	7	28	35
	Risk	0.81	0.78	0.79
75+	Dead	13	64	77
	Alive	0	0	0
	Risk	1.00	1.00	1.00

of women who were passing through their teenage or young adult years became
smokers. The result was strikingly different age distributions for the female smokers and nonsmokers of Whickham. Were this difference in the age distribution
ignored, one might conclude erroneously that smoking was not related to a higher
risk of death. In fact, smoking is related to a higher risk of death, but confounding
by age has obscured this relation in the crude data of Table 1–1. In Chapter 10,
I will return to these data and show how to calculate the effect of smoking on
the risk of death after removal of the age confounding.

Confounding is a problem that pervades many epidemiologic studies, but it is
by no means the only issue that bedevils epidemiologic inferences. One day, readers of the Boston Globe opened the paper to find a feature story about orchestra
conductors. The point of the article was that conducting an orchestra is salubrious,
as evinced by the fact that so many well-known orchestra conductors have lived
to be extremely old. Common sense suggests that if the people in an occupation
tend to live long lives, the occupation must be good for health. Unfortunately,
what appeared to be common sense for the author of the article is not very sensible from an epidemiologic point of view. The long-lived conductors who were
cited in the article were mentioned because they lived to be old. Citing selected
examples in this way constitutes anecdotal information, which can be extremely
misleading. For all we know, the reporter searched specifically for examples of

elderly conductors and overlooked other conductors who might have died at an earlier age. Most epidemiologists would not even classify anecdotal information as epidemiologic data at all.

Furthermore, the reporter's observation had problems that went beyond the reliance on anecdotes instead of a formal evaluation. Suppose that the reporter had identified all orchestra conductors who worked in the United States during the past 100 years and studied their longevity. This approach avoids relying on hand-picked examples, but it still suffers from an important problem that leads to an incorrect answer. The problem is that orchestra conductors are not born as orchestra conductors. They become conductors at a point in their careers when they may have already attained a respectable age. If we start with a group of people who are 40 years old, on the average they are likely to survive to an older age than the typical person who was just born. Why? Because they have a 40-year head start; if they had died before age 40, they could not have been part of a group in which everyone is 40 years old. To determine whether conducting an orchestra is beneficial to health, one should compare the risk of death among orchestra conductors with the risk of death among other people who have attained the same age as the conductors. Simply noting the average age at death of the conductors gives the wrong answer, even if all orchestra conductors in a population are studied.

Here is another example that makes this point clearly. Suppose that we study two groups of people over a period of 1 year, and we look at the average age at death among those who die during that year. Suppose that in group A the average age at death is 4 years and in group B it is 38 years. Can we say that being a member of group A is riskier than being a member of group B? We cannot, for the same reason that the age at death of orchestra conductors was misleading. Suppose that group A comprises nursery school students and group B comprises firefighters. It would be no surprise that the average age at death of people who are currently firefighters is 38 years or that the average age at death of people who are currently nursery school students is 4 years. Still, we suspect that being a firefighter is riskier than being a nursery school student and that these data on the average age at death do not address the issue of which of these groups faces a greater risk of death. When one looks at the average age at death, one looks only at those who actually die and ignores all those who survive. Consequently, the average age at death does not reflect the risk of death but only expresses a characteristic of those who die.

In a study of factory workers, an investigator inferred that the factory work was dangerous because the average age at onset of a particular kind of cancer was lower in these workers than among the general population. But just as for the nursery students and firefighters, if these workers were young, the cancers that occurred among them would have to be occurring in young people. Furthermore, the age at onset of a disease does not take into account what proportion of people get the disease. It may have been that the number of workers who developed the cancer was no greater, or was even smaller, than the number expected to do so based on the risk of cancer in the general population. Looking at the age at which cancer develops among those who get cancer cannot address the question of risk for cancer.

These examples reflect the fallacy of comparing the average age at which death or disease strikes, rather than comparing the risk of death between groups of the same age. In later chapters, I will explore the proper way to make epidemiologic comparisons. The point of these examples is to illustrate that what may appear to be a commonsense approach to a simple problem can be overtly wrong until we educate our common sense to appreciate better the nature of the problem. Any sensible person can understand epidemiology, but without considering the principles outlined in this book, even a sensible person using what appears to be common sense is apt to go astray. By mastering a few fundamental epidemiologic principles, it is possible to refine our common sense to avoid these traps.

QUESTIONS

1. Age is a variable that is often responsible for confounding in epidemiology, in part because the occurrence of many diseases changes with age. The change in disease risk with age is often referred to as the effect of age. Does it make sense to think of age as having an effect on disease risk, or is it more sensible to think that the effect of age is itself confounded by other factors?

2. More people in Los Angeles die from cardiovascular disease each year than do people in San Francisco. What is the most important explanation for this difference? What additional factors would you consider to explain the difference in the number of deaths?

3. In Table 1–2, which age group would you say shows the greatest effect of smoking on the risk of death during the 20-year interval? How have you defined "greatest effect"? What other way could you have defined it? Does your answer depend on which definition you use?

4. On a piece of graph paper, use the data in Table 1–2 to plot the 20-year risk of death against age. Put age on the horizontal axis and the 20-year risk of death on the vertical axis. Describe the shape of the curve. What biological forces account for the shape?

5. A physician who was interested in jazz studied the age at death of jazz musicians, whom he identified from an encyclopedia of jazz. He found that the average age at death of the jazz musicians was about the same as that in the general population. He concluded that this finding refuted the prevailing wisdom that jazz musicians tended to live dissolute lives and therefore experienced greater mortality than other people. Explain his error.

6. A researcher determined that being left-handed was dangerous, because he found that the average age at death of left-handers was lower than that of right-handers. Was he correct? Why or why not?

7. What is the underlying problem in comparing the average age at death, or the average age at which a person gets a specific disease, between two populations? How should you avert this problem?

REFERENCES

1. MacMahon B, Pugh TF. *Epidemiology: Principles and Methods.* Boston: Little, Brown; 1970:137–198,175–184.
2. Gaylord Anderson, as cited in: Cole P. The evolving case-control study. *J Chron Dis.* 1979;32:15–27.
3. Appleton DR, French JM, Vanderpump MPJ. Ignoring a covariate: an example of Simpson's paradox. *Am Statistician.* 1996;50:340–341.
4. Turnbridge WMG, Evered DC, Hall R, et al. The spectrum of thyroid disease in a community. *Clin Endocrinol.* 1977;7:481–493.
5. Vanderpump MPJ, Turnbridge WMG, French JM, et al. The incidence of thyroid disorders in the community: a twenty-year follow-up of the Whickham survey. *Clin Endocrinol.* 1995;43:55–69.

2

Pioneers in Epidemiology and
Public Health

*Throughout human history, the major problems of health that men have
faced have been concerned with community life, for instance, the control of
transmissible disease, the control and improvement of the physical environment (sanitation), the provision of water and food of good quality and in
sufficient supply, the provision of medical care, and the relief of disability and
destitution. The relative emphasis placed on each of these problems has varied
from time to time, but they are all closely related, and from them has come
public health as we know it today.*

GEORGE ROSEN, *A History of Public Health,* 1958[1]

ORIGINS OF PUBLIC HEALTH

Public health may be defined as the community effort to protect, maintain, and
improve the health of a population by organized means, including preventive programs, hygiene, education, and other interventions. Preventive medicine and health
care are important components of public health, but the reach of public health
extends beyond medicine to clean water, sanitation, housing, sex education, and
other areas that affect the health of communities. Among the fields that contribute to public health, epidemiology plays a crucial role, but many other disciplines
are involved. Public-health efforts may involve contributions from fields as diverse
as engineering, architecture, biology, social science, ecology, and economics.

The origin of public health dates from the first aggregation of small clans into
larger, settled communities. Some basic needs, such as provision of potable water
and disposal of bodily waste, were best addressed as community concerns. Public
wells that provided clean water for drinking and aqueducts that transported water
from mountain springs or creeks into towns, cities, and agricultural fields were
community efforts that had obvious health benefits. Fountains, public baths,

and water delivery systems supplying individual homes were features of ancient civilizations in the Indus River valley, Mesopotamia, Persia, Troy, and China.

Treatment of drinking water in settling basins and purification with chemicals was practiced in many early civilizations. Sanitary removal of human and animal waste is a fundamental public-health concern, one that became more challenging as settlements increased in size. The construction of sewers to remove waste materials was also common in antiquity. In ancient Rome, water delivery and sanitation were sophisticated engineering feats. Roman aqueducts brought mountain water from sources as far away as 100 km or more to the city, using trenches, arched bridges, walls, tunnels, and siphons to traverse varied landscapes. The water supplied a few wealthy homes, public baths, and public fountains, from which it overflowed to flush the streets. Excess water collected into a remarkable sewer system, culminating in the *cloaca maxima* (literally, "greatest sewer"), which conveyed effluent from the city into the Tiber River, facilitating hygiene for the city, though at the expense of polluting the river. Parts of the cloaca maxima are still connected to the Roman sewage system in the 21st century. Water supply and sanitation remain essential concerns for large communities and rank as top priorities for public health today. Among those still afflicted by poverty, and with the planet facing continued population growth and mounting environmental concerns, the basic public-health needs of clean water and sanitation are unlikely to recede in importance.

Another basic public-health priority has been control of transmissible diseases. Historically, community efforts to prevent the spread of communicable disease were often hampered by inadequate understanding of effective means to control transmission. The microbial origin of many transmissible diseases became evident only during the latter part of the 19th century. Nevertheless, concern about disease transmission and measures to control it has deep roots. In the Middle Ages, the growth of cities in Europe was accompanied by epidemics of leprosy, plague, and other scourges that stirred frightened populations into drastic actions, not often successful. The Black Death was a pandemic of what is believed to be bubonic plague that swept Europe in the mid–14th century. Although its cause was not clear to medieval populations, who tended to see epidemics as divine wrath, it was considered transmissible, which led communities to bar entry to foreigners from plague-ridden areas and to isolate patients and all their contacts. During periods when plague threatened Venice, an important shipping port, all vehicles, goods, and travelers were isolated for a period of time. This procedure, today called *quarantine* (from the Italian phrase *quaranta dei*, meaning "40 days"), is still invoked occasionally. It was used to notable advantage during the outbreak of severe acute respiratory syndrome (SARS) in 2003[2] (see Chapter 6).

FROM HIPPOCRATES TO SNOW AND THE MODERN DAY

Although public health has its origins in antiquity and epidemiology is considered by many to be the fundamental science of public health, epidemiology did not develop noticeably as a scientific discipline until the 20th century. Nonetheless, certain signal contributions to public health and epidemiology represented long-lasting, important increments to our outlook and understanding. Here we review highlights from some of the key contributors to the foundation of public health.

Hippocrates (~460–370 BC)

Hippocrates was a Greek physician who had a profound influence on the practice of medicine as well as on public health. Scholars believe that many of the surviving writings that are nominally attributed to Hippocrates were authored by others, probably his students. Nevertheless, these writings were undoubtedly influenced by Hippocrates and reflect a revolutionary approach to health and disease that Hippocrates helped to bring about. The prevailing view in the time of Hippocrates was that disease was the result of demonic possession or divine displeasure. Hippocrates turned attention to earthly causes. Greek physicians in Hippocrates' day were itinerant. Hippocrates advised these physicians to consider what environmental factors in each community might affect locally occurring diseases. For example, in *Airs, Waters, and Places,* the influence of the environment on disease occurrence was stressed for the first time in a scholarly treatise[3]:

> Whoever wishes to investigate medicine properly, should proceed thus: in the first place to consider the seasons of the year, and what effects each of them produces for they are not at all alike, but differ much from themselves in regard to their changes. Then the winds, the hot and the cold, especially such as are common to all countries, and then such as are peculiar to each locality. We must also consider the qualities of the waters, for as they differ from one another in taste and weight, so also do they differ much in their qualities. In the same manner, when one comes into a city to which he is a stranger, he ought to consider its situation, how it lies as to the winds and the rising of the sun; for its influence is not the same whether it lies to the north or the south, to the rising or to the setting sun. These things one ought to consider most attentively, and concerning the waters which the inhabitants use, whether they be marshy and soft, or hard, and running from elevated and rocky situations, and then if saltish and unfit for cooking; and the ground, whether it be naked and deficient in water, or wooded and well watered, and whether it lies in a hollow, confined situation, or is elevated and cold; and the mode in which the inhabitants live, and what are their pursuits, whether they are fond of drinking and eating to excess, and given to indolence, or are fond of exercise and labor, and not given to excess in eating and drinking ...
>
> And in particular, as the season and the year advances, he can tell what epidemic diseases will attack the city, either in summer or in winter, and what each individual will be in danger of experiencing from the change of regimen. For knowing the changes of the seasons, the risings and settings of the stars, how each of them takes place, he will be able to know beforehand what sort of a year is going to ensue. Having made these investigations, and knowing beforehand the seasons, such a one must be acquainted with each particular, and must succeed in the preservation of health, and be by no means unsuccessful in the practice of his art.

Many of the specific theories espoused in the writings that are attributed to Hippocrates would seem strange to modern readers. He believed it important to study astrology, with each astrological sign being associated with a part of the body. He also embraced the theory of humors, which held that when one of the four humors (black bile, phlegm, yellow bile, and blood) was out of balance, disease resulted. Although such theories are not in accord with modern views of disease, Hippocrates fostered a sea change away from mysticism and religion toward observation and reason as means of understanding the causes of disease.

Avicenna (Ibn Sina) (980–1037)

Avicenna, or Ibn Sina, a Persian philosopher, scientist, and physician, lived during the time that Europe was plodding through the Dark Ages, with science in full retreat. But in the Islamic world, it was a golden age of knowledge, to which Avicenna was a major contributor. A prolific genius, he wrote on many topics, foremost among them medicine and health. He is not identified specifically with public health, but, like Hippocrates, his contributions to the understanding of disease causation and his emphasis on empirical evidence had an enormous influence on both medicine and public health. His 14-volume *Canon of Medicine* is perhaps the most renowned textbook of medicine ever written. It was translated into Latin in 1187 and had a long-lasting influence in both the East and the West. In Europe, it was the primary medical text for centuries and was still in use as late as 1650.

Avicenna emphasized the need for bringing experimentation and quantification into the study of physiology and medicine. He inferred from his observations that some infectious diseases were spread by contagion, and he suggested the use of quarantine to limit their spread. The following excerpt from the introduction to Avicenna's *Canon of Medicine* shows the influence of Hippocrates and his embrace of scientific study. In it, one can easily see the foreshadowing of modern epidemiologic theory[4]:

> The knowledge of anything, since all things have causes, is not acquired or complete unless it is known by its causes. Therefore in medicine we ought to know the causes of sickness and health. And because health and sickness and their causes are sometimes manifest, and sometimes hidden and not to be comprehended except by the study of symptoms, we must also study the symptoms of health and disease. Now it is established in the sciences that no knowledge is acquired save through the study of its causes and beginnings, if it has had causes and beginnings; nor completed except by knowledge of its accidents and accompanying essentials. ... These are the subjects of the doctrine of medicine; whence one inquires concerning the disease and curing of the human body. One ought to attain perfection in this research; namely, how health may be preserved and sickness cured. And the causes of this kind are rules in eating and drinking, and the choice of air, and the measure of exercise and rest; and doctoring with medicines and doctoring with the hands. All this with physicians is according to three species: the well, the sick, and the medium of whom we have spoken.

Fracastoro (1478–1553)

The Renaissance physician and poet Fracastoro, from Verona, extended the concept of contagion by suggesting a theory about how contagious disease spreads. In his master work, *De contagione et contagiosis morbis et curatione*, which was published in 1546, he described many diseases, such as plague, typhus, and syphilis, that were transmitted from person to person, and he suggested a theory that disease was spread through self-replicating particles. He postulated that these particles, which he called *seminaria*, or seeds, were too small to see and were specific for each disease. His theory was the forerunner of the germ theory, although he had no concept that the seminaria were alive. He suggested that seminaria could infest an environment and could spread disease by direct person-to-person contact, by indirect contact with articles he called *fomites* (a term still in use for contaminated articles), and by transmission at a distance (eg, through air or water).

He thought that atmospheric conditions could influence the ability of the seminaria to spread and cause epidemics, an idea that traces back to Hippocrates, although for Hippocrates the causal role of airs and waters was more definitive.

Despite the importance of *De contagione*, Fracastoro is best known for his earlier epic poem *Syphilis sive morbus Gallicus* ("Syphilis or the French Disease"). This Latin verse was one of the most celebrated poems of the Renaissance, but at the same time it was a clinical dissertation on this new disease that had spread rapidly through Europe in the early years of the 16th century. He discussed the known treatments for syphilis, which included mercury and a New World treatment called *guaiacum*. The poem includes a detailed discussion of Columbus' voyage of discovery, not because of Columbus' possible role in importing syphilis to Europe but because the source of guaiacum was the New World that Columbus had explored.

John Graunt (1620–1674)

A London haberdasher by trade, John Graunt is known as the world's first epidemiologist and demographer. His avocation as a scientist led him to focus on an available data resource, the weekly *Bills of Mortality*, which summarized data collected in the parishes of London and later throughout England, originally to monitor deaths from the plague. The list included baptisms and deaths by cause in each parish. The collection of these data had begun late in the 15th century (uninterruptedly from 1603), and continued until the 19th century, when they were superseded by a more formal registration system (see section on William Farr). Graunt realized that much could be learned from a compilation of the data, thus setting a tradition for epidemiologists who still seek to use already collected data for epidemiologic research.

He published only one work based on his research, but this small volume contained an impressive number of original findings. The book had the unwieldy title *Natural and Political Observations Mentioned in a Following Index, and Made Upon the Bills of Mortality*. It included the first observation that more boys are born than girls. It presented the first actuarial table. It included the first reports of time trends for various diseases, adjusting for population size. He noted that some diseases changed in frequency because of changes in disease classification, as opposed to natural phenomena. He gave the first estimate of the population of London, demonstrating that it was growing rapidly through immigration rather than by an increase in births. He offered evidence to refute the theory that plague epidemics accompany the crowning of a new king. And he noted that physicians see more female patients than male patients.

Although Graunt was an amateur scientist, he had a natural appreciation for the fine points of epidemiology. For example, he was meticulous in describing the method of data collection for the *Bills of Mortality*[5]:

These *Bills* were Printed and published, not onely every week on *Thursdays*, but also a general Accompt of the whole Year given in, upon the *Thursday* before *Christmas Day*: which said general Accompts have been presented in the several manners following, *viz.* from the Year 1603, to the Year 1624, *inclusive* ...

We have hitherto described the several steps, whereby the *Bills of Mortality* are come up to their present state; we come next to shew how they are made, and composed, which is in this manner, *viz.*

When any one dies, then, either by tolling, or ringing of a Bell, or by bespeaking of a Grave of the *Sexton*, the same is known to the *Searchers*, corresponding with the said *Sexton*.

The *Searchers* hereupon (who are antient Matrons, sworn to their Office) repair to the place, where the dead Corps lies, and by view of the same, and by other enquiries, they examine by what *Disease*, or *Casualty* the Corps died. Hereupon they make their Report to the *Parish-Clerk*, and he, every *Tuesday* night, carries in an Accompt of all the *Burials*, and *Christnings*, hapning that Week, to the *Clerk* of the *Hall*. On *Wednesday* the general Accompt is made up, and Printed, and on *Thursdays* published and dispersed to the several Families, who will pay four shillings *per Annum* for them.

The classification of deaths in the *Bills of Mortality* would seem strange to the modern eye. For example, categories of death included "Suddenly," "Killed by Several Accidents," and "Found Dead in the Streets." Nevertheless, Graunt's concern about possible misclassification of the events that were tabulated in the *Bills of Mortality* was very modern. He suspected, for example, that plague deaths were underascertained, because in years that had more plague deaths, there were also more deaths from other causes. He inferred that about 20% of plague deaths were mistakenly recorded as deaths attributable to other causes and on that basis produced a refined estimate of mortality from the plague. This was the first recorded example of correction for misclassification error. He also considered the reasons for misclassification of deaths. The matrons who served as searchers could recognize a corpse as well as anyone and could easily establish whether a death should be attributed to hanging, leprosy, drowning, or other obvious causes. But some causes of death were more difficult to ascertain. With respect to consumption (ie, tuberculosis), he noted[5] that

> ... all dying thereof so emaciated and lean (their *Ulcers* disappearing upon Death) that the Old-women *Searchers* after the mist of a cup of *Ale*, and the bribe of a two-groat fee, instead of one, given them, cannot tell whether this emaciation, or leanness were from a *Phthisis*, or from an *Hectic Fever*, *Atrophy*, &c or from an Infection of the *Spermatick* parts.

Graunt's work provides several lessons that still apply to good epidemiologic work.[6] Among these are the following:

1. He was succinct. His short work contained many original findings and yet had an ample description of methods and results.
2. He provided clear explanations for his reasoning, for example with the calculations showing the underestimation of plague deaths.
3. He subjected his theories and novel findings to repeated tests. For example, he estimated the population of London to be 384,000, but he derived this figure using five different approaches.
4. He invited readers to criticize his work, to "correct my *Positions*, and raise others of their own: For herein I have, like a silly Scholeboy, coming to say my Lesson to the World (that Peevish, and Tetchie Master) brought a bundle of Rods wherewith to be whipt, for every mistake I have committed."[5] Such humility is less common nowadays.
5. He described how he had revised his opinions in the light of new data.
6. He relied on estimation, a quantitative approach to his subject matter rather than a qualitative approach, such as the presence or absence of statistical significance, which infests much of today's research (see Chapter 8).

Bernardino Ramazzini (1633–1714)

Ramazzini was born in Carpi, Italy, in the year when Galileo was interrogated by the Inquisition. He was a polymath who became a pioneer in epidemiology and especially in the field of occupational medicine. As a physician, he was noted as an early proponent for the use of cinchona bark (a source of quinine) to treat malaria. His crowning achievement, however, was the text *De morbis artificum diatriba* ("On Artificially Caused Disease"), the first comprehensive work on occupational diseases and industrial hygiene. Published in 1700, it described risks related to dozens of occupational hazards. He counseled physicians to inquire about the work activities and workplace exposures of their patients[7]:

> "When you come to a patient's house, you should ask him what sort of pains he has, what caused them, how many days he has been ill, whether the bowels are working and what sort of food he eats." So says Hippocrates in his work *Affections*. I may venture to add one more question: what occupation does he follow?

He gave detailed descriptions of specific occupational diseases, including a review of existing knowledge and suggestions for prevention and treatment. He was also concerned with the physical demands of specific occupations and with repetitive physical tasks. His interest in ergonomics can be seen in this excerpt[8]:

> Nowadays women sit to weave, but in such a posture that they somehow look as though they were standing. This kind of work is certainly very fatiguing, for the whole body is tasked, both hands, arms, feet, and back, so that every part of the body at once shares in the work.... Now an occupation so fatiguing naturally has its drawbacks, especially for women, for if pregnant they easily miscarry and expel the fetus prematurely and in consequence incur many ailments later on. It follows that women weavers, I mean those who are engaged wholly in this occupation, ought to be particularly healthy and robust, otherwise they break down from overwork and as they get on in years are compelled to abandon this trade. ... Therefore in work so taxing moderation would be the best safeguard against these maladies, for men and women alike; for the common maxim "Nothing to excess" is one that I excessively approve.

In 1982, an international group of public-health scientists founded the Collegium Ramazzini, headquartered in Carpi. The Collegium was founded to advance the study of environmental and occupational disease and, according to its bylaws, to be "a bridge between the world of scientific discovery and those social and political centers which must act on these discoveries to conserve life and to prevent disease."[9]

William Farr (1807–1883)

Farr was the first Compiler of Abstracts at the General Register Office in England. The General Register Office was created by an act of Parliament in 1836 to record the civil registration of births, deaths, and marriages in England and Wales. Around that time, information on cause of death was collected along with age and occupation for all deaths. Farr's appointment began in 1839, and he remained in the General Register Office for 40 years, where he continued the tradition that began with John Graunt of using routinely collected vital statistics to learn about disease occurrence.

Farr occupied himself with many of the same issues that Graunt addressed. He studied demographic issues of population size, sex ratio at birth, fecundity, and time trends. He tested the theories that had been proposed by Malthus on population growth. He constructed actuarial tables, examined infant mortality, and, following in the footsteps of Ramazzini, studied the relation between specific occupations and mortality. He was famously engaged in a series of analyses of the cholera epidemics that struck London in the mid–19th century, in which he determined that local and comparatively small changes in altitude were strongly related to mortality from cholera. At first, he attributed the effect of altitude to atmospheric influences, consistent with the then-popular theory that foul air was the medium by which cholera was spread. In this, he was in conflict with John Snow, who attributed the spread of cholera to contaminated water (see next section). But eventually his own data persuaded Farr to change his mind, and he became a champion of Snow's theory that sewage contaminated with excreta from cholera victims perpetuated the epidemics.

Farr's work defined the field of vital statistics and had a lasting influence on epidemiology and public health. He was a dispassionate scientist, but he also saw the harsh social burden of industrialization and was an ardent reformer as well as a member of the sanitary movement. On the fundamental role of epidemiology in public health, Farr remarked, "Diseases are more easily prevented than cured and the first step to their prevention is the discovery of their exciting causes."[10]

John Snow (1813–1858)

Esteemed for his meticulous research on cholera as well as his pioneering work in the use of anesthetic gases, John Snow is considered the founding father of both epidemiology and anesthesiology. His renown as an anesthetist stems from his study of anesthetic gases, the design of inhalers to control the flow of these gases, and the sensational administration of chloroform to Queen Victoria during delivery. His renown as an epidemiologist stems from his investigation of the London cholera epidemics in the mid–19th century and his famous persuasion of the Board of Guardians of Saint James' Parish to remove the pump handle from the Broad Street pump in Golden Square, so as to contain the epidemic of cholera that raged there in the summer of 1854.

The popularization of the dramatic vignette of the pump handle has Snow's intervention stopping the epidemic cold. As I describe in Chapter 4, however, the epidemic was already waning when the pump handle was removed, and it is not clear that any cholera cases were prevented by its removal. On the other hand, it is possible that removal of the handle may have prevented a second outbreak. The likely index case of the outbreak was an infant who lived near the pump and whose mother soaked the soiled diapers of the infant in pails and dumped them into a cesspool near the pump. Later investigation showed that the brickwork around the pump was defective and water from the cesspool could enter the pump. The infant's father developed cholera the day that the pump handle was removed and therefore might have ignited a second epidemic had the pump still been in operation.[11,12]

The real story was not so much the removal of the pump handle but Snow's meticulous investigations that demonstrated the connection between consuming fouled water and risk of cholera. By 1854, Snow had already been pursuing for several years the theory that cholera was transmitted by ingestion of an agent that was spread through fecal contamination of drinking water. He brought many lines of inquiry to bear on his research. At the time, the germ theory was not accepted—most experts still believed that miasmas were the means for spreading communicable diseases. Farr, for example, believed in miasmas, despite his own analyses that showed that altitude in the London area was a strong determinant of cholera risk. Altitude could affect the flow of bad air, so Farr and others thought that the altitude data supported the miasma theory. But altitude is also related to the flow of water, with individuals living at lower altitudes much more likely to be drinking water containing the sewage of those at higher elevations. Snow noted that inhalation of bad air would make more sense if the cholera patient developed a respiratory disease, but he saw that clinically the disease begins as a gastrointestinal affliction. Snow marshaled a wide array of facts to make his case. For example, he noted that miners experienced a greater risk of cholera than those in any other occupation. Miners also spent long hours underground, with no access to privies, and carried food along that they ate with bare hands that they were unable to wash adequately.

Although the incident with the Broad Street pump is iconic, Snow's most important contribution to epidemiology was his groundbreaking work on the relation between water supply and cholera conducted in certain neighborhoods of London. The key study was one in which water pipes from two competing companies, one carrying clean water and the other water that was contaminated with London sewage, supplied the same neighborhood. Most residents did not even know which company supplied their apartment, because landlords typically contracted to provide water. This situation, elegantly described by Snow as being better than any experiment that could have been devised, became known as a *natural experiment*. It is described in greater detail in Chapters 4 and 5. Snow is celebrated today by epidemiologists even more for being a pioneer of epidemiologic study design than for his seminal work on the mode of cholera transmission.

Ignasz Semmelweis (1818–1865)

Today recognized as a pioneering epidemiologist and revered as a hero in his native Hungary, in his time Semmelweis was an outcast who was widely spurned by the medical profession. He was born in Budapest and studied medicine and practiced obstetrics in Vienna at a time when puerperal fever raged throughout the maternity hospitals of Europe with no satisfactory explanation. The Vienna Maternity Hospital was the largest hospital of its kind in the world. Patients were admitted on alternate days to each of its two obstetrics clinics. Medical students were taught in the first clinic and midwives in the second. During the period 1840–1846, the risk of maternal death during delivery was about 10% for women admitted to the first clinic but less than 4% in the second clinic, where the midwives trained. Almost all maternal deaths were from puerperal fever. The mortality rate was so high in the first clinic that women who could afford to do so gave birth at home rather than risk being assigned to the first clinic.

Semmelweis investigated a theory that doctors themselves were the source of disease for their patients. In the first clinic, when a woman died with puerperal fever, students and their teachers would conduct an autopsy, and from there they would proceed back to the clinic to examine other patients. Semmelweis noted that when he left Vienna for a sabbatical, puerperal fever deaths in the first clinic declined, but they rose again after his return. He also noted that a colleague who nicked himself with a scalpel during an autopsy died of a disease that resembled puerperal fever. From these and other observations, Semmelweis theorized that the source of disease, the "morbid matter," was being spread by doctors and students from cadavers in the morgue to patients on the ward. Semmelweis instituted a policy of washing hands in a chlorinated lime disinfectant before returning to the wards, and the risk of puerperal fever in the first clinic was reduced to the same level as in the second clinic.

Unfortunately, the germ theory of disease was not yet accepted. Most physicians believed that miasmas, or bad air, were the source of communicable disease. Semmelweis was also handicapped by his own personality. He was slow to publish, loath to accept criticism, quick to anger, and dogmatic.[13] Consequently, he was not effective in persuading others to take his theory seriously, despite the remarkable evidence that he assembled. After a series of professional setbacks, he died young and ignominiously while hospitalized in a mental institution, and his work was forgotten. Eventually, the English surgeon Joseph Lister, influenced by Pasteur, introduced antiseptic technique to surgery practice, and from there it was carried over to maternity clinics. All this happened without any influence from Semmelweis, whose reputation rose only after his work was rediscovered.

Florence Nightingale (1820–1910)

Nightingale is best known for her contribution to nursing, but she also was an accomplished epidemiologist and statistician who made major contributions to the field of public health.[14,15] Born to a wealthy family, she entered the nursing profession as a calling to work for the public good, facing parental opposition and societal roadblocks. Her early professional efforts were aimed at caring for people in poverty, helping to improve medical care available to the poor, and working to reform the Poor Law of the United Kingdom. In 1854, she was asked by the British Secretary of War to go to the British front where the Crimean war was being waged. She went with a staff of trained volunteer nurses and discovered that poor nutrition and hygiene, lack of medicines, and indifference were responsible for more deaths among soldiers than battlefield injuries. She instigated improvements such as better sewage and ventilation. Death rates soon dropped in the military field hospital.

Nightingale's efforts in the Crimea brought her fame and with it a mandate to continue her efforts in public health. She wrote a treatise on health conditions in the Crimea, for which she invented a diagram now known as a *polar-area diagram* or *coxcomb* (Fig. 2–1). It plotted monthly deaths attributable to preventable and unpreventable causes (deaths were proportional to area, not to radius); the

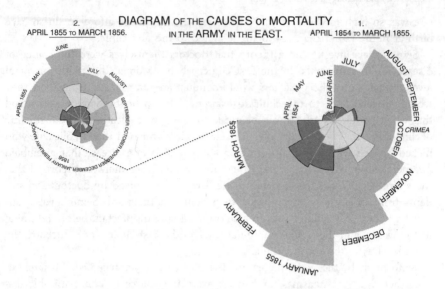

Figure 2–1. Diagram of mortality by cause during the Crimean war, by Florence Nightingale, 1858. Each wedge represents one month. The area of the outer wedges is proportional to death from "preventable or mitigable zymotic diseases," the area of the white wedges represents deaths from wounds, and the area from the dark shaded wedges represents deaths from all other causes. The graph shows that sickness took a much greater toll than injuries, and deaths were much greater during the first year than the second.

data revealed that most deaths were preventable and showed clear time trends. Back in England, she noted that the poor nutrition and hygiene she had found at the front also afflicted military men stationed at home. She wrote a report that sparked an overhaul of medical care of soldiers and led to the establishment of a medical school for the army. Later, she turned her attention to sanitation in rural India and became a voice for improvement of public health throughout India. Her work was characteristically meticulous, grounded in carefully collected data, and presented in compelling graphics.

Janet Lane-Claypon (1877–1967)

Another female British pioneer in epidemiology, who has been largely overlooked despite her seminal contribution, is the inventor of the modern case-control study. Lane-Claypon, like Nightingale, was a public-health leader who became an innovator in epidemiology in pursuit of her public-health objectives. In 1912, she published the results of a study that examined breast feeding versus bottle feeding in relation to weight gain during infancy and secondarily compared the effect of boiled versus raw cow's milk among the bottle-fed infants. This study has been described as the first retrospective cohort study,[16] although one could argue that the earlier studies of Snow on cholera or of Semmelweiss on puerperal fever were retrospective cohort studies. Regardless of priority, Lane-Claypon's work was ahead of its time, not only for the basic study design but also for her attention to both systematic and random error. She excluded sick infants to prevent confounding, and she wrote about possible confounding by social class, a factor that was not controlled and could affect the data she reported.

Her seminal work came in 1926 with the publication of results from the first modern case-control study, which was aimed at evaluating risk factors for breast cancer.[17] She selected 500 cases and an equal number of controls from hospitals in London and Glasgow. Exposure information was obtained by interview using a questionnaire designed for the study. Her analyses laid the groundwork for breast cancer epidemiology, establishing the relation of age at first pregnancy, age at menopause, number of children, and surgically induced menopause to breast cancer risk. Although it was not recognized at the time, this study introduced a novel study design that has since become a hallmark of modern epidemiology. Lane-Claypon seemed well aware, however, of the strengths and weaknesses of the method. She discussed the possibility of recall bias, long considered an important source of error in case-control studies that rely on interviews to gather data. She also acknowledged possible problems stemming from the facts that cases were survivors and that cases and controls were drawn from a set of hospitals. Many decades before the principles of epidemiologic study design were codified and discussed, Lane-Claypon had the insight to describe many of the important issues in both cohort and case-control studies.[18,19]

Wade Hampton Frost (1880–1938)

Wade Hampton Frost was the first professor of epidemiology in the first university department of epidemiology, at the Johns Hopkins School of Hygiene and Public Health (now known as the Johns Hopkins Bloomberg School of Public Health).[20] After graduating with a degree in medicine from the University of Virginia in 1903, Frost chose to pursue a career in public health. (One speculative view suggests that Frost chose a career in public health because he contracted tuberculosis while a student and was consequently advised to avoid working in general practice.) At the start of the 20th century, the germ theory of disease was still new, and the control of disease spread by infectious agents was in its infancy. Soon after graduation, Frost was called to New Orleans to investigate an outbreak of yellow fever. The role of the mosquito vector, *Aedes aegypti*, in the transmission of yellow fever had only recently been established. Frost and a team of colleagues spent weeks eliminating breeding spots for the mosquito and eventually stopped the outbreak after 459 people had died. It marked the first time that a yellow fever outbreak in the United States was halted before the arrival of winter, and it was also the last epidemic of yellow fever in the United States.

Frost's subsequent work and teaching were influenced by the classic investigations by William Budd on typhoid fever and by Snow on cholera. His later work focused on typhoid, poliomyelitis, meningococcal meningitis, tuberculosis, and influenza. His studies on polio led to the understanding that paralytic cases constitute only a small proportion of those infected by the virus and that childhood infection with the virus confers lasting immunity. His influenza research documented the spread of the global pandemic of 1918–1919, showed that the effects of influenza epidemics could be tracked using death rates for pneumonia, and revealed that the case-fatality rate for influenza during the pandemic had a bimodal age distribution, hitting hard among young adults and the very old. His work on tuberculosis was an early and elegant demonstration of the power of analyzing mortality rates by birth cohort, a method first used a decade earlier by the Norwegian physician Kristian Andvord. Frost is also known for his collaboration with Lowell Reed in developing the elegant Reed-Frost mathematical model for infectious disease transmission and the development of herd immunity (see Chapter 6).

ALSO NOTEWORTHY

The contributions of these pioneers highlight only a few of the important milestones in the history of epidemiology and public health. Many others could easily have been mentioned—William Budd, Edward Goldberger, Major Greenwood, Joseph Jenner, James Lind, Pierre Louis, Peter Panum, Geoffrey Rose, and Edgar Sydenstricker, to suggest a few. By the mid–20th century, epidemiology research and teaching had expanded rapidly. It had also extended its purview to include an ever-widening range of disease foci, such as psychiatric illness, violent behavior, and obesity. Leaders such as Austin Bradford-Hill, Richard Doll, Brian MacMahon, Abraham Lilienfeld, John Cassel, and many others nurtured the growth of epidemiology during this period, influencing others through their teaching but even more so by the quality of their work. The surge in epidemiologic activity has continued through the 20th century and into the present.

QUESTIONS

1. Although epidemiologic research is greatly facilitated by computers, its conduct is based on enumerating events in populations and is not especially dependent on technology. The ideas needed to conduct epidemiologic research could have been developed and applied long ago. Speculate as to why epidemiologic research did not become commonplace until the middle of the 20th century.

2. Both Snow and Semmelweiss conducted research that showed how one might prevent infectious disease before the germ theory was accepted. Yet the existence of microorganisms had been known for almost 200 years, since van Leeuwenhoek first described what he saw under a microscope. Speculate on the nature of social and scientific thinking of the time that hindered the scientists of the 19th century from accepting the role of microorganisms in disease.

3. Graunt and Farr advanced the field of epidemiology by studying public records and vital statistics, setting examples for generations of epidemiologists. Others, such as Snow and Semmelweiss, devised studies to collect their own data, which required considerable time and effort but was possible as an

independent effort. Today, collection of ad hoc epidemiologic data is expensive and often requires collaborative efforts and substantial funding that must be approved in a peer-review process. It appears that peer review, had it been necessary, might have been an obstacle to Snow and Semmelweiss. Give arguments listing the strengths and weaknesses of a system of peer review for funding of scientific research.

ADDITIONAL READING

Buck C, Llopis A, Nájera E, Terris M. *The Challenge of Epidemiology: Issues and Selected Readings.* Pan American Health Organization Scientific Publication No. 505. Geneva: World Health Organization, 1988.

REFERENCES

1. Rosen G. *History of Public Health.* Expanded edition. Baltimore: Johns Hopkins University Press; 1993.
2. Svoboda T, Henry B, Shulman L, et al. Public health measures to control the spread of the severe acute respiratory syndrome during the outbreak in Toronto. *N Engl J Med.* 2004;350:2352–2361.
3. Hippocrates. *On Airs, Waters, and Places.* Adams F, trans. http://classics.mit.edu/Hippocrates/airwatpl.html. Accessed September 30, 2011.
4. Horne CF, ed. *The Sacred Books and Early Literature of the East.* Vol VI: Medieval Arabia. New York: Parke, Austin, & Lipscomb; 1917:90–91.
5. Graunt J. *Natural and Political Observations Mentioned in a Following Index, and Made Upon the Bills of Mortality.* Facsimile edition. New York: Arno Press; 1975.
6. Rothman KJ. Lessons from John Graunt. *Lancet.* 1996;347:37–39.
7. Ramazzini B. Diseases of workers. *The Classics of Medicine Library.* Special edition. Chicago: University of Chicago Press; 1983.
8. Franco G, Franco F. Bernardino Ramazzini: The father of occupational medicine. *Am J Publ Health.* 2001;91:1380–1382.
9. Bylaws of the Collegium Ramazzini. http://www.collegiumramazzini.org/download/Bylaws.pdf. Accessed September 30, 2011.
10. Farr W. Letter to the Registrar General. In: *First Annual Report of the Registrar General.* London: Her Majesty's Stationery Office; 1839.
11. Vinten-Johansen P, Brody H, Paneth N, et al. *Cholera, Chloroform, and the Science of Medicine: A Life of John Snow.* New York: Oxford University Press; 2003.
12. Rothman KJ. My interview with John Snow. *Epidemiology.* 2004;15:640–644.
13. Nuland SB. *The Doctors' Plague: Germs, Childbed Fever, and the Strange Story of Ignac Semmelweis.* New York: WW Norton; 2003.
14. Winkelstein W. Florence Nightingale: founder of modern nursing and hospital epidemiology. *Epidemiology.* 2009;20:311.
15. Cook E. *The Life of Florence Nightingale.* Vol 2. London: Macmillan; 1913.
16. Winkelstein W Jr. Vignettes of the history of epidemiology: three firsts by Janet Elizabeth Lane-Claypon. *Am J Epidemiol.* 2004;160:97–101.
17. Lane-Claypon JE. *A Further Report on Cancer of the Breast, With Special Reference to Its Associated Antecedent Conditions.* Reports on Public Health and Medical

Subjects No. 32, Ministry of Health. London: His Majesty's Stationery Office; 1926.

18. Winkelstein W Jr. Janet Lane-Claypon, a forgotten epidemiologic pioneer. *Epidemiology.* 2006;17:705.

19. Paneth N, Susser E, Susser M. Origins and early development of the case-control study. Part 2: The case-control study from Lane-Claypon to 1950. *Social Prev Med.* 2002;47:359–365.

20. Daniel TM. *Wade Hampton Frost, Pioneer Epidemiologist 1880–1938.* Rochester, NY: University of Rochester Press; 2004.

3

What Is Causation?

The acquired wisdom that certain conditions or events bring about other conditions or events is an important survival trait. Consider an infant whose first experiences are a jumble of sensations that include hunger, thirst, color, light, heat, cold, and many other stimuli. Gradually, the infant begins to perceive patterns in the jumble and to anticipate connections between actions such as crying and effects such as being fed. Eventually, the infant assembles an inventory of associated perceptions. Along with this growing appreciation for specific causal relations comes the general idea that some events or conditions can be considered causes of other events or conditions.

Thus, our first appreciation of the concept of causation is based on our own observations. These observations typically involve causes with effects that are immediately apparent. For example, changing the position of a light switch on the wall has the instant effect of causing the light to go on or off. There is, however, more to the causal mechanism for getting the light to shine than turning the light switch to the on position. If the electric lines to the building are down because of a storm, turning on the switch will have no effect. If the bulb is burned out, manipulating the switch also will have no effect. One cause of the light going on is having the switch in the proper place, but along with it we must include a supply of power to the circuit, a working bulb, and intact wiring. When all other factors are in place, turning the switch will cause the light to go on, but if one or more of the other factors is not playing its causal role, the light will not go on when the switch is turned. There is a tendency to consider the switch as the unique cause of turning on the light, but we can define a more intricate causal mechanism in which the switch is one component of several. The tendency to identify the switch as the unique cause stems from its usual role as the final factor that acts in the causal mechanism. The wiring can be considered part of the causal mechanism, but after it is installed, it seldom warrants further attention. The switch is typically the only part of the mechanism that needs to be activated to turn on the light. The effect usually occurs immediately after turning the switch, and as a result, we tend to identify the switch as a unique cause. The inadequacy of this assumption is emphasized when the bulb fails and must be replaced before the light will go on.

THE CAUSAL PIE MODEL

Causes of disease can be conceptualized in the same way as the causes of turning on a light. A helpful way to think about causal mechanisms for disease is depicted in Figure 3–1.[1] Each *pie* in the diagram represents a theoretical *causal mechanism* for a given disease, sometimes called a *sufficient cause*. The three pies illustrate that there are multiple mechanisms that cause any type of disease. Each individual instance of disease occurs through a single mechanism or sufficient cause. A given causal mechanism requires the joint action of many component factors, or *component causes*. Each component cause is an event or a condition that plays a necessary role in the occurrence of some cases of a given disease. For example, the disease may be cancer of the lung, and in the first mechanism in Figure 3–1, factor C may be cigarette smoking. Other factors include genetic traits or other environmental exposures that play a causal role in cancer of the lung. Some component causes presumably act in many different causal mechanisms. (Terminology note: the *causal pie model* has also been described as the *sufficient-component cause model*.)

Implications of the Causal Pie Model

MULTICAUSALITY

The model of causation shown in Figure 3–1 illuminates several important principles of causation, the most important of which is that every causal mechanism involves the joint action of a multitude of component causes. Consider as an example the cause of a broken hip. Suppose that someone experiences a traumatic injury to the head that leads to a permanent disturbance in equilibrium. Many years later, faulty equilibrium plays a causal role in a fall that occurs while the person is walking on an icy path. The fall results in a broken hip. Other factors

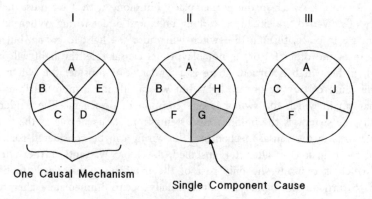

Figure 3–1 Three sufficient causes of a disease.

playing a causal role for the broken hip may include the type of shoe the person was wearing, the lack of a handrail along the path, a sudden gust of wind, and the weight of the person. The complete causal mechanism involves a multitude of factors. Some factors, such as the earlier injury that resulted in the equilibrium disturbance and the weight of the person, reflect earlier events that have had a lingering effect. Some causal components of the broken hip are *genetic*. Genetic factors affect the person's weight, gait, behavior, and recovery from the earlier trauma. Other factors, such as the force of the wind, are *environmental* (nongenetic). There usually are some genetic and some environmental component causes in every causal mechanism. Even an event such as a fall on an icy path that results in a broken hip is part of a complicated causal mechanism that involves many component causes.

GENETIC VERSUS ENVIRONMENTAL CAUSES

It is a strong assertion that every case of every disease has both genetic and environmental causes. Nevertheless, if all genetic factors that determine disease are taken into account, essentially 100% of disease can be said to be inherited, in the sense that nearly all cases of disease have some genetic component causes. What would be the genetic component causes of someone who gets drunk and is killed in an automobile after colliding with a tree? Genetic traits may lead to psychiatric problems such as alcoholism, which may lead to drunk driving and consequent fatality. It is also possible to claim that essentially 100% of any disease is environmentally caused, even diseases that often are considered to be purely genetic. Phenylketonuria, for example, is considered by many to be purely genetic. Nonetheless, if we consider the disease that phenylketonuria represents to be the mental retardation that may result from it, we can prevent the disease by appropriate dietary intervention. The disease therefore has environmental determinants, and its causes are both environmental and genetic. Although it may seem like an exaggeration to claim that 100% of cases of any disease are environmental and genetic at the same time, it is a good approximation. It may seem counterintuitive, because we cannot manipulate many of the causes in most situations and the ones that can be controlled are usually solely environmental causes, as in the manipulation of diet to prevent the mental retardation of phenylketonuria.

STRENGTH OF CAUSES

It is common to think that some component causes play a more important role than other factors in the causation of disease. One way this concept is expressed is by the strength of a causal effect. We say that smoking has a strong effect on lung cancer risk because smokers have about 10 times the risk of lung cancer as nonsmokers. We say that smoking has a weaker effect on myocardial infarction because the risk of a heart attack is only about twice as great in smokers as in nonsmokers. With respect to an individual case of disease, however, every component cause that played a role was necessary to the occurrence of that case.

According to the causal pie model, for a given case of disease, there is no such thing as a strong cause or a weak cause. There is only a distinction between factors that were causes and factors that were not causes.

To understand what epidemiologists mean by *strength* of a cause, we need to shift from thinking about an individual case to thinking about the total burden of cases occurring in a population. We can then define a *strong cause* to be a component cause that plays a causal role in a large proportion of cases and a *weak cause* to be a causal component in a small proportion of cases. Because smoking plays a causal role in a high proportion of the lung cancer cases, we call it a strong cause of lung cancer. For a given case of lung cancer, smoking is no more important than any of the other component causes for that case; but on the population level, it is considered a strong cause of lung cancer because it causes such a large proportion of cases.

The strength of a cause defined in this way necessarily depends on the prevalence of other causal factors that produce disease. As a result, the concept of a strong or weak cause cannot be a universally accurate description of any cause. Suppose we say that smoking is a strong cause of lung cancer because it plays a causal role in a large proportion of cases. Exposure to ambient radon gas is considered to be a weaker cause because it has a causal role in a much smaller proportion of lung cancer cases. Imagine that society eventually succeeds in eliminating tobacco smoking, with a consequent reduction in smoking-related cases of lung cancer. One result is that a much larger proportion of the lung cancer cases that continue to occur will be caused by exposure to radon gas; eliminating smoking would strengthen the causal effect of radon gas on lung cancer. This example illustrates that *strength of effect* is not a biologically stable characteristic of a factor. From a biologic perspective, the causal role of a factor in producing disease is neither strong nor weak; the biology of causation corresponds to the identity of the component causes in a causal mechanism and the ways in which they interact to produce disease. The proportion of the population burden of disease that a factor causes, which we use to define the strength of a cause, can change from population to population and over time if there are changes in the distribution of other causes of the disease. The strength of a cause does not portray the biology of causation.

INTERACTION BETWEEN CAUSES

The causal pie model posits that several causal components act in concert to produce an effect. *Acting in concert* does not imply that factors must act at the same time. Consider the earlier example of the person who sustained trauma to the head that resulted in an equilibrium disturbance, which led years later to a fall on an icy path. The earlier head trauma played a causal role in the later hip fracture, as did the weather conditions on the day of the fracture. If both factors played a causal role in the hip fracture, they interacted with one another to cause the fracture, despite the fact that their time of action was many years apart. We would say that any and all of the factors in the same causal mechanism interact with one another to cause disease. The head trauma interacted with the weather conditions and with the other component causes, such as the type of footwear, the absence of a handhold, and any other conditions that were necessary to the causal mechanism of the fall and the broken hip that resulted. Each causal pie can be considered as a set of interacting causal components. This model provides a biologic basis for the concept of interaction that differs from the more traditional statistical view of interaction. The implication of this difference is discussed in Chapter 11.

SUM OF ATTRIBUTABLE FRACTIONS

Consider the data in Table 3–1, which shows the rates of head and neck cancer according to smoking status and alcohol exposure. Suppose that the differences in the rates reflect causal effects, so that confounding can be ignored. Among those who are smokers and alcohol drinkers, what proportion of the cases of head and neck cancer that occur is attributable to the effect of smoking? We know that the rate for these people is 12 cases per 10,000 person-years. If these same people were not smokers, we can infer that their rate of head and neck cancer would be 3 cases per 10,000 person-years. If this difference reflects the causal role of smoking, we can infer that 9 of every 12 cases (75%) are attributable to smoking among those who smoke and drink alcohol. If we turn the question around and ask what proportion of disease among these same people is attributable to alcohol drinking, we would be able to attribute 8 of every 12 cases (67%) to alcohol drinking.

Can we attribute 75% of the cases to smoking and 67% to alcohol drinking among those who are exposed to both? The answer is yes, because some cases are counted more than once as a result of the interaction between smoking and alcohol consumption. These cases are attributable to both smoking and alcohol drinking because both factors played a causal role in producing them. One consequence of interaction is that the proportions of disease attributable to various component causes do not sum to 100%.

A widely discussed but unpublished paper from the 1970s written by scientists at the National Institutes of Health proposed that as much as 40% of cancer is attributable to occupational exposures. Many scientists thought that this fraction was an overestimate and argued against this claim.[2,3] One of the arguments used in rebuttal was as follows: x percent of cancer is caused by smoking, y percent by diet, z percent by alcohol, and so on; when all of these percentages are summed, only a small percentage, much less than 40%, is left for occupational causes. This rebuttal, however, is fallacious because it is based on the naive view that every case of disease has a single cause and that two causes cannot both contribute to the same case of cancer. Because diet, smoking, asbestos, and various occupational exposures and other factors interact with one another and with genetic

Table 3–1 HYPOTHETICAL RATES
OF HEAD AND NECK CANCER
(CASES PER 10,000 PERSON-YEARS)
ACCORDING TO SMOKING STATUS
AND ALCOHOL DRINKING

Smoking Status	Alcohol Drinking	
	No	Yes
Nonsmoker	1	3
Smoker	4	12

factors to cause cancer, each case of cancer can be attributed repeatedly to many separate component causes. The sum of disease attributable to various component causes has no upper limit.

INDUCTION TIME

Because the component causes in a given causal mechanism do not act simultaneously, there usually is a period of time between the action of a component cause and the completion of a sufficient cause. The only exception is the last component cause to act in a given causal mechanism. The last-acting component cause completes the causal mechanism, and we can say that disease begins concurrently with its action. For earlier-acting component causes, we can define the *induction period* as the time interval that begins concurrently with the action of a component cause and ends when the final component cause acts and the disease occurs. For example, in the illustration of the fractured hip, the induction time between the head trauma that resulted in an equilibrium disturbance and the later hip fracture was many years. The induction time between the decision to wear nongripping shoes and the hip fracture might have been a matter of minutes or hours. The induction time between the gust of wind that triggered the fall and the hip fracture might have been seconds or less.

In an individual instance, we usually cannot know the exact length of an induction period, because we cannot be sure of the causal mechanism that produces disease in an individual instance nor when all the relevant component causes in that mechanism exerted their causal action. With research data, however, we can learn enough to characterize the induction period that relates the action of a single component cause to the occurrence of disease in general. An example of a lengthy induction time is the cause-effect relation between exposure of a female fetus to diethylstilbestrol (DES) and her subsequent development of adenocarcinoma of the vagina. The cancer generally occurs after the age of 15 years. Because the causal exposure to DES occurs during gestation, there is an induction time of more than 15 years for carcinogenesis. During this time, other causes presumably operate; some evidence suggests that hormonal action during adolescence may be part of the mechanism.[4]

The causal pie model makes it clear that it is incorrect to characterize a disease itself as having a lengthy or brief induction time. The induction time can be conceptualized only in relation to a specific component cause. We can say that the induction time relating DES to clear cell carcinoma of the vagina is at least 15 years, but we cannot say that 15 years is the minimum induction time for clear cell carcinoma in general. Because each component cause in any causal mechanism can act at a time different from the other component causes, each can have its own induction time. For the component cause that acts last, the induction time always equals zero. If another component cause of clear cell carcinoma of the vagina that acts during adolescence were identified, it would have a much shorter induction time than that of DES. Induction time characterizes a specific cause-effect pair rather than only the effect.

In carcinogenesis, the terms *initiator* and *promoter* are used to refer to component causes of cancer that act early and late, respectively, in the causal mechanism. Cancer itself has often been characterized as a disease process with a long induction time, but this characterization is a misconception. Any late-acting component in the causal process, such as a promoter, will have a short induction time, and the induction time will always be zero for the last component cause (eg, the gust of wind causing the broken hip in the earlier example), because after the final causal component acts, disease has occurred. At that point, however, the presence of disease is not necessarily apparent. A broken hip may be apparent immediately, but a cancer that has just been caused may not become noticed or diagnosed for an appreciable time. The time interval between disease occurrence and its subsequent detection, whether by medical testing or by the emergence of symptoms, is called the *latent period*.[4] The length of the latent period can be reduced by improved methods of disease detection. The induction period, however, cannot be reduced by early detection of disease, because there is no disease to detect until after the induction period is over. Practically, it may be difficult to distinguish between the induction period and the latent period, because there may be no way to establish when the disease process began if it is not detected until later. Diseases such as slow-growing cancers may appear to have long induction periods with respect to many causes, in part because they have long latent periods.

Although it is not possible to reduce the induction period by earlier detection of disease, it may be possible to observe intermediate stages of a causal mechanism. The increased interest in biomarkers such as DNA adducts is an example of focusing on causes that are more proximal to the disease occurrence. Biomarkers may reflect the effects on the organism of agents that have acted at an earlier time.

IS A CATALYST A CAUSE?

Some agents may have a causal action by shortening the induction time of other agents. Suppose that exposure to factor A leads to epilepsy after an average interval of 10 years. It may be that exposure to drug B can shorten this interval to 2 years. Is B acting as a catalyst or as a cause of epilepsy? The answer is both; a catalyst *is* a cause. Without B, the occurrence of epilepsy comes 8 years later than it comes with B, so we can say that B causes the epilepsy to occur earlier. It is not sufficient to argue that the epilepsy would have occurred anyway and therefore that B is not a cause of its occurrence. First, it would not have occurred at that time, and the time of occurrence is considered part of the definition of an event. Second, epilepsy will occur later only if the person survives an additional 8 years, which is not certain. Agent B therefore determines when the epilepsy occurs, and it can determine whether it occurs at all. For this reason, we consider any agent that acts as a catalyst of a causal mechanism, shortening the induction period for other agents, to be a cause. Similarly, any agent that postpones the onset of an event, drawing out the induction period for another agent, we consider to be a preventive. It should not be too surprising to equate postponement with prevention; we routinely use such an equation when we employ the euphemism that we prevent death, which can only be postponed. We prevent death at a given time in favor of death at a later time. Similarly, slowing the process of atherosclerosis can result in postponement (and thereby prevention) of cardiovascular disease and death.

THE PROCESS OF SCIENTIFIC INFERENCE

Much epidemiologic research is aimed at uncovering the causes of disease. Now that we have a conceptual model for causes, how do we determine whether a given relation is causal? Some scientists refer to checklists for causal inference, and others focus on complicated statistical approaches, but the answer to this question is not to be found in checklists or statistical methods. The question itself is tantamount to asking how we apply the scientific method to epidemiologic research. This question leads directly to the philosophy of science, a topic that goes well beyond the scope of this book. Nevertheless, it is worthwhile to summarize two of the major philosophic doctrines that have influenced modern science.

Induction

Since the rise of modern science in the 17th century, scientists and philosophers have puzzled over the question of how to determine the truth about assertions that deal with the empirical world. From the time of the ancient Greeks, deductive methods have been used to prove the validity of mathematic propositions. These methods enable us to draw airtight conclusions because they are self-contained, starting with a limited set of definitions and axioms and applying rules of logic that guarantee the validity of the method. Empirical science is different, however. Assertions about the real world do not start from arbitrary axioms, and they involve observations on nature that are fallible and incomplete. These stark differences from deductive logic led early modern empiricists, such as Francis Bacon, to promote what they considered a new type of logic, which they called *induction* (not to be confused with the concept of an induction period). *Induction* was an indirect method used to gain insight into what has been metaphorically described as the fabric of nature.

The method of induction starts with observations on nature. To the extent that the observations fall into a pattern, they are said to induce in the mind of the observer a suggestion of a more general statement about nature. The general statement can range from a simple hypothesis to a more profound natural law or natural relation. The statement about nature is reinforced with further observations or refuted by contradictory observations. For example, suppose an investigator in New York conducts an experiment to determine the boiling point of water and observes that the water boils at 100°C. The experiment is repeated many times, each time showing that the water boils at about 100°C. By induction, the investigator concludes that the boiling point of water is 100°C. The induction itself involves an inference beyond the observations to a general statement that describes the nature of boiling water. As induction became popular, it was seen to differ considerably from deduction. Although not as well understood as deduction, the approach was considered a new type of logic, *inductive logic*.

Although induction, with its emphasis on observation, represented an important advance over the appeal to faith and authority that characterized medieval scholasticism, it was not long before the validity of the new logic was questioned. The sharpest criticism came from the skeptical philosopher David Hume, who pointed out that induction had no logical force. Rather, it amounted to the assumption that what had been observed in the past would continue to occur in the future. When supporters of induction argued that induction was a valid process because it had been seen to work on numerous occasions, Hume countered that the argument was an example of circular reasoning that relied on induction to justify itself. Hume was so profoundly skeptical that he distrusted any inference based on observation because observations depend on sense perceptions and are therefore subject to error.

Refutationism

Hume's criticisms of induction have been a powerful force in modern scientific philosophy. The most influential reply to Hume was offered by Karl Popper. Popper accepted Hume's point that in empirical science one cannot prove the validity of a statement about nature in any way that is comparable with a deductive proof. Popper's philosophy, known as *refutationism*, held that statements about nature can be "corroborated" by evidence, but corroboration does not amount to a logical proof. On the other hand, Popper also asserted that statements about nature can be refuted by deductive logic. To grasp the point, consider the earlier example of observing the boiling point of water. The refutationist view is that the repeated experiments showing that water boils at 100°C corroborate the hypothesis that water boils at this temperature, but they do not prove it.[5] A colleague of the New York researcher who works in Denver, a city located at high altitude, would find that water there boils at 94°C. This single contrary observation carries more weight regarding the hypothesis about the boiling point of water than thousands of repetitions of the initial experiment at sea level.

The asymmetric implications of a refuting observation compared with supporting observations are the essence of the refutationist view. This school of thought encourages scientists to subject a new hypothesis to rigorous tests that may falsify the hypothesis in preference to repetitions of the initial observations that add little beyond the weak corroboration that replication can supply. The implication for the method of science is that hypotheses should be evaluated by subjecting them to crucial tests. If a test refutes a hypothesis, a new hypothesis needs to be formulated that can then be subjected to further tests. After finding that water boils in Denver at a lower temperature than it boils in New York, the investigator must discard the hypothesis that water boils at 100°C and replace it with a more refined hypothesis, such as one that will explain the difference in boiling points under different atmospheric pressures. This process describes an endless cycle of *conjecture and refutation*. The conjecture, or hypothesis, is the product of scientific insight and imagination. It requires little justification except that it can account for existing observations. A useful approach is to pose competing hypotheses to explain existing observations and to test them against one another. The refutationist philosophy postulates that all scientific knowledge is tentative because it may one day need to be refined or even discarded. In this philosophy, what we call scientific knowledge is a body of currently unrefuted hypotheses that appear to explain existing observations.

How can an epidemiologist apply refutationist thinking to his or her work? If causal mechanisms are stated specifically, an epidemiologist can construct crucial tests of competing hypotheses. For example, when toxic shock syndrome was first studied, there were two competing hypotheses about the origin of the toxin. In one, the toxin responsible for the disease was a chemical in the tampon, and women using tampons were exposed to the toxin directly from the tampon. In the other hypothesis, the tampon acted as a culture medium for staphylococci that produced the toxin. Both hypotheses explained the correlation of toxic shock occurrence and tampon use. The two hypotheses, however, led to opposite predictions about the relation between the frequency of changing tampons and the risk of toxic shock. If chemical intoxication were the cause, more frequent tampon changes would lead to more exposure to the toxin and possible absorption of a greater overall dose. This hypothesis predicted that women who changed tampons more frequently would have a higher risk of toxic shock syndrome than women who changed tampons infrequently. The culture-medium hypothesis predicted that the women who change tampons frequently would have a lower risk than those who left the tampon in for longer periods, because a short duration of use for each tampon would prevent the staphylococci from multiplying enough to produce a damaging dose of toxin. Epidemiologic research, which showed that infrequent changing of tampons was associated with greater risk of toxic shock, refuted the chemical theory.

Critics of refutationism point out that refutation is not logically certain because it depends on theories, assumptions, and observations, all of which are susceptible to error. In epidemiology, for example, any study result may be influenced by an obscure bias, which is an inescapable source of uncertainty. Among the dissenting philosophic views is that of Thomas Kuhn,[6] who held that it is ultimately the collective beliefs of the community of scientists that determines what is accepted as truth about nature. According to Kuhn, the truth is not necessarily objective but rather something determined by consensus. Feyerabend,[7] another skeptic, held that science proceeds through intellectual anarchy, without any coherent method. A more moderate although still critical view was taken by Haack.[8,9] She saw science as an extension of everyday inquiry, employing pragmatic methods that she likened to solving a crossword puzzle, integrating clues with other answers in a trial-and-error approach. Despite these criticisms, refutationism has been a positive force in science by encouraging bold, testable theories and then fostering a valuable skeptical outlook by subjecting those theories to rigorous challenges.

Causal Criteria

Earlier we said that there is no simple checklist that can determine whether an observed relation is causal. Nevertheless, attempts at such checklists have appeared. Most of these lists stem from the canons of inference described by John Stuart Mill.[10] The most widely cited list of causal criteria, originally posed as a list of standards, is attributed to Hill,[11] who adapted them from the U.S. Surgeon General's 1964 report on Smoking and Health.[12] The Hill standards, often labeled the Hill criteria, are listed in Table 3–2, along with some problems related to each of the criteria.

Although Hill did not propose these criteria as a checklist for evaluating whether a reported association could be interpreted as causal, many others have

Table 3–2 CAUSAL CRITERIA OF HILL

Criterion	Problems with the Criterion
1. Strength	Strength depends on the prevalence of other causes; it is not a biologic characteristic and can be confounded.
2. Consistency	Causal relations have exceptions that are understood best with hindsight.
3. Specificity	A cause can have many effects.
4. Temporality	It may be difficult to establish the temporal sequence between cause and effect.
5. Biologic gradient	It can be confounded; threshold phenomena would not show a progressive relation.
6. Plausibility	Too subjective
7. Coherence	How does it differ from consistency or plausibility?
8. Experimental evidence	Not always available
9. Analogy	Analogies abound.

attempted to apply them in that way. Admittedly, the process of causal inference as described earlier is difficult and uncertain, making the appeal of a simple checklist undeniable. Unfortunately, this checklist, like all others with the same goal, fails to deliver on the hope of clearly distinguishing causal from noncausal relations. Consider the first criterion, strength. It is tempting to believe that strong associations are more likely to be causal than weak ones, but as we saw in our discussion of causal pies, not every component cause has a strong association with the disease that it produces; strength of association depends on the prevalence of other factors. Some causal associations, such as the association between cigarette smoking and coronary heart disease, are weak. Furthermore, a strong association can be noncausal, a confounded result stemming from the effect of another risk factor for the disease that is highly correlated with the one under study. For example, birth order is strongly associated with the occurrence of Down syndrome, but it is a confounded association that is completely explained by the effect of maternal age. If weak associations can be causal and strong associations can be noncausal, it does not appear that strength of association can be considered a criterion for causality.

The third criterion (see Table 3–2), specificity, suggests that a relation is more likely to be causal if the exposure is related to a single outcome rather than myriad outcomes. This criterion is misleading because it implies, for example, that the more diseases with which smoking is associated, the greater the evidence that smoking is not causally associated with any of them. The fifth criterion, biologic gradient, is often taken as a sign of a causal relation, but it can just as well result from confounding or other biases as from a causal connection. The relation between Down syndrome and birth order, mentioned earlier, shows a biologic gradient despite being completely explained by confounding from maternal age.

Other criteria from Hill's list are vague (eg, consistency, plausibility, coherence, analogy) or do not apply in many settings (eg, experimental evidence). The only characteristic on the list that is truly a causal criterion is temporality, which implies that the cause comes before the effect. This criterion, which is part of the definition of a cause, is a useful one, although it may be difficult to establish the proper time sequence for cause and effect. For example, does stress lead to overeating, or does overeating lead to stress? It usually is better to avoid a checklist approach to causal inference and instead consider approaches such as conjecture and refutation. Checklists lend a deceptive kind of mindless authority to an inherently imperfect and creative process. In contrast, causal inference based on conjecture and refutation fosters a highly desirable critical scrutiny.

Although checklists may not be appropriate for causal inference, the points laid out by Hill are still important considerations. The criteria may be useful when applied in the context of specific hypotheses. For example, Weiss observed that the specificity of effects might be important in inferring the beneficial effect of sigmoidoscopy in screening for colorectal cancer if the association between sigmoidoscopy and reduced death from colorectal cancer is stronger for cancer occurring at sites within reach of a sigmoidoscope.[13]

Generalization in Epidemiology

A useful way to think of scientific generalization is to consider a generalization to be the elaboration of a scientific theory. A given study may test the viability of one or more theories. Theories that survive such tests can be viewed as general statements about nature that tell us what to expect in people or settings that were not studied. Because theories can be incorrect, scientific generalization is not a perfect process. Formulating a theory is not a mathematical or statistical process, and generalization should not be considered a statistical exercise. It is the process of causal inference itself.

Many people believe that generalizing from an epidemiologic study involves a mechanical process of making an inference about a target population of which the study population is considered a sample. This type of generalization does exist, in the field of survey sampling. In survey sampling, researchers draw samples from a population to avoid the expense of studying the entire population, which makes the statistical representativeness of the sample the main concern for generalizing to the source population.

Although survey sampling is an important tool for characterizing a population efficiently and may be used in some epidemiologic applications, such as prevalence surveys, it is a mechanical tool that does not always share the same goals as science. Survey sampling is useful for problems such as trying to predict how a population will vote in an election or what type of laundry soap the people in a region prefer. These are characteristics that depend on attitudes and for which there is little coherent biologic theory on which to base a scientific generalization. Survey results may be quickly outdated (eg, election polls may be repeated weekly or even daily) and do not apply outside the populations from which the surveys were conducted. (Disclaimer: I am not saying that social science is not science or that we cannot develop theories about social behavior. I am saying only that surveys about the current attitudes of a specific group of people are not the same as social theories.) Even if survey sampling is used to characterize the prevalence of disease or the medical needs of a population, the objectives are pragmatic rather than scientific and may not apply outside the study population. Scientific results from epidemiologic studies, in contrast, seldom need to be repeated weekly to see if they still apply. An epidemiologic study conducted in Chicago showing that exposure to ionizing radiation causes cancer does not need to be repeated in Houston to determine whether ionizing radiation also causes cancer in people living in Houston. Generalization about ionizing radiation and cancer is based on understanding of the underlying biology rather than on statistical sampling.

It may be helpful to consider the problem of scientific generalization about causes of cancer from the point of view of a biologist studying carcinogenesis in mice. Most researchers who study cancer in animals do so because they would like to understand better the causes of human cancer. If scientific generalization depended on having studied a statistically representative sample of the target population, researchers studying mice would have nothing to contribute to the understanding of human cancer. Mouse researchers obviously do not study representative samples of people; they do not even study representative samples of mice. Instead, they seek mice that have uniformly similar genes and perhaps certain biologic characteristics. In choosing mice to study, they have to consider mundane issues such as the cost of the mice. Although researchers studying animals are unlikely to worry about whether their mouse or rabbit subjects are statistically representative of all mice or rabbits, they may consider whether the biology of the animal population they are studying is similar to (and representative of) that of humans. This type of representativeness, however, is not statistical representativeness based on sampling from a source population; it is a biologic representativeness based on scientific knowledge. Despite the absence of statistical representativeness, no one seriously doubts the contribution that animal research can make to the understanding of human disease.

Many epidemiologic activities, such as measuring the prevalence of patients in need of dialysis, do require surveys to characterize a specific population, but these activities are usually examples of applied epidemiology rather than the science of epidemiology. The activities of applied epidemiology involve taking already established epidemiologic knowledge and applying it to specific settings, such as preventing malaria transmission by reducing the mosquito vector population or reducing lung cancer and cardiovascular disease occurrence by implementing an antismoking campaign. The activities of epidemiologic research, as in laboratory science, move away from the specific toward the general. We make specific observations in research studies and then hope to generalize from them to a broader base of understanding. This process is based more on scientific knowledge, insight, and conjecture about nature than it is on the statistical representativeness of the actual study participants. This principle has important implications for the design and interpretation of epidemiologic studies (see Chapter 7).

QUESTIONS

1. Criticize the following statement: The cause of tuberculosis is infection with the tubercle bacillus.

2. A trait in chickens called yellow shank occurs when a specific genetic strain of chickens is fed yellow corn. Farmers who own only this strain of chickens

observe the trait to depend entirely on the nature of the diet, specifically whether they feed their chickens yellow corn. Farmers who feed all of their chickens only yellow corn but own several strains of chicken observe the trait to be genetic. What argument could you use to explain to both kinds of farmer that the trait is both environmental and genetic?

3. A newspaper article proclaims that diabetes is neither genetic nor environmental but multicausal. Another article announces that one half of all colon cancer cases are linked to genetic factors. Criticize both messages.

4. Suppose a new treatment for a fatal disease defers the average time before onset of death among those with the disease for 20 years beyond the time when they would have otherwise died. Is it proper to say that this new treatment reduces the risk of death, or does it merely postpone death?

5. It is typically more difficult to study an exposure-disease relation that has a long induction period than one that has a short induction period. What difficulties ensue because the exposure-disease induction period is long?

6. Suppose that both A and B are causes of a disease that is always fatal, so that the disease can occur only once in a single person. Among people exposed to both A and B, what is the maximum proportion of disease that can be attributed to either A or B? What is the maximum for the sum of the amount attributable to A and the amount attributable to B? Suppose that A and B exert their causal influence only in different causal mechanisms, so that they never act through the same mechanism. Would that change your answer?

7. Adherents of induction claim that we all use this method of inference every day. We assume, for example, that the sun will rise tomorrow as it has in the past. Critics of induction claim that this knowledge is based on belief and assumption and that it is no more than a psychological crutch. Why should it matter to a scientist whether scientific reasoning is based on induction or on a different approach, such as conjecture and refutation?

8. Give an example of competing hypotheses for which an epidemiologic study would provide a refutation of at least one.

9. Could a causal association fail to show evidence of a biologic gradient (ie, Hill's fifth criterion)? Explain.

10. Suppose you are studying the influence of socioeconomic factors on cardiovascular disease. Would the study be more informative if (1) the study participants had the same distribution of socioeconomic factors as the general population or (2) the study participants were recruited so that there were equal numbers of participants in each category of the socioeconomic variables? Why?

REFERENCES

1. Rothman KJ. Causes. *Am J Epidemiol.* 1976;104:587–592.
2. Higginson J. Proportion of cancer due to occupation. *Prev Med.* 1980;9:180–188.
3. Ephron E. *The Apocalyptics. Cancer and the Big Lie.* New York: Simon & Schuster, 1984.
4. Rothman KJ: Induction and latent period. *Am J Epidemiol.* 1981;114:253–259.
5. Magee B. *Philosophy and the Real World. An Introduction to Karl Popper.* La Salle, Illinois, Open Court, 1985.
6. Kuhn T. *The Structure of Scientific Revolutions.* Chicago: University of Chicago Press, 1962.
7. Feyerabend P. *Against Method.* New York: New Left Books, 1975.
8. Haack S. *Defending Science Within Reason.* Amherst: Prometheus Books, 2003.
9. Haack S. Trial and error: the Supreme Court's philosophy of science. *Am J Public Health.* 2005;95(suppl 1):S66-S73.
10. Mill JS. *A System of Logic, Ratiocinative and Inductive.* 5th ed. London: Parker, Son & Bowin, 1862.
11. Hill AB. The environment and disease: Association or causation? *Proc R Soc Med.* 1965;58:295–300.
12. U.S. Department of Health, Education and Welfare. *Smoking and Health: Report of the Advisory Committee to the Surgeon General of the Public Health Service.* Public Health Service Publication No. 1103. Washington, DC: Government Printing Office, 1964.
13. Weiss NS. Can the "specificity" of an association be rehabilitated as a basis for supporting a causal hypothesis? *Epidemiology.* 2002;13:6–8.

4

Measuring Disease Occurrence and Causal Effects

As with most sciences, measurement is a central feature of epidemiology, which has been defined as the study of the occurrence of illness.[1] The broad scope of epidemiology demands a correspondingly broad interpretation of illness, to include injuries, birth defects, health outcomes, and other health-related events and conditions. The fundamental observations in epidemiology are measures of the occurrence of illness. In this chapter, I discuss several measures of disease frequency, including *risk, incidence rate,* and *prevalence.* I also examine how these fundamental measures can be used to obtain derivative measures that aid in quantifying potentially causal relations between exposure and disease.

MEASURES OF DISEASE OCCURRENCE

Risk and Incidence Proportion

The concept of *risk* for disease is widely used and reasonably well understood by many people. It is measured on the same scale and interpreted in the same way as a *probability.* Epidemiologists sometimes speak about risk applying to an individual, in which case they are describing the probability that a person will develop a given disease. It is usually pointless, however, to measure risk for a single person, because for most diseases, the person simply either does or does not contract the disease. For a larger group of people, we can describe the proportion who developed the disease. If a population has N people and A people of the N develop disease during a period of time, the proportion A/N represents the average risk of disease in the population during that period:

$$\text{Risk} = \frac{A}{N} = \frac{\text{Number of subjects developing disease during a time period}}{\text{Number of subjects followed for the time period}}$$

The measure of risk requires that all of the N people are followed for the entire time during which the risk is being measured. The average risk for a group is also referred to as the *incidence proportion*. The word *risk* often is used in reference to a single person, and *incidence proportion* is used in reference to a group of people (Table 4–1). Because averages taken from populations are used to estimate the risk for individuals, the two terms often are used synonymously. We can use risk or incidence proportion to assess the onset of disease, death from a given disease, or any event that marks a health outcome.

One of the primary advantages of using risk as a measure of disease frequency is the extent to which it is readily understood by many people, including those who have little familiarity with epidemiology. To make risk useful as a technical or scientific measure, however, we need to clarify the concept. Suppose you read in the newspaper that women who are 60 years old have a 2% risk of dying of cardiovascular disease. What does this statement mean? If you consider the possibilities, you may soon realize that the statement as written cannot be interpreted. It is certainly not true that a typical 60-year-old woman has a 2% chance of dying of cardiovascular disease within the next 24 hours or in the next week or month. A 2% risk would be high even for 1 year, unless the women in question have one or more characteristics that put them at unusually high risk compared with most 60-year-old women. The risk of developing fatal cardiovascular disease over the remaining lifetime of 60-year-old women, however, would likely be well above 2%. There might be some period over which the 2% figure would be correct, but any other period of time would imply a different value for the risk.

The only way to interpret a risk is to know the length of time over which the risk applies. This period may be short or long, but without identifying it, risk values are not meaningful. Over a very short time period, the risk of any particular disease is usually extremely low. What is the probability that a given person will develop a given disease in the next 5 minutes? It is close to zero. The total risk over a period of time may climb from zero at the start of the period to a maximum theoretical limit of 100%, but it cannot decrease with time. Figure 4–1 illustrates two different possible patterns of risk during a 20-year interval. In pattern A, the risk climbs rapidly early during the period and then plateaus, whereas in pattern B, the risk climbs at a steadily increasing rate during the period.

How might these different risk patterns occur? As an example, a pattern similar to A could occur if a person who is susceptible to an infectious disease becomes immunized, in which case the leveling off of risk is sudden, not gradual. Pattern A also could occur if those who come into contact with a susceptible person become immunized, reducing the susceptible person's risk of acquiring the disease. A pattern similar to B could occur if a person who has been exposed to a cause

Table 4–1 COMPARISON OF INCIDENCE PROPORTION (RISK)
AND INCIDENCE RATE

Property	Incidence Proportion	Incidence Rate
Smallest value	0	0
Greatest value	1	Infinity
Units (dimensionality)	None	1/time
Interpretation	Probability	Inverse of waiting time

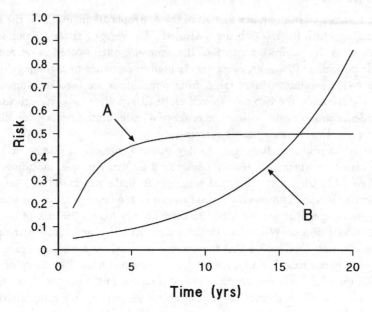

Figure 4–1   Two possible patterns of disease risk with time.

is nearing the end of the typical induction time for the causal action, such as risk of adenocarcinoma of the vagina among young women who were exposed to diethylstilbestrol (DES) while they were fetuses, as discussed in Chapter 3. In that example, the shape of the curve is similar to that of B in Figure 4–1, but the actual risks are much lower than those in Figure 4–1. Another phenomenon that can give rise to pattern B is the aging process, which often leads to sharply increasing risks as people progress beyond middle age.

Risk is a cumulative measure. For a given person, risk increases with the length of the risk period. For a given risk period, however, risks for a person can rise or fall with time. Consider the 1-year risk of dying in an automobile crash for a driver. For any one person during a period of 1 year, the risk cumulates steadily from zero at the beginning of the year to a final value at the end of that year. Nevertheless, the 1-year risk is greater for most drivers in their teenage years than for the same drivers when they reach their 50s.

Risk carries an important drawback as a tool for assessing the occurrence of illness; over any appreciable time interval, it is usually technically impossible to measure risk. The reason is a practical one: For almost any population followed for a sufficient time, some people in the population will die from causes other than the outcome under study.

Suppose that you are interested in measuring the occurrence of domestic violence in a population of 10,000 married women over a 30-year period. Unfortunately, not all 10,000 women will survive the 30-year period. Some may die from extreme instances of domestic violence, but many more are likely to die from cardiovascular disease, cancer, infection, vehicular injury, or other causes. What if a woman died after 5 years of being followed without having been a victim of domestic violence? We could not say that she would not have been a victim of domestic violence during the subsequent 25 years. If we count her as part of the denominator, N, we will obtain an underestimate of the risk of domestic violence for a population of women who do survive 30 years. To understand why, imagine that there are many women who do not survive the 30-year follow-up period. It is likely that among them there are some women who would have experienced domestic violence if they had instead survived. If we count the women who die during the follow-up period in the denominator, N, of a risk measure, then the numerator, A, which gives the number of cases of domestic violence, will be underestimated because A is supposed to represent the number of victims of domestic violence among a population of women who were followed for a full 30 years.

This phenomenon of people being removed from a study through death from other causes is sometimes referred to as *competing risks*. There is one outcome for which there can be no competing risk: the outcome of death from any cause. If we study all deaths, there is no possibility of someone dying of a cause that we are not measuring. For any other outcome, it will always be possible for someone to die before the end of the follow-up period without experiencing the event that we are measuring. Therefore, unless we are studying all deaths, competing risks become a consideration.

Over a short period of time, the influence of competing risks usually is small. It is not unusual for studies to ignore competing risks if the follow-up period is short. For example, in the experiment in 1954 in which the Salk vaccine was tested, hundreds of thousands of schoolchildren were given either the Salk vaccine or a placebo. All of the children were followed for 1 year to assess the vaccine's efficacy. Because only a small proportion of school-age children died of competing causes during the year of the study, it was reasonable to report the results of the Salk vaccine trial in terms of the observed risks. When study participants are older or are followed for longer periods, competing risks are greater and may need to be taken into account. One way to remove competing risks is to measure incidence rates instead, and convert these to risk measures, and another is to use a life-table analysis. Both approaches are described later in this chapter.

A related issue that affects long-term follow-up is *loss to follow-up*. Some people may be hard to track to assess whether they have developed disease. They may move away or choose not to participate further in a research study. The difficulty in interpreting studies in which there have been considerable losses to follow-up is sometimes similar to the challenge of interpreting studies in which there are strong competing risks. In both situations, the researcher lacks complete follow-up of a study group for the intended period of follow-up.

Because of competing risks, it is often useful to think of risk or incidence proportion as hypothetical measures in the sense that they usually cannot be directly observed in a population. If competing risks did not occur and all losses to follow-up could be avoided, we could measure incidence proportion directly in a population by dividing the number of observed cases by the number of people in the population followed. As mentioned earlier, if the outcome of interest is death from any cause, there will be no competing risk; any death that occurs represents an outcome that will count in the numerator of the risk measure. Most attempts to measure disease risk are focused on outcomes more specific than death from any cause, such as death from a specific cause (eg, cancer, multiple sclerosis, infection) or the occurrence of a disease rather than death. For these outcomes, there is always the possibility of competing risks. In reporting the fraction A/N, which is the observed number of cases divided by the number of people who were initially being followed, the incidence proportion that would have been observed had there been no competing risk will be underestimated, because competing risks will have removed some people from the at-risk population before their disease developed.

ATTACK RATE AND CASE-FATALITY RATE

A term for risk or incidence proportion that is sometimes used in connection with infectious outbreaks is *attack rate*. An attack rate is the incidence proportion, or risk, of contracting a condition during an epidemic period. For example, if an influenza epidemic has a 10% attack rate, 10% of the population will develop the disease during the epidemic period. The time reference for an attack rate is usually not stated but is implied by the biology of the disease being described. It is usually short, typically no more than a few months, and sometimes much less. A *secondary attack rate* is the attack rate among susceptible people who come into direct contact with *primary cases*, the cases infected in the initial wave of an epidemic (see Chapter 6).

Another version of the incidence proportion that is encountered frequently in clinical medicine is the *case-fatality rate*, which is described in greater detail in Chapter 13. The case-fatality rate is the proportion of people dying of the disease (fatalities) among those who develop the disease (cases). Thus, the population at risk when a case-fatality rate is used is the population of people who have already developed the disease. The event being measured is not development of the disease but rather death from the disease (sometimes all deaths among patients, rather than only deaths from the disease, are counted). Like an attack rate, the case-fatality rate is seldom accompanied by a specific time referent, and this lack of time specificity can make it difficult to interpret. It is typically used and easiest to interpret as a description of the proportion of people who succumb to an infectious disease, such as measles. The case-fatality rate for measles in the United States is about 1.5 deaths per 1000 cases. The period for this risk of death is the comparatively short time frame during which measles infects an individual, ending in recovery, death, or some other complication. For diseases that continue to affect a person over long periods, such as multiple sclerosis, it is more difficult to interpret a measure such as case-fatality rate, and other types of mortality or survival measures are used instead.

Incidence Rate

To address the problem of competing risks, epidemiologists often resort to a different measure of disease occurrence, the *incidence rate*. This measure is similar to incidence proportion in that the numerator is the same. It is the number of cases,

A, that occur in a population. The denominator is different. Instead of dividing the number of cases by the number of people who were initially being followed, the incidence rate divides the number of cases by a measure of time. This time measure is the summation across all individuals of the time experienced by the population being followed.

$$\text{Incidence rate} = \frac{A}{\text{Time}} = \frac{\text{Number of subjects developing disease}}{\text{Total time experienced for the subjects followed}}$$

One way to obtain this measure is to sum the time that each person is followed for every member of the group being followed. If a population was followed for 30 years and a given person died after 5 years of follow-up, that person would have contributed only 5 years to the sum for the group. Others might have contributed more or fewer years, up to a maximum of the full 30 years of follow-up.

For people who do not die during follow-up, there are two methods of counting the time during follow-up. These methods depend on whether the disease or event can recur. Suppose that the disease is an upper respiratory tract infection, which can occur more than once in the same person. Because the numerator of an incidence rate could contain more than one occurrence of an upper respiratory tract infection from a single person, the denominator should include all the time during which each person was at risk for getting any of these bouts of infection. In this situation, the time of follow-up for each person continues after that person recovers from an upper respiratory tract infection. On the other hand, if the event were death from leukemia, a person would be counted as a case only once. For someone who dies of leukemia, the time that would count in the denominator of an incidence rate would be the interval that begins at the start of follow-up and ends at death from leukemia. If a person can experience an event only once, the person ceases to contribute follow-up time after the event occurs.

In many situations, epidemiologists study events that can occur more than once in an individual, but they count only the first occurrence of the event. For example, researchers may count the occurrence of the first heart attack in an individual and ignore (or study separately) second or later heart attacks. If only the first occurrence of a disease is of interest, the time contribution of a person to the denominator of an incidence rate will end when the disease occurs. The unifying concept in regard to tallying the time for the denominator of an incidence rate is simple: The time that goes into the denominator corresponds to the time experienced by the people being followed during which the disease or event being studied could have occurred. For this reason, the time tallied in the denominator of an incidence rate is often referred to as the *time at risk for disease*. The time in the denominator of an incidence rate should include every moment during which a person being followed is at risk for an event that would get tallied in the numerator of the rate. For events that cannot recur, after a person experiences the event, he or she will have no more time at risk for the disease, and therefore the follow-up for that person ends with the disease occurrence. The same is true of a person who dies from a competing risk.

Figure 4–2 illustrates the time at risk for five hypothetical people being followed to measure the mortality rate of leukemia. A *mortality rate* is an incidence

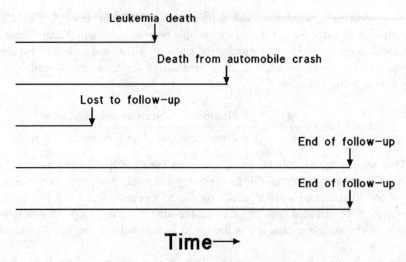

Figure 4-2   Time at risk for leukemia death for five people.

rate in which the event being measured is death. Only the first of the five people died of leukemia during the follow-up period. This person's time at risk ended with his or her death from leukemia. The second person died in an automobile crash, after which he or she was no longer at risk for dying of leukemia. The third person was lost to follow-up early during the follow-up period. After a person is lost, even if that person dies of leukemia, the death will not be counted in the numerator of the rate because the researcher would not know about it. Therefore the time at risk to be counted as a case in the numerator of the rate ends when a person becomes lost to follow-up. The last two people were followed for the complete follow-up period. The total time tallied in the denominator of the mortality rate for leukemia for these five people corresponds to the sum of the lengths of the five line segments in Figure 4–2.

Incidence rates treat one unit of time as equivalent to another, regardless of whether these time units come from the same person or from different people. The incidence rate is the ratio of cases to the total time at risk for disease. This ratio does not have the same simple interpretability as the risk measure.

A comparison of the risk and incidence rate measures (Table 4–1) shows that, whereas the incidence proportion, or risk, can be interpreted as a probability, the incidence rate cannot. Unlike a probability, the incidence rate does not have the range of $[0,1]$. Instead, it can theoretically become extremely large without numeric limit. It may at first seem puzzling that a measure of disease occurrence can exceed 1; how can more than 100% of a population be affected? The answer is that the incidence rate does not measure the proportion of the population that is affected. It measures the ratio of the number of cases to the time at risk for disease. Because the denominator is measured in time units, we can always imagine that the denominator of an incidence rate could be smaller, making the rate larger. The numeric value of the incidence rate depends on what time unit is chosen.

Suppose that we measure an incidence rate in a population as 47 cases occurring in 158 months. To make it clear that the time tallied in the denominator of an incidence rate is the sum of the time contribution from various people, we often refer to these time values as *person-time*. We can express the incidence rate as

$$\frac{47\,\text{cases}}{158\,\text{person-months}} = \frac{0.30\,\text{cases}}{\text{person-month}}$$

We could also restate this same incidence rate using person-years instead of person-months:

$$\frac{47\,\text{cases}}{13.17\,\text{person-years}} = \frac{3.57\,\text{cases}}{\text{person-year}}$$

These two expressions measure the same incidence rate; the only difference is the time unit chosen to express the denominator. The different time units affect the numeric values. The situation is much the same as expressing speed in different units of time or distance. For example, 60 miles/hr is the same as 88 ft/sec or 26.84 m/sec. The change in units results in a change in the numeric value.

The analogy between incidence rate and speed is helpful in understanding other aspects of incidence rate as well. One important insight is that the incidence rate, like speed, is an instantaneous concept. Imagine driving along a highway. At any instant, you and your vehicle have a certain speed. The speed can change from moment to moment. The speedometer gives you a continuous measure of the current speed. Suppose that the speed is expressed in terms of kilometers per hour. Although the time unit for the denominator is 1 hour, it does not require an hour to measure the speed of the vehicle. You can observe the speed for a given instant from the speedometer, which continuously calculates the ratio of distance to time over a recent short interval of time. Similarly, an incidence rate is a momentary rate at which cases are occurring within a group of people. Measuring an incidence rate takes a nonzero amount of time, as does measuring speed, but the concepts of speed and incidence rate can be thought of as applying at a given instant. If an incidence rate is measured, as is often the case, with person-years in the denominator, the rate nevertheless may characterize only a short interval, rather than a year. Similarly, speed expressed in kilometers per hour does not necessarily apply to an hour but perhaps to an instant. It may seem impossible to get an instantaneous measure of incidence rate, but in a situation analogous to use of the speedometer, current incidence or mortality for a sufficiently large population can be measured by counting, for example, the cases occurring in 1 day and dividing that number by the person-time at risk during that day. Time units can be measured in days or hours but may be expressed in years by dividing by the number of days or hours in a year. The unit of time in the denominator of an incidence rate is arbitrary and has no implication for the period of time over which the rate is actually measured, nor does it communicate anything about the actual time to which it applies.

Incidence rates commonly are described as *annual incidence* and expressed in the form of "50 cases per 100,000." This is a clumsy description of an incidence rate, equivalent to describing an instantaneous speed as an "hourly distance." Nevertheless, we can translate this phrasing to correspond with what we have already described for incidence rates. We can express this rate as 50 cases per 100,000 person-years, or $50/100,000 \text{ yr}^{-1}$. The negative 1 in the exponent means inverse, implying that the denominator of the fraction is measured in units of years.

Whereas the risk measure typically transmits a clear message to epidemiologists and nonepidemiologists alike (provided that a time period for the risk is specified), the incidence rate may not. It is more difficult to conceptualize a measure of occurrence that uses the ratio of events to the total time in which the events occur. Nevertheless, under certain conditions, there is an interpretation that we can give to an incidence rate. The dimensionality of an incidence rate is that of the reciprocal of time, which is another way of saying that in an incidence rate, the only units involved are time units, which appear in the denominator. Suppose we invert the incidence rate. Its reciprocal is measured in units of time. To what time does the reciprocal of an incidence rate correspond?

Under steady-state conditions—a situation in which the rates do not change with time—the reciprocal of the incidence rate equals the average time until an event occurs. This time is referred to as the *waiting time*. Take as an example the incidence rate described earlier, 3.57 cases per person-year. This rate can be written as 3.57 yr^{-1}; the cases in the numerator of an incidence rate do not have units. The reciprocal of this rate is $1/3.57$ years $= 0.28$ years. This value can be interpreted as an average waiting time of 0.28 years until the occurrence of an event.

As another example, consider a mortality rate of 11 deaths per 1000 person-years, which could also be written as $11/1000 \text{ yr}^{-1}$. If this is the total mortality rate for an entire population, the waiting time that corresponds to it will represent the average time until death. The average time until death is also referred to as the *expectation of life* or *expected survival time*. Using the reciprocal of $11/1000 \text{ yr}^{-1}$, we obtain 90.9 years, which can be interpreted as the expectation of life for a population in a steady state that has a mortality rate of $11/1000 \text{ yr}^{-1}$. Because mortality rates typically change with time over the time scales that apply to this example, taking the reciprocal of the mortality rate for a population is not a practical method for estimating the expectation of life. Nevertheless, it is helpful to understand what kind of interpretation we may assign to an incidence rate or a mortality rate, even if the conditions that justify the interpretation are often not applicable.

CHICKEN AND EGG

An old riddle asks, "If a chicken and one half lay an egg and one half in a day and one half, how many eggs does one chicken lay in 1 day?" This riddle is a rate problem. The question amounts to asking, "What is the rate of egg laying expressed in eggs per chicken-day?" To get the answer, we express the rate as the number of eggs in the numerator and the number of chicken-days in the denominator: 1.5 eggs/[(1.5 chickens) • (1.5 days)] = 1.5 eggs/2.25 chicken-days. This calculation gives a rate of 2/3 egg per chicken day.

The Relation Between Risk and Incidence Rate

Because the interpretation of risk is so much more straightforward than the interpretation of incidence rate, it is often convenient to convert incidence rate measures into risk measures. Fortunately, this conversion usually is not difficult. The simplest formula to convert an incidence rate to a risk is as follows:

$$\text{Risk} \approx \text{Incidence rate} \times \text{Time} \qquad [4\text{--}1]$$

For Equation 4–1 and other such formulas, it is a good habit to confirm that the dimensionality on both sides of the equation is equivalent. In this case, risk is a proportion, and therefore has no dimensions. Although risk applies for a specific period of time, the time period is a descriptor for the risk but not part of the measure itself. Risk has no units of time or any other quantity built in; it is interpreted as a probability. The right side of Equation 4–1 is the product of two quantities, one of which is measured in units of the reciprocal of time and the other of which is time itself. Because this product has no dimensionality, the equation holds as far as dimensionality is concerned.

In addition to checking the dimensionality, it is useful to check the range of the measures in an equation such as Equation 4–1. The risk is a pure number in the range $[0,1]$; values outside this range are not permitted. In contrast, incidence rate has a range of $[0,\infty]$, and time also has a range of $[0,\infty]$. The product of incidence rate and time does not have a range that is the same as risk, because the product can exceed 1. This analysis shows that Equation 4–1 is not applicable throughout the entire range of values for incidence rate and time. In general terms, Equation 4–1 is an approximation that works well as long as the risk calculated on the left is less than about 20%. Above that value, the approximation deteriorates.

For example, suppose that a population of 10,000 people experiences an incidence rate of lung cancer of 8 cases per 10,000 person-years. If we followed the population for 1 year, Equation 4–1 suggests that the risk of lung cancer is 8 in 10,000 for the 1-year period (ie, 8/10,000 person-years × 1 year), or 0.0008. If the same rate applied for only 0.5 year, the risk would be one half of 0.0008, or 0.0004. Equation 4–1 calculates risk as directly proportional to both the incidence rate and the time period, so as the time period is extended, the risk becomes proportionately greater.

Now suppose that we have a population of 1000 people who experience a mortality rate of 11 deaths per 1000 person-years for a 20-year period. Equation 4–1 predicts that the risk of death over 20 years will be $11/1000 \text{ yr}^{-1} \times 20 \text{ yr} = 0.22$, or 22%. In other words, Equation 4–1 predicts that among the 1000 people at the start of the follow-up period, there will be 220 deaths during the 20 years. The 220 deaths are the sum of 11 deaths that occur among 1000 people every year for 20 years. This calculation neglects the fact that the size of the population at risk shrinks gradually as deaths occur. If the shrinkage is taken into account, fewer than 220 deaths will have occurred at the end of 20 years.

Table 4–2 describes the number of deaths expected to occur during each year of the 20 years of follow-up if the mortality rate of $11/1000 \text{ yr}^{-1}$ is applied to a population of 1000 people for 20 years. The table shows that at the end of

Table 4-2 NUMBER OF EXPECTED DEATHS OVER 20 YEARS AMONG
1000 PEOPLE WITH A MORTALITY RATE OF 11 DEATHS PER 1000
PERSON-YEARS

Year	Expected Number Alive at Start of Year	Expected Deaths	Cumulative Deaths
1	1000.000	10.940	10.940
2	989.060	10.820	21.760
3	978.240	10.702	32.461
4	967.539	10.585	43.046
5	956.954	10.469	53.515
6	946.485	10.354	63.869
7	936.131	10.241	74.110
8	925.890	10.129	84.239
9	915.761	10.018	94.257
10	905.743	9.909	104.166
11	895.834	9.800	113.966
12	886.034	9.693	123.659
13	876.341	9.587	133.246
14	866.754	9.482	142.728
15	857.272	9.378	152.106
16	847.894	9.276	161.382
17	838.618	9.174	170.556
18	829.444	9.074	179.630
19	820.370	8.975	188.605
20	811.395	8.876	197.481

20 years, about 197 deaths have occurred, rather than 220, because a steadily smaller population is at risk of death each year. The table also shows that the prediction of 11 deaths per year from Equation 4–1 is a good estimate for the early part of the follow-up but the number of deaths expected each year gradually becomes considerably lower than 11. Why is the number of expected deaths not quite 11 even for the first year, in which there are 1000 people being followed at the start of the year? As soon as the first death occurs, the number of people being followed is less than 1000, which influences the number of expected deaths in the first year. As is seen in Table 4–2, the expected deaths decline gradually throughout the period of follow-up.

If we extended the calculations in the table further, the discrepancy between the risk calculated from Equation 4–1 and the actual risk would grow. Figure 4–3 graphs the cumulative total of deaths that would be expected and the number projected from Equation 4–1 over 50 years of follow-up. Initially, the two curves are close, but as the cumulative risk of death rises, they diverge. The bottom curve in the figure is an exponential curve, related to the curve that describes *exponential decay*. If a population experiences a constant rate of death, the proportion remaining alive follows an exponential curve with time. This exponential decay is the same curve that describes radioactive decay. If a population of radioactive atoms converts from one atomic state to another at a constant rate, the proportion of atoms left in the initial state follows the curve of exponential decay. The lower

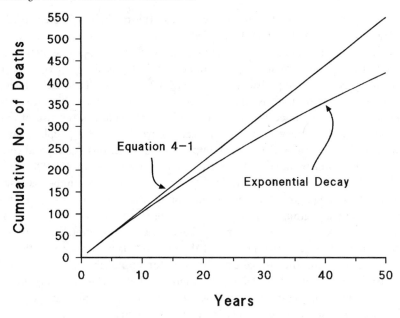

Figure 4–3 Cumulative number of deaths among 1000 people with a mortality rate of 11 deaths per 1000 person-years, presuming no population shrinkage (see Equation 4–1) and taking the population shrinkage into account (ie, exponential decay).

curve in Figure 4–3 is actually the complement of an exponential decay curve. Instead of showing the decreasing number remaining alive (ie, the curve of exponential decay), it shows the increasing number who have died, which is the total number in the population minus the number remaining alive. Given enough time, this curve gradually flattens, and the total number of deaths approaches the total number of people in the population. In contrast, the curve based on Equation 4–1 continues to predict 11 deaths each year regardless of how many people remain alive, and it eventually would predict a cumulative number of deaths that exceeds the original size of the population.

Clearly, Equation 4–1 cannot be used to calculate risks that are large, because it provides a poor approximation in such situations. For many epidemiologic applications, however, the calculated risks are reasonably small, and Equation 4–1 is quite adequate for converting incidence rates to risks.

Equation 4–1 calculates risk for a time period over which a single incidence rate applies. The calculation assumes that the incidence rate, an instantaneous concept, remains constant over the time period. What if the incidence rate changes with time, as is often the case? In that event, risk can still be calculated, but it should be calculated first for separate subintervals of the time period. Each of the time intervals should be short enough so that the incidence rate that applies to it could be considered approximately constant. The shorter the intervals, the better the overall accuracy of the risk calculation, although the intervals should not be so short that there are inadequate data to obtain meaningful incidence rates for each interval.

The method of calculating risks over a time period with changing incidence rates is known as *survival analysis*. It can also be applied to nonfatal risks, but the approach originated from data related to deaths. The method is implemented by creating a table similar to Table 4–2, called a *life table*. The purpose of a life table is to calculate the probability of surviving through each successive time interval that constitutes the period of interest. The overall survival probability is equal to the cumulative product of the probabilities of surviving through each successive interval, and the overall risk of death is equal to 1 minus the overall probability of survival.

Table 4–3 is a simplified life table that enables calculation of the risk of dying of a motor vehicle injury in a hypothetical cohort of 100,000 people followed from birth through age 85.[2] In this example, the time periods correspond to age intervals. The number initially at risk has been arbitrarily set to 100,000 people. The life-table calculation is strictly hypothetical, because the number at risk at the start of each age group is reduced only by deaths from motor vehicle injury in the previous age group, ignoring all other causes of death. With this assumption that there are no competing risks, the results are interpretable as risks or survival probabilities that would result if the only risk faced by a population was the one under study. The risk of dying of a motor vehicle injury for each of the age intervals is calculated by taking the number of deaths in each age interval (column 3) and dividing it by the number who are at risk during that age interval (column 2). The survival probability in column 5 is equal to 1 minus the risk for that age category. The cumulative survival probability (column 6) is the product of the age-specific survival probabilities up to that age. The bottom number in column 6 is the probability of surviving to age 85 without dying of a motor vehicle injury, assuming that there are no competing risks (ie, assuming that without a motor vehicle injury, the person would survive to age 85).

Subtracting the final cumulative survival probability from 1 gives the total risk, from birth until the 85th birthday, of dying of a motor vehicle injury. This risk is $1 - 0.98378 = 1.6\%$. Because this calculation is based on the assumption that everyone will live to their 85th birthday except those who die of motor vehicle accidents, it overstates the actual proportion of people who will die in a motor vehicle accident before they reach age 85. Another assumption in the calculation is that these mortality rates, which have been gathered from a cross section of the population at a given time, can be applied to a group of people over the course of 85 years of life. If the mortality rates changed with time, the risk estimated from the life table would be inaccurate.

Table 4–3 LIFE TABLE FOR DEATH FROM MOTOR VEHICLE INJURY FROM BIRTH THROUGH AGE 85[a]

Age	Number at Risk	Deaths in Interval	Risk of Dying	Survival Probability	Cumulative Survival Probability
0–14	100,000	70	0.00070	0.99930	0.99930
15–24	99,930	358	0.00358	0.99642	0.99572
25–44	99,572	400	0.00402	0.99598	0.99172
45–64	99,172	365	0.00368	0.99632	0.98807
65–84	98,807	429	0.00434	0.99566	0.98378

[a]Mortality rates are deaths per 100,000 person-years.
Adapted from Iskrant and Joliet, Table 24.[2]

Table 4–3 shows a hypothetical cohort being followed for 85 years. If this had been an actual cohort, there would have been some people lost to follow-up and some who died of other causes. When follow-up is incomplete for either of these reasons, the usual approach is to use the information that is available for those with incomplete follow-up; their follow-up is described as *censored* at the time that they are lost or die of another cause.

Table 4–4 shows what the same cohort experience would look like under the more realistic situation in which many people have incomplete follow-up. Two new columns have been added with hypothetical data on the number that are censored because they were lost to follow-up or died of other causes (column 4) and the effective number at risk (column 5). The effective number at risk is calculated by taking the number at risk in column 2 and subtracting one half of the number who are censored (column 4). Subtracting one half of those who are censored is based on the assumption that the censoring occurred uniformly throughout each age interval. If there is reason to believe that the censoring tended to occur nonuniformly within the interval, the calculation of the effective number at risk should be adjusted to reflect that belief.

Point-Source and Propagated Epidemics

An *epidemic* is an unusually high occurrence of disease. The definition of *unusually high* depends on the circumstances, and there is no clear demarcation between an epidemic and a smaller fluctuation. The high occurrence may represent an increase in the occurrence of a disease that still occurs in the population in the absence of an epidemic, although less frequently than during the epidemic, or it may represent an *outbreak*, which is a sudden increase in the occurrence of a disease that is usually absent or nearly absent (Fig. 4–4).

If an epidemic stems from a single source of exposure to a causal agent, it is considered a *point-source epidemic*. Examples of point-source epidemics are food poisoning of restaurant patrons who have been served contaminated food and cancer occurrence among survivors of the atomic bomb blasts in Hiroshima

Table 4–4 Life Table for Death from Motor Vehicle Injury from Birth Through Age 85[a]

Age	At Risk	Motor Vehicle Injury Deaths in Interval	Lost to Follow-up or Died of Other Causes	Effective Number at Risk	Risk of Dying	Survival Probability	Cumulative Survival Probability
0–14	100,000	67	9,500	95,250	0.00070	0.99930	0.99930
15–24	90,433	301	12,500	84,183	0.00358	0.99642	0.99572
25–44	77,632	272	20,000	67,632	0.00402	0.99598	0.99172
45–64	57,360	156	30,000	42,360	0.00368	0.99632	0.98807
65–84	27,204	64	25,000	14,704	0.00435	0.99565	0.98377

[a]Mortality rates are deaths per 100,000 person-years.

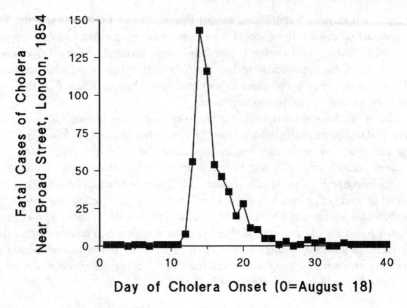

Figure 4–4 Epidemic curve for fatal cholera cases during the Broad Street outbreak in London in 1854.

and Nagasaki. Although the time scales of these epidemics differ dramatically, along with the nature of the diseases and their causes, all people in both cases were exposed to the same causal component that produced the epidemic— contaminated food in the restaurant or ionizing radiation from the bomb blast. The exposure in a point-source epidemic is typically newly introduced into the environment, thus accounting for the epidemic.

Typically, the shape of the epidemic curve for a point-source epidemic shows an initial steep increase in the incidence rate followed by a more gradual decline in the incidence rate; this pattern is often described as a log-normal distribution. The asymmetry of the curve stems partly from the fact that biologic curves with a meaningful zero point tend to be asymmetric because there is less variability in the direction of the zero point than in the other direction. For example, the distribution of recovery times for healing of a wound is log-normal. Similarly, the distribution of induction times until the occurrence of illness after a common exposure is log-normal. If the zero point is sufficiently far from the modal value, the asymmetry may not be apparent. For example, birth weight has a meaningful zero point, but the zero point is far from the center of the distribution, and the distribution is almost symmetric.

An example of an asymmetric epidemic curve is that of the 1854 cholera epidemic described by John Snow.[3] In that outbreak, exposure to contaminated water in the neighborhood of the water pump at Broad Street in London produced a log-normal epidemic curve (see Fig. 4–4). Snow is renowned for having convinced local authorities to remove the handle from the pump, but they only did so on September 8 (day 21), when the epidemic was well past its peak and the number of cases was almost back to zero.

The shape of an epidemic curve also may be affected by the way in which the curve is calculated. It is common, as in Figure 4–4, to plot the number of new cases instead of the incidence rate among susceptible people. People who have already succumbed to an infectious disease may no longer be susceptible to it for some period of time. If a substantial proportion of a population is affected by the outbreak, the number of susceptible people will decline gradually as the epidemic progresses and the attack rate increases. This change in the susceptible population leads to a more rapid decline over time in the number of new cases compared with the incidence rate in the susceptible population. The incidence rate declines more slowly than the number of new cases because in the incidence rate, the declining number of new cases is divided by a dwindling amount of susceptible person-time.

A *propagated epidemic* is one in which the causal agent is transmitted through a population. Influenza epidemics are propagated by person-to-person transmission of the virus. The epidemic of lung cancer during the 20th century was a propagated epidemic attributable to the spread of tobacco smoking through many cultures and societies. The curve for a propagated epidemic tends to show a more gradual initial rise and a more symmetric shape than for a point-source epidemic because the causes spread gradually through the population. Transmission of infectious disease within a population is discussed further in Chapter 6, which also presents the Reed-Frost model, a simple model that describes transmission of an infectious disease in a closed population.

Although we may think of point-source epidemics as occurring over a short time span, they are not always briefer than propagated epidemics. The epidemic of cancer attributable to exposure to the atomic bombs detonated in Hiroshima and Nagasaki was a point-source epidemic that began a few years after the explosions and continues into the present. Another possible point-source epidemic that occurred over decades was an apparent outbreak of multiple sclerosis in the Faroe Islands that followed the occupation of those islands by British troops during the Second World War[4] (although this interpretation of the data has been questioned[5]). Propagated epidemics can occur over extremely short time spans. An example is epidemic hysteria, a disease often propagated from person to person in minutes. An example of an epidemic curve for a hysteria outbreak is depicted in Figure 4–5. In this epidemic, 210 elementary school children developed symptoms of headache, abdominal pain, and nausea. These symptoms were attributed by the investigators to hysteric anxiety.[6]

Prevalence Proportion

Incidence proportion and incidence rate are measures that assess the frequency of disease onsets. The numerator of either measure is the frequency of events that are defined as the occurrence of disease. In contrast, *prevalence proportion,* often referred to simply as *prevalence,* does not measure disease onset. Instead, it is a measure of disease status.

The simplest way of considering disease status is to consider disease as being either present or absent. The prevalence proportion is the proportion of people in a population who have disease. Consider a population of size N, and suppose that P individuals in the population have disease at a given time. The prevalence proportion is P/N. For example, suppose that among 10,000 women residents of a town on July 1, 2001, 1200 have hypertension. The prevalence proportion of hypertension among women in that town on that date is $1200/10,000 = 0.12$,

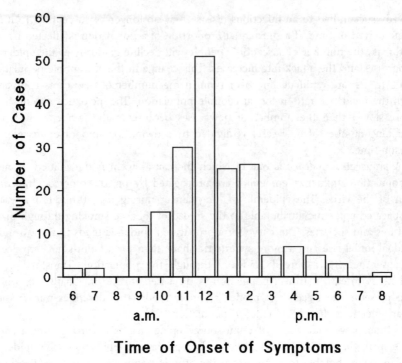

Time of Onset of Symptoms

Figure 4–5 Epidemic curve for an outbreak of hysteria among elementary school children on November 6, 1985.

or 12%. This prevalence applies only to a single point in time, July 1, 2001. Prevalence can change with time as the factors that affect prevalence change.

What factors affect prevalence? Clearly, disease occurrence affects prevalence. The greater the incidence of disease, the more people there are who have it. Prevalence is also related to the length of time that a person has disease. The longer the duration of disease, the higher the prevalence. Diseases with short duration may have a low prevalence even if the incidence rate is high. One reason is that if the disease is benign, there may be a rapid recovery. For example, the prevalence of upper respiratory infection may be low despite a high incidence, because after a brief period, most people recover from the infection and are no longer in the disease state. Duration may also be short for a grave disease that leads to rapid death. The prevalence of aortic hemorrhage would be low even with a high incidence because it usually leads to death within minutes. The low prevalence means that, at any given moment, only an extremely small proportion of people are suffering from an aortic hemorrhage. Some diseases have a short duration because either recovery or death ensues promptly; appendicitis is an example. Other diseases have a long duration because, although a person cannot recover from them, they are compatible with a long survival time (although survival is often shorter than it would be without the disease). Diabetes, Crohn's disease, multiple sclerosis, parkinsonism, and glaucoma are examples.

Because prevalence reflects both incidence rate and disease duration, it is not as useful as incidence alone for studying the causes of disease. It is extremely useful, however, for measuring the disease burden on a population, especially if those who have disease require specific medical attention. For example, the prevalent number of people in a population with end-stage renal disease predicts the need in that population for dialysis facilities.

In a *steady state*, which is the situation in which incidence rates and disease duration are stable over time, the prevalence proportion, P, has the following relation to the incidence rate:

$$\frac{P}{1 - P} = I\bar{D} \qquad [4\text{–}2]$$

In Equation 4–2, I is the incidence rate and $\bar{D}$ is the average duration of disease. The quantity $P/(1 - P)$ is known as the *prevalence odds*. In general, when a proportion, such as prevalence proportion, is divided by 1 minus the proportion, the resulting ratio is referred to as the *odds* for that proportion. If a horse is a 3-to-1 favorite at a racetrack, it means that the horse is thought to have a probability of winning of 0.75. The odds of the horse winning is $0.75/(1 - 0.75) = 3$, usually described as 3 to 1. Similarly, if a prevalence proportion is 0.75, the prevalence odds would be 3, and a prevalence of 0.20 would correspond to a prevalence odds of $0.20/(1 - 0.20) = 0.25$. For small prevalences, the value of the prevalence proportion and that of the prevalence odds are close because the denominator of the odds expression is close to 1. For small prevalences (eg, <0.1), we can rewrite Equation 4–2 as follows:

$$P \approx I\bar{D} \qquad [4\text{–}3]$$

Equation 4–3 indicates that, given a steady state and a low prevalence, prevalence is approximately equal to the product of the incidence rate and the mean duration of disease. Note that this relation does not hold for age-specific prevalences. In that case, $\bar{D}$ corresponds to the duration of time spent within that age category rather than the total duration of time with disease.

As we did earlier for risk and incidence rate, we should check this equation to make certain that the dimensionality and ranges of both sides of the equation are satisfied. For dimensionality, the right-hand sides of Equations 4–2 and 4–3 involve the product of a time measure, disease duration, and an incidence rate, which has units of reciprocal of time. The product is dimensionless, a pure number. Prevalence proportion, like risk or incidence proportion, is also dimensionless, which satisfies the dimensionality requirement for the two equations, 4–2 and 4–3. The range of incidence rate and that of mean duration of illness is $[0,\infty]$, because there is no upper limit to an incidence rate or the duration of disease. Therefore Equation 4–3 does not satisfy the range requirement, because the prevalence proportion on the left side of the equation, like any proportion, has a range of $[0,1]$. For this reason, Equation 4–3 is applicable only for small values of prevalence. The measure of prevalence odds in Equation 4–2, however, has a range of $[0,\infty]$, and it is applicable for all values, rather than just for small values of the prevalence proportion. We can rewrite Equation 4–2 to solve for the prevalence proportion as follows:

$$P = \frac{I\bar{D}}{1 + I\bar{D}} \qquad [4\text{–}4]$$

Prevalence measures the disease burden in a population. This type of epidemiologic application relates more to administrative areas of public health than to causal research. Nevertheless, there are research areas in which prevalence measures are used more commonly than incidence measures, even to investigate causes. Examples are birth defects and birth-related phenomena such as birth weight or preterm birth. We use a prevalence measure when describing the occurrence of congenital malformations among liveborn infants in terms of the proportion of these infants who have a malformation. For example, the proportion of infants who are born alive with a defect of the ventricular septum of the heart is a prevalence. It measures the status of liveborn infants with respect to the presence or absence of a ventricular septal defect. Measuring the incidence rate or incidence proportion of ventricular septal defects would require ascertainment of a population of embryos who were at risk for developing the defect and measurement of the defect's occurrence among these embryos. Such data are usually not obtainable, because many pregnancies end before the pregnancy is detected, and the population of embryos is not readily identified. Even when a woman knows she is pregnant, if the pregnancy ends early, information about the pregnancy may never come to the attention of researchers. For these reasons, incidence measures for birth defects are uncommon. Prevalence at birth is easier to assess and often is used as a substitute for incidence measures. Although prevalence measures are easier to obtain, they have a drawback when used for causal research: Factors that increase prevalence may do so not by increasing the occurrence of the condition but by increasing the duration of the condition. For example, a factor associated with the prevalence of ventricular septal defect at birth could be a cause of ventricular septal defect, but it could also be a factor that does not cause the defect but instead enables embryos that develop the defect to survive until birth. On the other hand, there may be practical interest in understanding the factors that are related to being born alive with the defect.

Prevalence is sometimes used in research to measure diseases that have insidious onset, such as diabetes or multiple sclerosis. These are conditions for which it may be difficult to define onset, and it therefore may be necessary in some settings to describe the condition in terms of prevalence rather than incidence.

Prevalence of Characteristics

Because prevalence measures status, it is often used to describe the status of characteristics or conditions other than disease in a population. For example, the proportion of a population that engages in cigarette smoking often is described as the prevalence of smoking. The proportion of a population exposed to a given agent is often referred to as the exposure prevalence. Prevalence can be used to describe the proportion of people in a population who have brown eyes, type O blood, or an active driver's license. Because epidemiology relates many individual and population characteristics to disease occurrence, it often employs prevalence measures to describe the frequency of these characteristics.

MEASURES OF CAUSAL EFFECTS

A central objective of epidemiologic research is to study the causes of disease. How should we measure the effect of exposure to determine whether exposure causes disease? In a courtroom, experts are asked to opine whether the disease of a given patient has been caused by a specific exposure. This approach of assigning causation in a single person is radically different from the epidemiologic approach, which does not attempt to attribute causation in any individual instance. The epidemiologic approach is to evaluate the proposition that the exposure is a cause of the disease in a theoretical sense, rather than in a specific person.

An elementary but essential principle to keep in mind is that a person may be exposed to an agent and then develop disease without there being any causal connection between the exposure and the disease. For this reason, we cannot consider the incidence proportion or the incidence rate among exposed people to measure a causal effect. For example, if a vaccine does not confer perfect immunity, some vaccinated people will get the disease that the vaccine is intended to prevent. The occurrence of disease among vaccinated people is not a sign that the vaccine is causing the disease, because the disease will occur even more frequently among unvaccinated people. It is merely a sign that the vaccine is not a perfect preventive. To measure a causal effect, we have to contrast the experience of exposed people with what would have happened in the absence of exposure.

The Counterfactual Ideal

It is useful to consider how to measure causal effects in an ideal way. People differ from one another in myriad ways. If we compare risks or incidence rates between exposed and unexposed people, we cannot be certain that the differences in risks or rates are attributable to the exposure. They could be attributable to other factors that differ between exposed and unexposed people. We may be able to measure and to take into account some of these factors, but others may elude us, hindering any definite inference. Even if we matched people who were exposed with similar people who were not exposed, they could still differ in inapparent ways. The ideal comparison would be the result of a thought experiment: the comparison of people with themselves, followed through time simultaneously in both an exposed and an unexposed state. Such a comparison envisions the impossible, because it requires each person to exist in two incarnations: one exposed and the other unexposed. If such an impossible goal were achievable, it would allow us to know the effect of exposure, because the only difference between the two settings would be the exposure. Because this situation is impossible, it is called *counterfactual*.

The counterfactual goal posits not only a comparison of a person with himself or herself but also a repetition of the experience during the same time period. Some studies do pair the experiences of a person under both exposed and unexposed conditions. The experimental version of such a study is called a *crossover study*, because the study subject crosses over from one study group to the other after a period of time. Although crossover studies come close to the ideal of a counterfactual comparison, they do not achieve it because a person can be in only one study group at a given time. The time sequence may affect the interpretation, and the passage of time means that the two experiences that are compared may differ by factors other than the exposure. The counterfactual setting is impossible, because it implies that a person lives through the same experience twice during the same time period, once with exposure and once without exposure.

In the theoretical ideal of a counterfactual study, each exposed person would be compared with his or her unexposed counterfactual experience. Everyone is exposed, and in a parallel universe everyone is also unexposed, with all other factors remaining the same. The effect of exposure could then be measured by comparing the incidence proportion among everyone while exposed with the incidence proportion while everyone is unexposed. Any difference in these proportions would have to be an effect of exposure. Suppose we observed 100 exposed people and found that 25 developed disease in 1 year, providing an incidence proportion of 0.25. We would theoretically like to compare this experience with the counterfactual, unobservable experience of the same 100 people going through the same year under the same conditions except for being unexposed. Suppose that 10 people developed disease in those counterfactual conditions. Then the incidence proportion for comparison would be 0.10. The difference, 15 cases in 100 during the year, or 0.15, would be a measure of the causal effect of the exposure.

EFFECT MEASURES

Because we can never achieve the counterfactual ideal, we strive to come as close as possible to it in the design of epidemiologic studies. Instead of comparing the experience of an exposed group with its counterfactual ideal, we must compare their experience with that of a real unexposed population. The goal is to find an unexposed population that would give a result that is close, if not identical, to that from a counterfactual comparison.

Suppose we consider the same 100 exposed people mentioned earlier, among whom 25 get the disease in 1 year. As a substitute for their missing counterfactual experience, we seek the experience of 100 unexposed persons who can provide an estimate of what would have occurred among the exposed had they not been exposed. This substitution is the crucial concern in many epidemiologic studies: Does the experience of the unexposed group actually represent what would have happened to the exposed group had they been unexposed? If we observe 10 cases of disease in the unexposed group, how can we know that the difference between the 25 cases in the exposed group and the 10 cases in the unexposed group is attributable to the exposure? Perhaps the exposure had no effect but the unexposed group was at a lower risk for disease than the exposed group. What if we had observed 25 cases in both the exposed and the unexposed groups? The exposure might have no effect, but it might also have had a strong effect that was balanced by the fact that the unexposed group had a higher risk for disease.

To achieve a valid substitution for the counterfactual experience, we resort to various design methods that promote comparability. One example is the crossover trial, which is based on comparison of the experience of each exposed person with himself or herself at a different time. But a crossover trial is feasible only for an exposure that can be studied in an experimental setting (ie, assigned by the investigator according to a study protocol) and only if it has a brief effect. A persistent exposure effect would distort the effect of crossing over from the exposed to the unexposed group. Another approach is a randomized experiment. In these studies, all participants are randomly assigned to the exposure groups. Given enough randomized participants, we can expect the distributions of other characteristics in the exposed and unexposed groups to be similar. Other approaches involve choosing unexposed study subjects who have the same or similar risk-factor profiles for disease as the exposed subjects. However the comparability is achieved, its success is the overriding concern for any epidemiologic study that aims to evaluate a causal effect.

If we can assume that the exposed and unexposed groups are otherwise comparable with regard to risk for disease, we can compare measures of disease occurrence to assess the effect of the exposure. The two most commonly compared measures are the incidence proportion, or risk, and the incidence rate. The *risk difference* (RD) is the difference in incidence proportion or risk between the exposed and the unexposed groups. If the incidence proportion is 0.25 for the exposed and 0.10 for the unexposed, the RD is 0.15. With an incidence rate instead of a risk to measure disease occurrence, we can likewise calculate the *incidence rate difference* (IRD) for the two measures. (Terminology note: In older texts, the RD is sometimes referred to as the *attributable risk*. The IRD also has been called the *attributable rate*.)

Difference measures such as RD and IRD measure the absolute effect of an exposure. It is also possible to measure the relative effect. As an analogy, consider how to assess the performance of an investment over a period of time. Suppose that an initial investment of $100 became $120 after 1 year. The difference in the value of the investment at the end of the year and the value at the beginning, $20, measures the absolute performance of the investment. The relative performance is obtained by dividing the absolute increase by the initial amount, which gives $20/$100, or 20%. Contrast this investment experience with that of another investment, in which an initial sum of $1000 grew to $1150 after 1 year. For the latter investment, the absolute increment is $150, far greater than the $20 from the first investment, but the relative performance of the second investment is $150/$1000, or 15%, which is worse than the first investment.

We can obtain relative measures of effect in the same manner. We first obtain an absolute measure of effect, which can be the RD or the IRD, and we then divide that by the measure of occurrence of disease among unexposed persons. For risks, the relative effect is given by the following equation:

$$\text{Relative effect} = \frac{\text{Risk difference}}{\text{Risk in unexposed}} = \frac{RD}{R_0}$$

where RD is the risk difference and R_0 is the risk among the unexposed. Because $RD = R_1 - R_0$ (R_1 being the risk among exposed persons), this expression can be rewritten as

$$\text{Relative effect} = \frac{RD}{R_0} = \frac{R_1 - R_0}{R_0} = RR - 1 \qquad [4\text{--}5]$$

In Equation 4–5, the *risk ratio* (RR) is defined as R_1/R_0. The relative effect is the risk ratio minus 1 $(RR - 1)$. This result is exactly parallel to the investment analogy, in which the relative success of the investment was the ratio of the value after investing divided by the value before investing minus 1. For the smaller of the two investments, this computation gives $(\$120/\$100) - 1 = 1.2 - 1 = 20\%$. If the risk in exposed people is 0.25 and that in unexposed people is 0.10, the relative effect is $(0.25/0.10) - 1$, or 1.5 (sometimes expressed as 150%). The RR is 2.5, and the relative effect is the part of the RR in excess of 1.0 (which is the value of the RR when there is no effect). By defining the relative effect in this way, we ensure that we have a relative effect of zero when the absolute effect is also zero.

Although the relative effect is $RR - 1$, it is common for epidemiologists to refer to the RR itself as a measure of relative effect, without subtracting 1. When the RR is used in this way, it is important to remember that a value of 1 corresponds to the absence of an effect. For example, an RR of 3 represents twice as great an effect as an RR of 2. Sometimes, epidemiologists refer to the percentage increase in risk to convey the magnitude of relative effect. For example, they may describe an effect that represents a 120% increase in risk. This increase is meant to describe a relative, not an absolute, effect, because we cannot have an absolute effect of 120%. Describing an effect in terms of a percentage increase in risk is the same as the relative effect defined previously. An increase of 120% corresponds to an RR of 2.2, which is $2.2 - 1.0 = 120\%$ greater than 1. The 120% is a description of the relative effect that subtracts the 1 from the RR. Usually, it is straightforward to determine from the context whether a description of relative effect is RR or $RR - 1$. If the effect is described as a fivefold increase in risk, for example, it means that the RR is 5. If the effect is described as a 10% increase in risk, it corresponds to an RR of 1.1, which is $1.1 - 1.0$.

Effect measures that involve the IRD and the incidence rate ratio are defined analogously to those involving the RD and the risk ratio. Table 4–5 compares absolute and relative measures constructed from risks and from rates.

The range of the RD measure derives from the range of risk itself, which is $[0,1]$. The lowest possible RD would result from an exposed group with zero risk and an unexposed group at 100% risk, giving −1 for the difference. Analogously, the greatest possible RD, 1, comes from an exposed group with 100% risk and an unexposed group with zero risk. RD has no dimensionality (ie, it has no units and is measured as a pure number) because the underlying measure, risk, is also dimensionless, and the dimensionality of a difference is the same as the dimensionality of the underlying measure.

Table 4–5 COMPARISON OF ABSOLUTE AND RELATIVE
EFFECT MEASURES

Measure	Numeric Range	Dimensionality
Risk difference	$[-1, +1]$	None
Risk ratio	$[0, \infty]$	None
Incidence rate difference	$[-\infty, +\infty]$	1/time
Incidence rate ratio	$[0, \infty]$	None

The risk ratio has a range that is never negative, because a risk cannot be negative. The smallest risk ratio occurs when the risk in the exposed group, the numerator of the risk ratio, is zero. The largest risk ratio occurs when the risk among the unexposed is zero, giving a ratio of ∞. Any ratio measure will be dimensionless if the numerator and denominator quantities have the same dimensionality, because the dimensions divide out. In the case of risk ratio, the numerator, the denominator, and the ratio are all dimensionless.

Incidence rates range from zero to infinity, and they have the dimensionality of 1/time. From these characteristics, it is straightforward to deduce the range and the dimensionality of the *IRD* and the incidence rate ratio.

WHEN TO USE ABSOLUTE AND RELATIVE EFFECT MEASURES

Absolute and relative effect measures provide different messages. When measuring the effect of an exposure on the health of a population, an absolute effect measure is needed. It reflects added or diminished disease burden in that population in terms of an increased risk or incidence rate or, for protective exposures, a decreased risk or incidence rate. The public-health implications of any exposure need to be assessed in terms of the absolute effect measures.

Relative effect measures convey a different message. The attributable fraction among exposed people, $(RR-1)/RR$, is purely a function of the relative effect measure, which gives a clue about the message of relative effect measures. These measures indicate the extent to which the exposure in question accounts for the occurrence of disease among the exposed people who get disease. The relative measure itself expresses this relation on a scale that goes from zero to infinity, and the attributable fraction converts it to a proportion, but both convey a message about the extent to which disease among the exposed population is a consequence of exposure.

It is important to realize that a relative effect may be extremely large but with little public-health consequence. If an exposure has a rate ratio of 10 for an extremely rare disease, the 10-fold increase in disease implies that the exposure accounts for almost all the disease among the exposed; however, even among exposed the disease may remain rare. Such an exposure may have less public-health consequence than another exposure that merely doubles the rate of a much more common disease.

In case-control studies (see Chapter 5), usually only relative effects are directly obtainable. Nevertheless, by taking into account the overall rate or risk of disease occurrence in a population, the relative measures obtained from case-control studies can be converted into absolute measures, which are needed to assess appropriately the public-health impact of an exposure.

Examples

Table 4–6 presents data on the risk of diarrhea among breast-fed infants during a 10-day period after their infection with *Vibrio cholerae 01* according to the level

Table 4-6 DIARRHEA DURING A 10-DAY FOLLOW-UP
PERIOD IN BREAST-FED INFANTS COLONIZED WITH
VIBRIO CHOLERA 01 ACCORDING TO THE LEVEL OF
ANTIPOLYSACCHARIDE ANTIBODY TITER IN THEIR
MOTHER'S BREAST MILK

| | Antibody Level | | |
	Low	High	Total
Diarrhea	12	7	19
No diarrhea	2	9	11
Total	14	16	30
Risk	0.86	0.44	0.63

Reproduced with permission from Glass RI et al.[7]

of antipolysaccharide antibody titers in their mother's breast milk.[7] The data show a substantial difference in the risk of developing diarrhea according to whether the mother's breast milk contains a low or a high level of antipolysaccharide antibody. The *RD* for infants exposed to milk with low compared with high levels of antibody is $0.86 - 0.44 = 0.42$. This *RD* reflects the additional risk of diarrhea among infants whose mother's breast milk has low antibody titers compared with the risk among infants whose mother's milk has high titers; it assumes that the infants exposed to low titers would have experienced a risk equal to that of those exposed to high titers were it not for the lower antibody levels.

We can also measure the effect of low titers on diarrhea risk in relative terms. The risk ratio, *RR*, is $0.86/0.44 = 1.96$. The relative effect is $1.96 - 1$, or 0.96, indicating a 96% greater risk of diarrhea among infants exposed to low antibody titers in breast milk. Commonly, we would describe the risk among the infants exposed to low titers as being 1.96 times the risk among infants exposed to high titers.

The calculation of effects from incidence rate data is analogous to the calculation of effects from risk data. Table 4-7 gives data for the incidence rate of breast cancer among women who were treated for tuberculosis early in the 20th century.[8] Some women received a treatment that involved repeated fluoroscopy of the lungs, with a resulting high dose of ionizing radiation to the chest.

Table 4-7 BREAST CANCER CASES AND PERSON-YEARS OF
OBSERVATION FOR WOMEN WITH TUBERCULOSIS WHO WERE
REPEATEDLY EXPOSED TO MULTIPLE X-RAY FLUOROSCOPIES AND
FOR UNEXPOSED WOMEN WITH TUBERCULOSIS

| | Radiation Exposure | | |
	Yes	No	Total
Breast cancer cases	41	15	56
Person-years	28,010	19,017	47,027
Rate (cases/10,000 person-years)	14.6	7.9	11.9

Reproduced with permission from Boice and Monson.[8]

The incidence rate among those exposed to radiation is 14.6/10,000 yr^{-1}, compared with 7.9/10,000 yr^{-1} among those unexposed. The *IRD* is (14.6 − 7.9)/10,000 yr^{-1} = 6.7/10,000 yr^{-1}. This difference reflects the rate of breast cancer among exposed women that can be attributed to the radiation exposure and assumes that the exposed women would have had a rate equal to that among the unexposed women were it not for the exposure. We can also measure the effect in relative terms. The incidence rate ratio is 14.6/7.9, or 1.86. The relative effect is 1.86 − 1, or 0.86, which can be expressed as an 86% greater rate of breast cancer among women exposed to the radiation. Alternatively, the incidence rate ratio can be described as indicating a rate of breast cancer among exposed women that is 1.86 times that of the rate among unexposed women.

ROUNDING: HOW MANY DIGITS SHOULD BE REPORTED?

A frequent question that arises in the reporting of results is how many digits of accuracy should be reported. In some published papers, a risk ratio may be reported as 4.1; in others, the same number may be reported as 4.0846. The number of digits should reflect the amount of precision in the data. The number 4.0846 implies that one is fairly sure that the data warrant a reported value that lies between 4.084 and 4.085. Only a truly large study can produce that level of precision. Nevertheless, it is surprisingly hard to offer a general rule for the number of digits that should be reported. For example, suppose that, for a given study, reporting should carry into the first decimal (eg, 4.1). If the study reported risk ratios and took on values lower than 1.0, the ratios would be rounded to values such as 0.7 or 0.8. This amount of rounding error is greater, in proportion to the size of the effect, than the rounding error in a reported value such as 4.1. Therefore, a simple rule such as one decimal place (for example) will not suffice.

How about the rule that suggests using a constant number of meaningful digits? With this rule, 4.1 would have the same reporting accuracy as 0.83. This rule may appear to be an improvement, but it breaks down near the value of 1.0 for ratio measures; it suggests that we should distinguish 0.98 from 0.99 but not 1.00 from 1.01: Both of the latter numbers would be rounded to 1.0, and the next reportable value would be 1.1. Because 1.0 is the zero point for ratio measures of effect, this rule treats positive effects near zero differently from negative effects. If all the risk ratios to be reported ranged from 0.9 to 1.1, this rule would make little sense.

No rule is needed as long as the writer uses good judgment and thinks about the number of digits to report. Values used in intermediate calculations should never be rounded; one should round only in the final step before reporting. Consider that rounding 1.41 to 1.4 is not a large error, but rounding 1.25 to 1.2 or to 1.3 is a rounding error that amounts to 20% of the effect for a rate ratio (keeping in mind that 1.0 equals no effect). Finally, when rounding a number ending in 5, it is customary to round upward, but it is preferable to use an unbiased strategy, such as rounding to the nearest even number. Under such a strategy, both 1.75 and 1.85 would be rounded to 1.8.

The Relation Between Risk Ratios and Rate Ratios

Risk data produce estimates of effect that are either risk differences or risk ratios, and rate data produce estimates of effect that are rate differences or rate ratios. Risks cannot be compared directly with rates (they have different units), and for the same reason, risk differences cannot be compared with rate differences. Under certain conditions, however, a risk ratio can be equivalent to a rate ratio. Suppose that we have incidence rates that are constant over time, with the rate among exposed people equal to I_1 and the rate among unexposed people equal to I_0. From Equation 4–1, we know that a constant incidence rate will result in a risk that is approximately equal to the product of the rate and the time period, provided that the time period is short enough so that the risk remains less than about 0.20. For greater values, the approximation does not work well. Assuming that we are dealing with short time periods, the ratio of the risk among the exposed to the risk among the unexposed, R_1/R_0, will be as follows:

$$\text{Risk ratio} = \frac{R_1}{R_0} \approx \frac{I_1 \times \text{time}}{I_0 \times \text{time}} = \frac{I_1}{I_0}$$

This relation shows that the risk ratio is nearly the same as the rate ratio, provided that the time period over which the risks apply is sufficiently short or the rates are sufficiently low for Equation 4–1 to apply. The shorter the time period or the lower the rates, the better the approximation represented by Equation 4–1 and the closer the value of the risk ratio to the rate ratio.

Over longer time periods (the length depending on the value of the rates involved), risks may become sufficiently great that the risk ratio will begin to diverge from the rate ratio. Because risks cannot exceed 1.0, the maximum value of a risk ratio cannot be greater than 1 divided by the risk among the unexposed. Consider the data in Table 4–6, for example. The risk in the high-titer antibody group (considered to be the unexposed group) is 0.44. With this risk for the unexposed group, the risk ratio cannot exceed 1/0.44, or 2.3. The observed risk ratio of 1.96 is not far below the maximum possible risk ratio. Incidence rate ratios are not constrained by this type of ceiling, and when risk among the unexposed is high, we can expect there to be a divergence between the incidence rate ratio and the risk ratio. Suppose the incidence rates that gave rise to the risks in Table 4–6 were constant over the 10-day follow-up period. If we take into account the exponential-decay relation between risk and rate, we can back-calculate from the risks in Table 4–6 to the underlying rates based on the exponential decay curve, and from that result, we can calculate that the ratio of those underlying rates is 3.4, compared with the 1.96 for the ratio of risks. This large discrepancy arises because the risks are large.

If the time period over which a risk is calculated approaches 0, the risk itself also approaches 0; the risk of a given person having a myocardial infarction may be 10% over a decade, but over the next 10 seconds, it will be extremely small, and its value will shrink along with the length of the time interval. Nevertheless, the ratio of two quantities that both approach 0 does not necessarily approach 0. In the case of the risk ratio calculated for risks that apply to shorter and shorter time intervals, as these risks approach 0, the risk ratio approaches the value of the incidence rate ratio. The incidence rate ratio is the limiting value for the risk ratio as the time interval over which the risks are taken approaches 0. We therefore can describe the incidence rate ratio as an *instantaneous risk ratio*. This equivalence of the two types of ratios for short time intervals has resulted in some confusion of terminology: Often, the phrase *relative risk* is used to refer to either an incidence rate ratio or a risk ratio. Either of the latter terms is preferable to the term relative risk, because they describe the nature of the data from which the ratio derives. Nevertheless, because the risk ratio and the rate ratio are equivalent for small risks, the more general term *relative risk* has some justification. The often-used notation *RR* is sometimes read to mean relative risk, which equally can be read as risk ratio or rate ratio, all of which are equivalent if the risks are sufficiently small.

WHEN RISK DOES NOT MEAN RISK

In referring to effects, some people inaccurately use the word *risk* in place of the word *effect*. For example, suppose that a study reports two risk ratios for lung cancer from asbestos exposure, 5.0 for young adults and 2.5 for older adults. These effect values may be described as follows: "The risk of lung cancer from asbestos exposure is not as great among older people as among younger people." This statement is incorrect. In fact, the *RD* between those exposed and those unexposed to asbestos is sure to be greater among older adults than younger adults, and the risk attributable to the effect of asbestos is greater in older adults. The risk ratio is smaller among older adults because the risk of lung cancer increases steeply with age, and the ratio for older adults is based on a larger denominator. The statement is wrong because the term *risk* has been used in place of the term *risk ratio* or the more general term *effect*. It is correct to describe the data as follows: "The risk ratio of lung cancer from asbestos exposure is not as great among older people as among younger people."

Attributable Fraction

If we take the *RD* between exposed and unexposed people, $R_1 - R_0$, and divide it by the risk in the unexposed group, we obtain the relative measure of effect (see Equation 4–5). We can also divide the *RD* by the risk in exposed people to get an expression that we refer to as the *attributable fraction*:

$$\text{Attributable fraction} = \frac{RD}{R_1} = \frac{R_1 - R_0}{R_1} = 1 - \frac{1}{RR} = \frac{RR - 1}{RR} \qquad [4\text{--}6]$$

If the *RD* reflects a causal effect that is not distorted by any bias, the attributable fraction is a measure that quantifies the proportion of the disease burden among exposed people that is caused by the exposure. Consider the hypothetical data in Table 4–8. The risk of disease during a 1-year period is 0.05 among the exposed and 0.01 among the unexposed. Suppose that this difference can

Table 4–8 HYPOTHETICAL DATA GIVING 1-YEAR
DISEASE RISKS FOR EXPOSED AND UNEXPOSED
PEOPLE

| | **Exposure** | | |
	No	**Yes**	**Total**
Disease	900	500	1,400
No disease	89,100	9,500	98,600
Total	90,000	10,000	100,000
Risk	0.01	0.05	0.014

be reasonably attributed to the effect of the exposure (because we believe that we have accounted for all substantial biases). The *RD* is 0.04, which is 80% of the risk among the exposed. We would then say that the exposure appears to account for 80% of the disease that occurs among exposed people during the 1-year period. Another way to calculate the attributable fraction is from the risk ratio: $(5 - 1)/5 = 80\%$. (Terminology note: The *attributable fraction* sometimes is referred to in older texts as the *attributable risk percent* or *attributable risk*.)

To calculate the attributable fraction for the entire population of 100,000 people in Table 4–8, we first calculate the attributable fraction for exposed people. To get the overall attributable fraction for the total population, the fraction among the exposed is multiplied by the proportion of all cases in the total population who are exposed. There are 1400 cases in the entire population, of whom 500 are exposed. The proportion of exposed cases is $500/1400 = 0.357$. The overall attributable fraction for the population is the product of the attributable fraction among the exposed and the proportion of cases who are exposed: $0.8 \times 0.357 = 0.286$; that is, 28.6% of all cases in the population are attributable to the exposure. This calculation is based on a straightforward idea: No case can be caused by exposure unless the person is exposed. Among all cases, only some of the exposed cases can be attributable to the exposure. There are 500 exposed cases, of whom we calculated that 400 represent excess cases caused by the exposure. None of the 900 cases among the unexposed is attributable to the exposure. Therefore, among the total of 1400 cases in the population, only 400 of the exposed cases are attributable to the exposure—the proportion $400/1400 = 0.286$, which is the same value that we calculated.

If the exposure is categorized into more than two levels, we can use the following equation, which takes into account each of the exposure levels:

$$\text{Total attributable fraction} = \sum_i (AF_i \times P_i) \qquad [4\text{–}7]$$

AF_i is the attributable fraction for exposure level i, P_i represents the proportion of all cases that falls in exposure category i, and $\sum$ indicates the sum of each of the exposure-specific attributable fractions. For the unexposed group, the attributable fraction is 0.

Equation 4–7 can be applied to the hypothetical data in Table 4–9, which describe risks for a population with three levels of exposure. The attributable fraction for the group with no exposure is 0. For the low-exposure group, the attributable fraction is 0.50, because the risk ratio is 2. For the high-exposure group,

Table 4–9 HYPOTHETICAL DATA GIVING 1-YEAR DISEASE RISKS FOR
PEOPLE AT THREE LEVELS OF EXPOSURE

| | Exposure | | | |
	None	Low	High	Total
Disease	100	1,200	1,200	2,500
No disease	9,900	58,800	28,800	97,500
Total	10,000	60,000	30,000	100,000
Risk	0.01	0.02	0.04	0.025
Risk ratio	1.00	2.00	4.00	
Proportion of all cases	0.04	0.48	0.48	

the attributable fraction is 0.75, because the risk ratio is 4. The total attributable fraction is

$$0 + 0.50(0.48) + 0.75(0.48) = 0.24 + 0.36 = 0.60$$

The same result can be calculated directly from the number of attributable cases at each of the exposure levels:

$$(0 + 600 + 900)/2500 = 0.60$$

Under certain assumptions, estimation of attributable fractions can be based on rates as well as risks. In Equation 4–6, which uses the risk ratio to calculate the attributable fraction, the rate ratio can be used instead, provided that the conditions are met for the rate ratio to approximate the risk ratio. If exposure results in an increase in disease occurrence at some levels of exposure and a decrease at other levels of exposure, compared with no exposure, the net attributable fraction will be a combination of the prevented cases and the caused cases at the different levels of exposure. The net effect of exposure in such situations can be difficult to assess and may obscure the components of the exposure effect. This topic is discussed in greater detail by Rothman, Greenland and Lash.[9]

QUESTIONS

1. Suppose that in a population of 100 people, 30 die. The risk of death can be calculated as 30/100. What is missing from this measure?

2. Can we calculate a rate for the data in question 1? If so, what is it? If not, why not?

3. Eventually, all people die. Why should we not state that the mortality rate for any population is always 100%?

4. If incidence rates remain constant with time and if exposure causes disease, which will be greater, the risk ratio or the rate ratio?

5. Why is it incorrect to describe a rate ratio of 10 as indicating a high risk of disease among the exposed?

6. A newspaper article states that a disease has increased by 1200% in the past decade. What is the rate ratio that corresponds to this level of increase?

7. Another disease has increased by 20%. What is the rate ratio that corresponds to this increase?

8. From the data in Table 4–6, calculate the fraction of diarrhea cases among infants exposed to a low antibody level that is attributable to the low antibody level. Calculate the fraction of all diarrhea cases attributable to exposure to low antibody levels. What assumptions are needed to interpret the result as an attributable fraction?

9. What proportion of the 56 breast cancer cases in Table 4–7 is attributable to radiation exposure? What are the assumptions?

10. Suppose you worked for a health agency and had collected data on the incidence of lower back pain among people in different occupations. What measures of effect would you choose to look at, and why?

11. Suppose that the rate ratio measuring the relation between an exposure and a disease is 3 in two different countries. Would this situation imply that exposed people have the same risk in the two countries? Would it imply that the effect of the exposure is the same magnitude in the two countries? Why or why not?

REFERENCES

1. Gaylord Anderson, as cited in Cole P. The evolving case-control study. *J Chron Dis.* 1979;32:15–27.
2. Iskrant AP, Joliet PV. *Accidents and Homicides.* Cambridge, MA: Harvard University Press; 1968.
3. Snow J. *On the Mode of Communication of Cholera.* 2nd ed. London: John Churchill; 1860. (Facsimile of 1936 reprinted edition by Hafner, New York, 1965.)
4. Kurtzke JF, Hyllested K. Multiple sclerosis in the Faroe Islands: clinical and epidemiologic features. *Ann Neurol.* 1979;5:6–21.
5. Poser CM, Hibberd PL, Benedikz J, Gudmundsson G. *Neuroepidemiology.* 1988;7:168–180.
6. Cole TB, Chorba TL, Horan JM. Patterns of transmission of epidemic hysteria in a school. *Epidemiology.* 1990;1:212–218.
7. Glass RI, Svennerholm AM, Stoll BJ, et al. Protection against cholera in breast-fed children by antibiotics in breast milk. *N Engl J Med.* 1983;308:1389–1392.
8. Boice JD, Monson RR. Breast cancer in women after repeated fluoroscopic examinations of the chest. *J Natl Cancer Inst.* 1977;59:823–832.
9. Rothman KJ, Greenland S, Lash TL. *Modern Epidemiology.* 3rd ed. Philadelphia, PA: Lippincott Williams & Wilkins; 2008.

5

Types of Epidemiologic Studies

Chapter 4 described measures of disease frequency, including risk, incidence rate, and prevalence; measures of effect, including risk and incidence rate differences and ratios; and attributable fractions. Epidemiologic studies may be viewed as measurement exercises undertaken to obtain estimates of these epidemiologic measures. The simplest studies aim only at estimating a single risk, incidence rate, or prevalence. More complicated studies aim at comparing measures of disease occurrence, with the goal of predicting such occurrence, learning about the causes of disease, or evaluating the impact of disease on a population. This chapter describes the two main types of epidemiologic study, the cohort study and the case-control study, along with several variants. More specialized study designs, such as two-stage designs and ecologic studies, are discussed in *Modern Epidemiology*.[1]

COHORT STUDIES

In epidemiology, a cohort is defined most broadly as "any designated group of individuals who are followed or traced over a period of time."[2] A cohort study, which is the archetype for all epidemiologic studies, involves measuring the occurrence of disease within one or more cohorts. Typically, a cohort comprises persons with a common characteristic, such as an exposure or ethnic identity. For simplicity, we refer to two cohorts, *exposed* and *unexposed*, in our discussion. In this context, we use the term *exposed* in its most general sense; for example, an exposed cohort may have in common the presence of a specific gene. The purpose of following a cohort is to measure the occurrence of one or more specific diseases during the period of follow-up, usually with the aim of comparing the disease rates for two or more cohorts.

The concept of following a cohort to measure disease occurrence may appear straightforward, but there are many complications involving who is eligible to be followed, what should count as an instance of disease, how the incidence rates or risks are measured, and how exposure ought to be defined. Before exploring these issues, we consider an example of an elegantly designed epidemiologic cohort study.

John Snow's Natural Experiment

In Chapter 4 we looked at data compiled by John Snow regarding the cholera outbreak in London in 1854 (see Fig. 4–4). In London at that time, there were several water companies that piped drinking water to residents. Snow's so-called natural experiment consisted of comparing the cholera mortality rates for residents subscribing to two of the major water companies, the Southwark and Vauxhall Company, which piped impure Thames water contaminated with sewage, and the Lambeth Company, which in 1852 changed its collection from opposite the Hungerford Market upstream to Thames Ditton, obtaining a supply of water free of the sewage of London. Snow[3] described it as follows:

> …the intermixing of the water supply of the Southwark and Vauxhall Company with that of the Lambeth Company, over an extensive part of London, admitted of the subject being sifted in such a way as to yield the most incontrovertible proof on one side or the other. In the subdistricts…supplied by both companies, the mixing of the supply is of the most intimate kind. The pipes of each company go down all the streets, and into nearly all the courts and alleys. A few houses are supplied by one company and a few by the other, according to the decision of the owner or occupier at the time when the Water Companies were in active competition. In many cases a single house has a supply different from that on either side. Each company supplies both rich and poor, both large houses and small; there is no difference in either the condition or occupation of the persons receiving the water of the different companies…it is obvious that no experiment could have been devised which would more thoroughly test the effect of water supply on the progress of cholera than this.
>
> The experiment, too, was on the grandest scale. No fewer than three hundred thousand people of both sexes, of every age and occupation, and of every rank and station, from gentle folks down to the very poor, were divided into two groups without their choice, and, in most cases, without their knowledge; one group being supplied with water containing the sewage of London, and amongst it, whatever might have come from the cholera patients, the other group having water quite free from impurity.
>
> To turn this experiment to account, all that was required was to learn the supply of water to each individual house where a fatal attack of cholera might occur…

From this natural experiment, Snow[3] was able to estimate the frequency of cholera deaths, using households as the denominator, separately for people in each of the two cohorts:

> According to a return which was made to Parliament, the Southwark and Vauxhall Company supplied 40,046 houses from January 1 to December 31, 1853, and the Lambeth Company supplied 26,107 houses during the same period; consequently, as 286 fatal attacks of cholera took place, in the first four weeks of the epidemic, in houses supplied by the former company, and only 14 in houses supplied by the latter, the proportion of fatal attacks to each 10,000 houses was as follows: Southwark and Vauxhall 71, Lambeth 5. The cholera was therefore fourteen times as fatal at this period, amongst persons having the impure water of the Southwark and Vauxhall Company, as amongst those having the purer water from Thames Ditton.

Snow also obtained estimates of the size of the population served by the two water companies, enabling him to report the attack rate of fatal cholera among

Table 5–1 ATTACK RATE OF FATAL CHOLERA AMONG
CUSTOMERS OF THE SOUTHWARK AND VAUXHALL COMPANY
(EXPOSED COHORT) AND THE LAMBETH COMPANY
(UNEXPOSED COHORT), LONDON, 1854

| | Water Company | |
	Southwark & Vauxhall	Lambeth
Cholera deaths	4,093	461
Population	266,516	173,748
Attack Rate	0.0154	0.0027

Data from Snow.[3]

residents of households served by them during the 1854 outbreak (Table 5–1). Residents whose water came from the Southwark and Vauxhall Company had an attack rate 5.8 times greater than that of residents whose water came from the Lambeth Company.

Snow saw that circumstance had created conditions that emulated an experiment, in which people who were otherwise alike in relevant aspects differed by their consumption of pure or impure water. In an actual experiment, the investigator assigns the study participants to the exposed and unexposed groups. In a natural experiment, as studies such as Snow's have come to be known, the investigator takes advantage of a setting that serves effectively as an experiment. It could be argued that the role of the investigator in a natural experiment requires more creativity and insight than in an actual experiment. In the natural experiment, the investigator has to see the opportunity for the research and define the study populations to capitalize on the setting. For example, Snow conducted his study within specific neighborhoods in London where the pipes from these two water companies were intermingled. In other districts, there was less intermingling of pipes from the various water companies that supplied water to dwellings. Comparing the attack rates across various districts of London would have been a less persuasive way to evaluate the effect of the water supply because many factors differed from one district to another. Within the area in which the pipes of the Southwark and Vauxhall and those of the Lambeth Companies were intermingled, however, Snow saw that there was little difference between those who consumed water from one company or the other, apart from the water supply itself. Part of his genius was identifying the precise setting in which to conduct the study.

Types of Experiments

Experiments are conceptually straightforward. Experiments are cohort studies, although not all cohort studies are experiments. In epidemiology, an experiment is a study in which the incidence rate or the risk of disease in two or more cohorts is compared after assigning the exposure to the people who constitute the cohorts. In an experiment, the reason for the exposure assignment is solely to suit the objectives of the study; if people receive their exposure assignment based on considerations other than the study protocol, it is not a true experiment. The *protocol* is the set of rules by which the study is conducted.

Among the several varieties of epidemiologic experiment, the main types are clinical trials, field trials, and community intervention trials. The word *trial* is used as a synonym for an epidemiologic experiment. Epidemiologic experiments are most frequently conducted in a clinical setting, with the aim of evaluating which treatment for a disease is better. These studies are known as *clinical trials*. In clinical trials, all study subjects have been diagnosed with a specific disease, but that disease is not the disease event that is being studied. Rather, it is some consequence of that disease, such as death or spread of a cancer, that becomes the "disease" event studied in a clinical trial. The aim of a clinical trial is to evaluate the incidence rate or risk of disease complications in the cohorts assigned to the different treatment groups. The primary outcome of interest is often a stage in the natural history of the disease, such as recurrence of cancer, or deaths among patients with cardiovascular disease. Alternatively, the outcome may be an adverse effect, ranging from transitory malaise to extreme outcomes such as liver failure or sudden death. In most trials, treatments are assigned by *randomization*, using random number assignment. Randomization tends to produce comparability between the cohorts with respect to factors that may affect the outcome under study.

To take full advantage of random assignment, the groups that should be compared in the analysis of an experiment are the groups that are classified according to their random assignment. Suppose 100 patients are randomly assigned to receive a new treatment in a clinical trial, and 100 patients are randomly assigned to receive an old treatment. To benefit maximally from the random assignment, the investigator should compare these two groups of 100, regardless of what treatments actually were given. It is not unusual for a patient to be assigned a treatment and not to take it as instructed. The patient may reject treatment for a variety of reasons or change his or her mind after the treatment assignment is made. Patients assigned to receive an old treatment may find a way to get the new treatment. Even if treatments are disguised in the form of coded medications that are not readily identified, patients may not be treated as assigned, because they react poorly to an assigned medication or otherwise ignore their assigned treatment. Thus, the assigned treatment may differ from the actual treatment for a proportion of study participants. Nevertheless, a standard approach in analyzing data from a clinical trial is to follow the principle of *intent to treat*, which means that the treatment assignment, rather than the actual treatment, determines the classification of participants in the data analysis. The intent-to-treat approach to the data analysis avoids problems that can arise if there is a tendency for patients who are at especially high or low risk for the outcome to fail to adhere to their assigned treatment. For example, if high-risk patients were more likely than low-risk patients to switch from the old treatment to the new treatment, the new treatment would appear to be worse than it should if the patients were compared according to the actual treatment that they received.

An intent-to-treat analysis may misclassify a substantial proportion of study participants with respect to their actual exposure. This misclassification of actual exposure leads to an underestimate of the treatment effect (see Chapter 7). Although the intent-to-treat approach is often desirable because it preserves the advantages of random assignment and therefore can lead to better comparability of the study groups, the fact that it will underestimate the treatment effect should be borne in mind. Underestimating the benefit of a new treatment may be considered a small problem, because adoption of the treatment will have even greater benefits than anticipated. If the randomized trial is intended to study adverse effects of treatment, however, underestimating the magnitude of those effects is a larger problem. In trials aimed at evaluating the safety (rather than efficacy) of a new treatment, the drawbacks of an intent-to-treat analysis may outweigh any advantages, and it may be preferable to analyze the data based on the actual exposure of participants, rather than the category determined by random assignment.

NATURAL EXPERIMENTS ARE NOT EXPERIMENTS

In John Snow's natural experiment, customers of the Southwark and Vauxhall and the Lambeth companies were not randomly assigned to their water supply, as they would be in an experiment. The *natural experiment* is not an actual experiment; it is a cohort study that simulates what would occur in an experiment. In Snow's description of the customers of the two water companies, he gives the impression that the comparability between them was nearly as good as might have been achieved by random assignment. Thus, we have an experiment created by "nature," or a natural experiment, which may be more accurately described as a cohort study designed by an ingenious epidemiologist.

The data in Table 5–2 come from a clinical trial of adult patients recently infected with human immunodeficiency virus (HIV) that was undertaken to determine whether early treatment with zidovudine was effective in improving the prognosis.[4] Patients were randomly assigned to receive zidovudine or placebo and then followed for an average of 15 months. The data show that the risk of getting an opportunistic infection during the follow-up period was low among those who received early zidovudine treatment but considerably higher among those who received a dummy (placebo) treatment.

Clinical trials may be the most common type of epidemiologic experiment, but they are not the only type. Epidemiologists also conduct *field trials*, which differ

Table 5–2 RANDOMIZED TRIAL COMPARING THE RISK OF OPPORTUNISTIC INFECTION AMONG PATIENTS WITH RECENT HIV INFECTION WHO RECEIVED EITHER ZIDOVUDINE OR PLACEBO

| | Treatment Group | |
	Zidovudine	Placebo
Opportunistic infection	1	7
Total patients	39	38
Risk	0.026	0.184

Data from Kinloch-de Loes et al.[4]

from clinical trials mainly in that the study participants are not patients. In a field trial, the goal is to study the primary prevention of a disease, rather than treatment of an existing disease. For example, experiments of new vaccines to prevent infectious illness are field trials because the study participants have not yet been diagnosed with a particular disease. In a clinical trial, the study participants can be followed through regular clinic visits, whereas in a field trial, it may be necessary to contact participants for follow-up directly at home, work, or school. The largest formal human experiment ever conducted, the Salk vaccine trial of 1954, is a prominent example of a field trial.[5] It was conducted to evaluate the efficacy of a new vaccine to prevent paralytic poliomyelitis, and it paved the way for the first widespread use of vaccination to prevent poliomyelitis.

Another type of experiment is a *community intervention trial*. In this type of study, the exposure is assigned to groups of people rather than singly. For example, the community fluoridation trials in the 1940s and 1950s that evaluated the effect of fluoride in a community water supply were community intervention trials. The data in Table 5–3 illustrate a community intervention trial that evaluated a program of home-based neonatal care and management of sepsis designed to prevent death among infants in rural India.[6] This trial, as is often the case for community intervention trials, did not employ random assignment. Instead, the investigators selected 39 villages targeted for the new program and 47 villages in which the new program was not introduced. The program consisted of frequent home visits after each birth in the village by health workers who were trained for the study to deal with problems in neonatal care. This program resulted in reduced neonatal mortality for each of the 3 years of its implementation, with the reductions increasing with time. The data in Table 5–3 show the results for the third of the 3 years.

Population at Risk

Snow's study on cholera defined two cohorts on the basis of their water supply. One was the customers of the Southwark and Vauxhall Company, which drew polluted water from the lower Thames River, and the other was the customers of the Lambeth Company, which drew its water from the comparatively pure upper

Table 5–3 NEONATAL MORTALITY IN THE
THIRD OF 3 YEARS AFTER INSTITUTING
A COMMUNITY INTERVENTION TRIAL OF
HOME-BASED NEONATAL CARE IN RURAL
INDIAN VILLAGES

| | Intervention Group | |
	Home Care	Usual Care
Infant deaths	38	64
Number of births	979	940
Risk	0.039	0.068

Data from Bang et al.[6]

Thames. Any person in either of these cohorts could have contracted cholera. Snow measured the rate of cholera occurrence among the people in each cohort.

EXPERIMENTS ARE AN IMPERFECT GOLD STANDARD

Randomized trials are commonly described as the gold standard of epidemiologic studies, with all that implies. The random assignment does confer an important advantage, usually preventing or at least reducing confounding by measured and unmeasured risk factors. Nevertheless, randomized trials are far from perfect:

- The full benefits of random assignment depend on conducting an intent-to-treat analysis, which comes with its own bias, leading to an underestimate of the effect.
- In small trials, random assignment can lead to large imbalances between groups, thus failing to balance risk factors as hoped.
- For practical and ethical reasons, many research questions do not lend themselves to being study in a randomized trial.
- Some trials evaluate treatments that are delivered more rigorously in the trial setting or differ in other ways from the real-world interventions that occur outside of trials.
- The expense of large trials may lead to substituting for the intended end point a more common intermediate end point, such as a change in a biomarker; this approach allows smaller studies, but the results may not correspond to the effect on the intended outcome.
- The small size of many trials leads to imprecise results that may not be replicable.

The gold standard does not necessarily provide certainty. If trials were perfect, trials of the same study question would always produce similar results, but that is seldom seen. Moreover, if the results of a trial and a non-experimental study differ, it is not guaranteed that the trial results are closer to the truth. Thorough consideration of the design and analysis of both studies is warranted to resolve discrepancies and is much more informative than simply assuming that results from randomized trials, being based on a supposed gold standard, are always correct.

To understand which people can belong to a cohort in an epidemiologic study, we must consider a basic requirement for cohort membership: Cohort members must meet the criteria for being at risk for disease. The members of a cohort to be followed are sometimes described as the *population at risk*. The term implies that all members of the cohort should be at risk for developing the specific diseases being measured. Determining who may be part of the population at risk may depend on which disease is being measured.

A standard requirement of any population at risk is that everyone be free of the disease being measured at the outset of follow-up. The reason is that a person usually cannot develop anew a disease that he or she currently has. Someone with diabetes cannot develop diabetes, and someone with schizophrenia cannot develop schizophrenia. To be at risk for disease also implies that everyone in the population at risk must be alive at the start of follow-up; dead people are not at risk of getting any disease. Being alive and free of the disease are straightforward eligibility conditions, but other eligibility conditions may not be as simple. Suppose that the outcome is the development of measles. Should people who have received a measles vaccination be included in the population at risk? If they are completely immunized, they are not at risk for measles, but how can we know whether the vaccine has conferred complete immunity? In a cohort being studied for the occurrence of breast cancer, should men be considered part of the population at risk? Men do develop breast cancer, but it is rare compared with its occurrence in women. One solution is to distinguish male and female breast cancer as different diseases. In that case, if female breast cancer is being studied, men would be excluded from the population at risk.

Some diseases occur only once in a person, whereas others can recur. Death is the clearest example of a disease outcome that can occur only once for a given person. Other examples include diabetes, multiple sclerosis, chicken pox, and cleft palate. Disease can occur only once if it is incurable (eg, diabetes, multiple sclerosis), if recovery confers complete lifetime immunity (eg, chicken pox), or if there is a period of vulnerability that a person passes through only once (eg, cleft palate). If the disease can only occur once, anyone in a cohort who develops the disease is no longer at risk for it again and therefore exits from the population at risk as soon as the disease occurs. Also, any person who dies during the follow-up period, for whatever reason, is no longer part of the population at risk. The members of the population at risk at any given time must be people in whom the disease can still occur.

It may be possible, however, for someone with a disease to recover from the disease and then develop it again. For example, someone with a urinary tract infection can recover and then succumb to another urinary tract infection. In that case, the person is not part of the population at risk while he or she has the urinary tract infection but can become part of the population at risk again at the time of recovery. Being part of a population at risk is a dynamic process. People may enter and leave a population at risk depending on their health and other possible eligibility criteria (eg, geography).

Cohort Study of Vitamin A During Pregnancy: An Example

To study the relation between diet and other exposures of pregnant women and the development of birth defects in their offspring, Milunsky and colleagues[7] interviewed more than 22,000 pregnant women early in their pregnancies. The original purpose was to study the potential effect of folate to prevent a class of birth defects known as neural tube defects. A later study, based on the same population of women, evaluated the role of dietary vitamin A in causing another class of birth defects that affect either the heart or the head, described as cranial neural crest defects.[8] For the latter study, the women were divided into cohorts according to the amount of vitamin A in their diet from food or supplements.

DISEASE-FREE DOES NOT IMPLY HEALTHY

Although a population at risk should be free of disease at the outset of follow-up, it is incorrect to conclude that the population at risk is healthy. The requirement to be free of disease does not imply health; it merely implies that the people being followed do not have the specific disease being measured. The search for a population that is healthy in the sense of being free of all disease is fruitless. If *disease* is defined broadly, virtually every person has some disease or disorder at any given time. Acne, periodontal disease, back ailments, allergies, vision deficits, obesity, asthma, and respiratory infection are examples of the prevalent conditions that make it almost impossible to find even one person who is completely healthy. Being free of disease and therefore a member of a population at risk implies only that the person is free of the specific disease being followed, not all diseases.

The data in Table 5–4 summarize the results of this cohort study and show that the prevalence of these defects increased steadily and substantially with increasing intake of vitamin A supplements by pregnant women.

Table 5–4 gives results for four separate cohorts of the study population, each defined according to the level of supplemental intake of vitamin A that the women reported in the interview. The occurrence of cranial neural crest defects increased substantially for women who took supplements of vitamin A in doses greater than 8000 IU/day.

Closed and Open Cohorts

Epidemiologists follow two types of cohorts. A *closed cohort* is one with a fixed membership. After it is defined and follow-up begins, no one can be added to a closed cohort. The initial roster may dwindle, however, as people in the cohort die, are lost to follow-up, or develop the disease. Randomized experiments are examples of studies of closed cohorts (Fig. 5–1); the follow-up begins at randomization, a common starting point for everyone in the study. Another example of a

Table 5–4 PREVALENCE OF CRANIAL NEURAL-CREST DEFECTS AMONG THE OFFSPRING OF FOUR COHORTS OF PREGNANT WOMEN, CLASSIFIED ACCORDING TO THEIR INTAKE OF SUPPLEMENTAL VITAMIN A DURING EARLY PREGNANCY

	Level of Vitamin A Intake from Supplements (IU/ Day)			
	0–5000	5001–8000	8001–10,000	≥10,001
Affected infants	51	54	9	7
Pregnancies	11,083	10,585	763	317
Prevalence	0.46%	0.51%	1.18%	2.21%

Data from Rothman et al.[8]

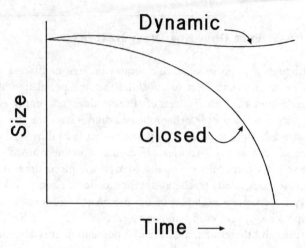

Figure 5–1   Size of hypothetical dynamic and closed cohorts over time.

closed cohort study is the landmark Framingham Heart Study, which was initiated in 1949 and is still ongoing.[9]

In contrast, an *open cohort*, also referred to as a *dynamic cohort* or a *dynamic population*, can take on new members as time passes (see Fig. 5–1). An example of an open cohort is the population of Connecticut, where one of the oldest cancer registries in the United States is found. The population studied in the Connecticut cancer registry may be considered a dynamic cohort that comprises the people of Connecticut. Cancer incidence rates over a period of time in Connecticut reflect the rate of cancer occurrence among a changing population as people move to or away from Connecticut. The population at risk at any given moment comprises current residents of Connecticut, but since residency may change, and in particular new residents may be added to the population, the population being described is dynamic, not closed. Another example of a dynamic population is the population of a school, with new students entering each year and others leaving. An extreme example of a dynamic cohort is the population of current U.S. presidents: whenever there is a new one sworn into office, the previous one leaves the cohort, and whenever one leaves, a new one takes over; the size of the population always remains constant at 1.

In contrast to a dynamic cohort, a closed cohort always becomes smaller with passing time. Ideally, investigators of a closed cohort attempt to track down cohort members if they leave the vicinity of the study. Members of a closed cohort constitute a group of people who remain members of the cohort even if they leave the area of the study. In a dynamic population that is defined geographically, people who leave the geographic boundaries of the study are leaving the cohort and will not be followed.

Counting Disease Events

In cohort studies, epidemiologists usually calculate incidence rates or risks by dividing the number of new *disease events* (ie, the number of disease onsets) by the appropriate denominator, based on the size of the population at risk. Usually there are one or more categories of disease that are of special interest, and new cases of those diseases are counted. Occasionally, however, some disease onsets are excluded, even if they represent the disease under study.

One reason to exclude a disease event might be that it is not the first occurrence of the disease in that person. For example, suppose a woman develops breast cancer in one breast and later develops breast cancer in the other breast. In many studies, the second onset of breast cancer would not be counted as a new case, despite all biologic indications that it represents a separate cancer rather than spread of the first cancer. Similarly, in many studies of myocardial infarction, only the first myocardial infarction is counted as a disease event, and subsequent heart attacks are excluded. Why should investigators make this distinction between the first occurrence of a disease and subsequent occurrences? First, it may be difficult to distinguish between a new case of disease and a recurrence or exacerbation of an earlier case. Second, recurrent disease may have a different set of causes than the primary occurrence. If the investigator limits his or her interest to the first occurrence of a disease, all subsequent occurrences will be excluded, but there will also have to be a corresponding adjustment in the population at risk. If only the first occurrence of disease is of interest, any person who develops the disease is removed from the at-risk population at the time the disease develops. This procedure is consistent with the requirement that members of the population at risk must be eligible to develop the disease. If only the first occurrence is counted, people who develop the disease terminate their eligibility to get disease at the point at which they develop disease.

If the epidemiologist is interested in measuring the total number of disease events, regardless of whether they are first or later occurrences, then a person who is in the cohort would remain as part of the population at risk even after getting the disease. In such an analysis, the first disease event would be counted just the same as a subsequent event, and there would be no way to distinguish the occurrence of first versus later events. The distinction can be made, however. One way is to calculate separate occurrence measures for first and subsequent events. For example, it is possible to calculate the incidence rate of first events, second events, third events, and so forth. The population at risk for second events would be those who have had a first event. On having a first event, a person would leave the population at risk for a first event and enter the population at risk for a second event.

Another reason not to count a disease event is that there was insufficient time for the disease to be related to an exposure. This issue is addressed in the "Exposure and Induction Time" section.

Measuring Incidence Rates or Risks

From a closed cohort, we can estimate a risk or an incidence rate to measure disease occurrence. Calculation of a risk is complicated by the problem of competing risks (see Chapter 4). Because of competing risks, the population at risk will not remain constant in size over time, which means that some people will be removed from the population at risk before they have experienced the entire period of follow-up. Despite this problem, there are many cohort studies in which risks are estimated directly. Usually, the period of follow-up is short enough or the competing risks are small enough in relation to the disease under study that there is relatively little distortion in the risk estimates. In these studies, the risk in each cohort is calculated by dividing the number of new disease events by the total number of people who are being followed in the closed cohort. This approach was used to calculate the risk for cholera in Snow's analysis depicted in Table 5–1. Essentially the same approach was used in the study of vitamin A and birth defects described earlier, although the measure reported is the prevalence, rather than the risk, of birth defects.

It is problematic to measure risk directly in a dynamic cohort, in which new people are added to the cohort during the follow-up period. To get around this problem, the investigator can take into account the amount of time that each person spends in the population at risk and calculate an incidence rate by dividing the number of new disease events by the amount of person-time experienced by the population at risk. The same approach can be applied to a closed cohort, addressing the problem of competing risks.

In the calculation of an incidence rate, the ideal situation is to have precise information on the amount of time that each person has been in the population at risk. Often, this time is calculated for each person in terms of days at risk, although the final results may be expressed in terms of years after converting the time units.

Cohort Study of X-Ray Fluoroscopy and Breast Cancer: An Example

The data in Table 4–6 (see Chapter 4) are taken from a cohort study of radiation exposure and breast cancer. As part of their treatment for tuberculosis, many of the women received substantial doses of x-rays for fluoroscopic monitoring of their lungs. Because the women were followed for highly variable lengths of time, it would not have been reasonable to calculate directly the risk of breast cancer; to do so requires a fixed length of follow-up or at least a minimum follow-up time for all the women in the cohort. (They could have calculated the risk of breast cancer for segments of the follow-up time using the life-table method described in Chapter 4.) Instead, the investigators measured the incidence rate of breast cancer among these women with x-ray exposure. They compared this rate with the rate of breast cancer among women treated during the same period for tuberculosis but not with x-rays. The data in Table 4–6 show that the women who received x-ray exposure had nearly twice the incidence rate of breast cancer as the women who did not receive x-ray exposure.

Exposure and Induction Time

After World War II, the United States and Japan jointly undertook a cohort study of the populations of Hiroshima and Nagasaki who survived the atomic bomb blasts. These populations have been followed for decades, initially under the aegis of the Atomic Bomb Casualty Commission and later under its successor, the Radiation Effects Research Foundation. A category of outcome that has been of primary interest to the researchers has been cancer occurrence. Leukemia is one of the types of cancer that or substantially increased in incidence by ionizing radiation. Consider the survivors of the bombs to constitute several closed cohorts, each corresponding to a different dose category of ionizing radiation. The main factors that determined the dose of exposure were the distance from the epicenter of the blast and the shielding provided by the immediate environment, such as buildings, at the time of the blast.

Suppose that we wish to measure the incidence rate of leukemia among atomic bomb survivors who received a high dose of ionizing radiation and compare this rate with the rate experienced by those who received little or no radiation exposure. The cohorts are defined as of the time of the blasts, and their subsequent experience is tracked as part of the cohort study. We might consider that those who received a high dose of ionizing radiation immediately entered the population at risk for leukemia. The difficulty with beginning the follow-up immediately after the exposure is that it does not allow a sufficient induction time for leukemia to develop as a result of the radiation exposure. For example, an exposed person who was diagnosed with leukemia 2 weeks after exposure is unlikely to have developed his or her leukemia as a consequence of the radiation exposure. After the exposure, disease does not occur until the induction period has passed (see Chapter 3). The induction period corresponds to the time that it takes for the causal mechanism to be completed by the action of the complementary component causes that act after radiation exposure. Suppose that the average time it takes before causal mechanisms that involve radiation are completed and leukemia occurs is 5 years and that few causal mechanisms if any are completed until 3 years have passed. After disease occurs, there is an additional interval, the latent period, during which disease exists but has not yet been diagnosed. It is important to consider the induction period and the latent period in the calculation of incidence rates. To measure the effect of radiation exposure most clearly, the investigator should define the time period at risk for leukemia among exposed people in a way that allows for the induction time and perhaps for the latent period. It would make more sense to allow exposed people to enter the population at risk for leukemia only after a delay of at least 3 years, if we assume that any case occurring before that time could not plausibly be related to exposure.

Typically, the investigator cannot be sure what the induction time is for a given exposure and disease. In that case, it may be necessary to hypothesize various induction times and reanalyze the data under each separate hypothesis. Alternatively, there are statistical methods that estimate the most appropriate induction time.[10]

Among exposed people, what happens to the person-time that is not related to exposure under the hypothesis of a specific induction time? Consider the previous example of studying the effect of radiation exposure from the atomic bomb blasts on the development of leukemia. If we hypothesize that no leukemia can occur as a result of the radiation until at least 3 years have elapsed since the blast, what happens to the first 3 years of follow-up for someone who was exposed? How should we treat the experience of exposed people before they are exposed? Although the induction time comes after exposure, it is a period during which the exposure is presumed not to have any effect and is therefore like the time that comes before exposure. There are two reasonable options for dealing with this time: ignore it or combine it with the follow-up time of people who were never exposed.

The hypothetical data in Figure 5–2 can be used to calculate incidence rates for exposed and unexposed cohorts in a cohort study. Figure 5–2 depicts the follow-up time for 10 people, 5 exposed and 5 unexposed, who were followed for up to 20 years after a point exposure. There are three ways in which follow-up can end: the person can be followed until the end of the study follow-up period of 20 years, the person can be lost to follow-up, or the person can get the disease. Those who are followed for the full 20 years are said to be withdrawn at the end of follow-up. We can calculate the incidence rate among exposed people during the 20 years after exposure. Figure 5–2 shows that the follow-up times for the first 5 people are 12, 20, 15, 2, and 10 years, which sum to 59 years. In this experience of 59 years, three disease events have occurred, for an incidence rate of 3 events per 59 years, or $3/59 \text{ yr}^{-1}$. We also can express this rate as 5.1 cases per 100 person-years, or $5.1/100 \text{ yr}^{-1}$. For the unexposed group, the follow-up times were 20, 18, 20, 11, and 20 years, for a total of 89 years, and there was only one disease event, for a rate of $1/89 \text{ yr}^{-1}$, or $1.1/100 \text{ yr}^{-1}$.

The rate for the exposed group, however, does not take into account the 3-year induction period for exposure to have an effect. To take that into account, we must ignore the first 3 years of follow-up for the exposed group. The follow-up times for the exposed cohort that comes after the induction period for exposure are 9, 17, 12, 0, and 7 years, for a total of 45 years, with only two disease events

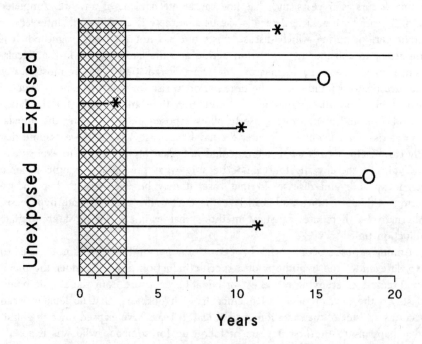

Figure 5–2 Follow-up data for 10 people in a hypothetical cohort study that followed 5 exposed people (top five lines) and 5 unexposed people (bottom five lines). The exposure was a point exposure that is hypothesized to have a minimum 3-year induction time (cross-hatched area) before any case of disease could result from it.

occurring during this follow-up experience. The rate after taking into account the 3-year induction period would be 2/45 yr^{-1}, or 4.4/100 yr^{-1}. There is no reason to exclude the first 3 years of follow-up for the unexposed group, because there is no induction period among those who are not exposed. An investigator may also consider including the first 3 years of follow-up for each exposed person as unexposed experience, because under the study hypothesis, this experience is not related to exposure. With that approach, the denominator of the rate for unexposed would include 14 additional years of follow-up and one additional event, giving a rate of 2/103 yr^{-1}, or 1.9/100 yr^{-1}.

The assumption that the induction time is 3 years is only a hypothesis, and it may be wrong. Other possible induction times can be considered as alternatives, leading to different results. Many epidemiologists ignore the issue of induction time and do not exclude any period of time following exposure. That practice is equivalent to assuming that the induction time is zero, which may be a reasonable assumption, but it may be unreasonable for many study questions. To the extent that the induction time hypothesis is incorrect, there will be nondifferential misclassification of exposure, which introduces a bias (see Chapter 7).

Eligibility Criteria, Exposure Classification, and Time Loops

In a prospective cohort study, the investigator selects subjects who meet the study eligibility criteria and then assigns them to exposure categories as they meet the conditions that define those categories. For example, in a prospective cohort study of smoking, subjects who meet age and other entry criteria may be invited into the cohort and then classified in appropriate smoking categories as they meet the definitions for those categories. A person classified as a nonsmoker at the start of the follow-up may be reclassified as a smoker if he takes up smoking during the follow-up, or a smoker who gives up smoking may be reclassified as an ex-smoker if he gives it up. In retrospective cohort studies, it is important to ensure that decisions about eligibility of participants and any exposure categorization are based on information that is known at the time to which these decisions or assignments pertain, rather than later. The investigator should only use information that would have been known at that time if the investigator had been conducting a prospective cohort study. If this rule is not observed, the result may be the formation of a "time loop," in which a decision is made to include or exclude or classify a study subject at a point in time before the information is known that the decision is based on. For example, suppose the intent is to exclude ex-smokers from the study. A smoker who gives up smoking during the follow-up and becomes an ex-smoker could not be prevented from enrolling in a prospective cohort study if the discontinuation of smoking is in the future at the time the study begins, because the information is not yet known. If the smoker becomes an ex-smoker during follow-up, it would create problems to exclude retroactively his already accumulated experience from the study. An investigator can, however, exclude or *censor* the person's future experience starting when he becomes an ex-smoker.

It is permissible to change the classification of a study participant as circumstances change during follow-up, but those changes should influence only the follow-up time that comes after the change. An unexposed person can become

WHICH MEASURES TO REPORT FROM COHORT STUDIES?

In a cohort study, the epidemiologist often has data that allow the calculation of a risk or a rate of disease. The choice depends on whether the denominators available are the number of people in the cohort, which gives risks, or the amount of person-time, which gives rates. To measure risks, everyone in the cohort should be followed for at least the length of the risk period. Risks are often reported in experimental studies, which usually aim for a uniform length of follow-up. If the follow-up time varies considerably from person to person, it may be preferable to use person-time as the denominator measure and report rates. In some cohort studies, the actual risks or rates in each cohort are not reported; instead, a risk or rate ratio is reported for one or more levels of the study exposure. Reporting only risk or rate ratios is a disservice to readers, who deserve to know the underlying risks or rates if these are obtainable. Ideally, the investigator should report the risk or rate for each level of exposure, as well as the numerators and denominators from which these risks or rates are calculated. The risk or rate differences are still of interest, although they are secondary to the actual risks or rates, because they can be derived from the risks or rates.

One reason that some studies report only ratio measures is that the investigators may have used a statistical model to analyze their data that only produces ratio measures. Nevertheless, it is not difficult to use stratification or other analytic methods to obtain the risks or rates themselves (see Chapter 10). Some cohort studies report odds ratios rather than risk ratios. Usually, odds ratios are reported because the statistical model used is a logistic model, which estimates odds ratios (see Chapter 12). Odds ratios are a fundamental measure in case-control studies, where they are used to estimate risk or rate ratios. In cohort studies, the risks or rates are obtainable directly, and there is little reason to consider an odds ratio. Although odds ratios are often reported in experiments, they should not be used, because in experiments, the outcome is typically frequent enough that the odds ratio is a poor estimate of the risk ratio, which could be obtained directly. Odds ratios are appropriate when analyzing case-control studies, but odds ratios usually have little reason to appear in cohort studies and should not be reported. If they are reported, it is better for readers to ignore them and look for information on the actual risks or rates.

exposed during the follow-up period of a cohort study. That information should not be used to change that person's categorization at the start of follow-up, when the person was unexposed. It can be used, however, to change the exposure category in which the person's follow-up time is tallied after the time he or she became exposed.

One example of the effect of a time loop is the creation of *immortal person-time*. Suppose we are conducting a cohort study of mortality among workers in a factory who are exposed to mercury vapor on the job. A common feature of many exposure measures for occupational (and other) exposures is that the measure is based on the amount of time exposed. For example, the number of years of employment for workers exposed to mercury vapor on the job is a crude index of cumulative exposure, especially if the exposure in the workplace has been relatively stable over time. It may seem reasonable to compare the mortality among workers who were employed for only a few years with the mortality among workers employed for longer periods. Consider classifying workers into the categories of 0 to 9 years, 10 to 19 years, and 20+ years of employment, which we hope will separate workers with different levels of exposure to mercury vapor. A worker who ends up in the category of 20+ years of employment must pass through the other two categories first. How do we tabulate the follow-up time for a worker at this factory, starting at the beginning of employment? For the first 10 years of employment, the follow-up time must be tallied in the category of 0–9 years and, for the next 10 years, in the second category. It is only after 20 years of employment that a worker can begin to contribute follow-up time to the third category of employment. If a worker with 40 years of employment had been inappropriately classified in the 20+ category with respect to all 40 years, the first 20 of those 40 years would constitute immortal person-time. Those long-term workers were not actually immortal during their first 20 years on the job, but if any of them had died before reaching the 20th anniversary of employment, he or she could not have reached the category of 20+ to contribute any time at all. Everyone in the category of 20+ would have had 20 years during which they could not have died, because those who did were not classified in this category. This mistake would lead to a severe underestimate of mortality among the longest employed workers and an overestimate of mortality for those employed for shorter periods. This kind of problem can be avoided by avoiding any time loops that come from using future information to classify person-time before that information could have been known.

Retrospective Cohort Studies

A prospective cohort study is one in which the exposure information is recorded at the beginning of the follow-up (with possible updates if exposure status changes), and the period of time at risk for disease runs concurrently with the conduct of the study. This is always the case with experiments and with many nonexperimental cohort studies. Nevertheless, a cohort study is not always prospective; cohort studies can also be retrospective. In a *retrospective cohort study* (also known as a *historical cohort study*), the cohorts are identified from recorded information, and the time during which they are at risk for disease occurred before the beginning of the study.

An outstanding example of a retrospective cohort study was conducted by Morrison et al.[11] They studied young women who were born in Florence in the 15th and 16th centuries and who were enrolled in a dowry fund soon after they were born. The dowry fund was an insurance plan that would pay the family a sizable return if an enrolled woman married. If the woman died or joined a convent first, the fund did not have to pay a dowry. The fund records contain the date of birth, date of investment, and date of dowry payment or death of 19,000 girls and women. More than 500 years after the first women were enrolled in the dowry fund, epidemiologists were able to use the fund records to chart waves of epidemic deaths from the plague and show how successive plague epidemics became milder over a period of 100 years. This retrospective cohort study, conducted centuries after the data were recorded, illustrates well that a cohort study need not be prospective.

Because a retrospective cohort study must rely on existing records, important information may be missing or otherwise unavailable. Nevertheless, when a retrospective cohort study is feasible, it offers the advantage of providing information that is usually much less costly than that from a prospective cohort study, and it may produce results much sooner because there is no need to wait for the disease to occur.

Tracing of Subjects

Cohort studies that span many years present a challenge with respect to maintaining contact with the cohort to ascertain disease events. Whether the study is retrospective or prospective, it is often difficult to locate people or their records many years after they have been enrolled in study cohorts. In prospective cohort studies, the investigator may contact study participants periodically to maintain current information on their location. Tracing subjects in cohort studies is a major component of their expense. If a large proportion of participants are lost to follow-up, the validity of the study may be threatened. Studies that trace less than about 60% of subjects usually are regarded with skepticism, but even follow-up of 70%, 80%, or more can be too low if the subjects lost to follow-up are lost for reasons related to both the exposure and the disease. Increasing access to the Internet may provide more efficient ways to enroll and trace participants in cohort studies.[12] We later consider the relative importance of successful tracing of subjects versus successful recruitment of subjects for cohort studies.

Special Exposure and General Population Cohorts

Cohort studies permit the epidemiologist to study many different disease end points at the same time. A mortality follow-up can be accomplished just as easily for all causes of death as for any specific cause. Health surveillance for one disease end point can sometimes be expanded to include many end points without much additional work. A cohort study can provide a comprehensive picture of the health effect of a given exposure. Cohort studies that focus on people who share a particular exposure are called *special-exposure cohort studies*. Examples of special-exposure cohorts include occupational cohorts exposed to substances in the workplace; soldiers exposed to Agent Orange in Vietnam; residents of the Love Canal area of Niagara, New York, exposed to chemical wastes; Seventh Day Adventists adhering to vegetarian diets; and atomic bomb victims exposed to ionizing radiation. Each of these exposures is uncommon; therefore, it is usually more efficient to study them by identifying a specific cohort of people who have sustained that exposure and comparing their disease experience with that of a cohort of people who lack the exposure.

In contrast, common exposures are sometimes studied through cohort studies that survey a segment of the population that is identified initially without regard to their exposure status. These *general-population cohorts* typically focus on exposures that a substantial proportion of people have experienced. Otherwise, there would be too few people in the study who are exposed to the factors of interest. After a general-population cohort is assembled, the cohort members can be classified according to smoking, alcoholic beverage consumption, diet, drug use, medical history, and many other factors of potential interest. The study described earlier of vitamin A intake in pregnant women and birth defects among their offspring[8] is an example of a general-population cohort study. No women in that study were selected for the study because they had vitamin A exposure. Their exposure to vitamin A was determined after they were selected for the study during the interview. Although the study was a general-population cohort study, a high level of vitamin A intake during pregnancy was not a common exposure. Table 5–4 shows that only 317 of the total of 22,058 women, or 1.4%, were in the highest category of vitamin A intake. Fortunately, the overall study population was large enough that the vitamin A analysis was feasible; it would have been difficult to identify or recruit a special-exposure cohort of women who had a high intake of vitamin A during pregnancy.

In both special-exposure and general-population cohort studies, the investigator must classify study participants into the exposure categories that form the cohorts. This classification is easier for some exposures than for others. When the female offspring of women who took diethylstilbestrol (DES) were assembled for a special population cohort study, defining their exposure was comparatively clear-cut, based on whether their mothers took DES while they were pregnant.[13] For other exposures, such as secondhand smoke or dietary intake of saturated fat, almost everyone is exposed to some extent, and the investigator must group people together according to their level of intake to form cohorts.

CASE-CONTROL STUDIES

The main drawback of conducting a cohort study is the necessity in many situations to obtain information on exposure and other variables from large populations to measure the risk or rate of disease. In many studies, however, only a tiny minority of those who are at risk for disease actually develop the disease. The case-control study aims at achieving the same goals as a cohort study, but more efficiently, using sampling. Properly carried out, case-control studies provide information that mirrors what could be learned from a cohort study, usually at considerably less cost and time.

Case-control studies are best understood by considering as the starting point a *source population*, which represents a hypothetical study population in which a cohort study might have been conducted. The source population is the population that gives rise to the cases included in the study. If a cohort study were undertaken, we would define the exposed and unexposed cohorts (or several cohorts), and from these populations obtain denominators for the incidence rates or risks that would be calculated for each cohort. We would then identify the number of cases occurring in each cohort and calculate the risk or incidence rate for each.

In a case-control study, the same cases are identified and classified according to whether they belong to the exposed or unexposed cohort. Instead of obtaining the denominators for the rates or risks, however, a control group is sampled from the entire source population that gives rise to the cases. Individuals in the control group are then classified into exposed and unexposed categories. The purpose of the control group is to determine the relative size of the exposed and unexposed components of the source population. Because the control group is used to estimate the distribution of exposure in the source population, the cardinal requirement of control selection is that the controls be sampled independently of exposure status.

Figure 5–3 shows the relation between a case-control study and the cohort study that it replaces. In the illustration, 25% of the 288 people in the source population are exposed. Suppose that the cases, illustrated at the right, arise during 1 year of follow-up. For simplicity, assume that the cases all occur at the end of the year; ordinarily they are spread out through time, which would necessitate discontinuing the person-time contribution to follow-up for each case at the time of the event. The rate of disease among exposed people is 8 cases occurring in 72 person-years, for a rate of 0.111 cases per person-year. Among the 216 unexposed people, 8 additional cases arise during the 1 year of follow-up, for a rate of 0.037 cases per person-year. In this hypothetical example, the incidence rate among the exposed cohort is three times the rate among the unexposed cohort. Now consider what would happen if a case-control study were conducted. The rectangle drawn around a portion of the source population represents a sample that could represent the control group. This sample must be taken independently of the exposure. Among the 48 people in the control group, 12 are exposed. If the sample is taken independently of the exposure, the same proportion of controls will be exposed as the proportion of people (or person-time) exposed in the original source population, apart from sampling error. The same cases that were included in the cohort study are also included in the case-control study as the case group. Later, we will see how the data in the case-control study can be used to estimate the ratio of the incidence rates in the source population, giving the same result for the incidence rate ratio that the cohort study provides.

Nested Case-Control Studies

It is helpful to think of every case-control study as being nested, or conducted, within cohorts of exposed and unexposed people, as illustrated in Fig. 5–3. Epidemiologists sometimes refer to specific case-control studies as *nested* case-control studies when the population within which the study is conducted is a well-defined cohort, but almost any case-control study can be thought of as nested within some source population. In many instances, this population may be identifiable, such as all residents of Rio de Janeiro during the year 2001; in other instances, the members of the source population may be hard to identify.

In occupational epidemiology, a commonly used approach is to conduct a case-control study nested within an occupational cohort that has already been enumerated. The reason for conducting a case-control study even when a cohort can be enumerated is usually that more information is needed than is readily

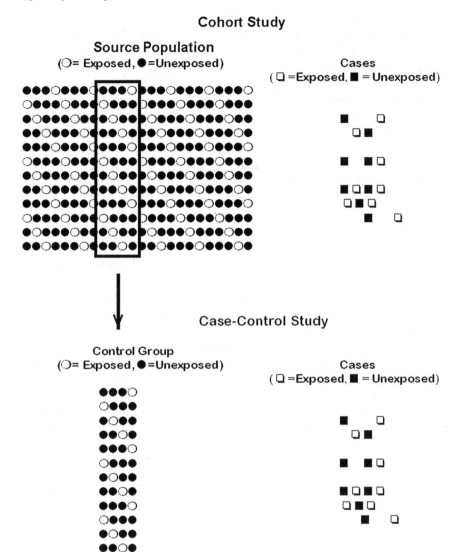

Cohort Study

Figure 5–3 Schematic of a cohort study and a nested case-control study within the cohort shows how the control group is sampled from the source population.

available from records and that it would be too expensive to seek this information for everyone in the cohort. A nested case-control study is then more efficient. In these studies, the source population is easy to identify. It is the occupational cohort. A control group can be selected by sampling randomly from this source population.

As an example of a case-control study in which the source population is hard to identify, consider one in which the cases are patients treated for severe psoriasis at the Mayo Clinic. These patients come to the Mayo Clinic from all corners of the world. What is the specific source population that gives rise to these cases? To answer this question, we need to know exactly who goes to the Mayo Clinic for severe psoriasis. We cannot identify this population because many people in it do not know themselves that they would go to or be referred to the Mayo Clinic for severe psoriasis unless they developed it. Nevertheless, we can still imagine a population spread around the world that constitutes the people who would go to the Mayo Clinic if they developed severe psoriasis. It is this population in which the case-control study is nested and from which the control series would ideally be drawn. (In practice, an investigator would likely draw the controls from other patients who attended the Mayo clinic, who might constitute a *proxy sample*, as discussed later.) From this perspective, almost any case-control study can be thought of as nested within a source population, and a description of this population corresponds to eligibility criteria for both cases and controls.

Basic Types of Case-Control Studies

Controls in a case-control study can be sampled in several ways, with each giving rise to a type of case-control study with slightly different implications for the design, analysis, and interpretation. The three basic types are density-based sampling, cumulative sampling, and case-cohort sampling. In density sampling, controls are sampled to represent the distribution of person-time in the source population with respect to exposure. In cumulative sampling, controls are sampled after the source population has gone through a period of risk, which is presumed to be over when the study is conducted. For example, a case-control study examining the effect of vaccination on the risk of influenza may be conducted at the end of the influenza season, when the annual epidemic has ended. In the cumulative case-control study, the control group is sampled from among those who did not become cases during the period of risk. If the cases were those who contracted influenza, the controls would be sampled from among those who remained free of influenza during the epidemic. In the case-cohort study, controls are sampled from the list of all people in the source population, regardless of whether they become cases. As a result, in a case-cohort study, some of the controls may also be included as cases. These three case-control designs are discussed further in the following sections.

Density Case-Control Studies

The phrase *density-based sampling* comes from the term *incidence density*, which is sometimes used as a synonym for incidence rate. The aim of this type of control sampling is to have the distribution of controls mirror the distribution of person-time in the source population with respect to exposure. If 20% of the person-time in the source population is classified as exposed person-time, the aim of a density case-control study will be to sample controls in such a way that 20% of them are exposed. In an actual study, we ordinarily do not know the exposure distribution in the source population, and we rely on our sampling methods to reveal it through our control series.

Suppose that we have a dichotomous exposure. We can consider the source population to have two subcohorts, exposed and unexposed, which we denote by the subscripts 1 and 0, respectively. During a given time period, the incidence rates for the exposed population would be

$$I_1 = \frac{a}{PT_1}$$

For the unexposed population, it would be

$$I_0 = \frac{b}{PT_0}$$

In these equations, I_1 and I_0 are the incidence rates among exposed and unexposed, respectively; a and b are the respective numbers of exposed and unexposed people who developed the disease; and PT_1 and PT_0 are the respective amounts of person-time at risk for the exposed and the unexposed cohorts.

In a case-control study with density-based sampling, the control series provides an estimate of the proportion of the total person-time for exposed and unexposed cohorts in the source population. Suppose that the control series sampled from the source population contains c exposed people and d unexposed people. The aim is to select the control series so that the following ratios are equal, apart from statistical sampling error:

$$\frac{c}{d} = \frac{PT_1}{PT_0}$$

Equivalently,

$$\frac{c}{PT_1} = \frac{d}{PT_0}$$

The ratios c/PT_1 and d/PT_0 are called the *control sampling rates* for the exposed and unexposed components of the source population. These sampling rates will be equal if the control sampling is conducted independently of exposure. If this goal is achieved, the incidence rate ratio can be readily estimated from the case-control data as follows:

$$\frac{I_1}{I_0} = \frac{a/PT_1}{b/PT_0} = \frac{a}{b} \times \frac{PT_0}{PT_1} = \frac{a}{b} \times \frac{d}{c} \quad \text{because} \quad \frac{d}{c} = \frac{PT_0}{PT_1}$$

The quantity ad/bc, which in a case-control study provides an estimate of the incidence rate ratio, is called the *cross-product ratio* or, more commonly, the *odds ratio*. Using the odds ratio in a case-control study with density-based sampling, an investigator can obtain a valid estimate of the incidence rate ratio in a population without having to obtain individual information on every person in the population.

What disadvantage is there in using a sample of the denominators rather than measuring the person-time experience for the entire source population? Sampling of the source population can lead to an inaccurate measure of the exposure distribution, giving rise to an incorrect estimate. A case-control study offers less statistical precision in estimating the incidence rate ratio than a cohort study of the same population. A loss in precision is to be expected whenever sampling is involved. This loss can be kept small if the number of controls selected per case is large. The loss is offset by the cost savings of not having to obtain information on everyone in the source population. The cost savings may allow the epidemiologist to enlarge the source population and therefore obtain more cases, resulting in a better overall estimate of the incidence rate ratio statistically and otherwise than would be possible using the same expenditures to conduct a cohort study.

DEFINING THE SOURCE POPULATION

The earlier discussion presumes that all people who develop the disease of interest in the source population are included as cases in the case-control study. The definition of the source population corresponds to the eligibility criteria for cases to enter the study. In theory, it is not necessary to include all cases occurring within an identifiable population, such as within a geographic boundary. The cases identified in a single clinic or treated by a single medical practitioner can be used for case-control studies. The corresponding source population for the cases treated in a clinic is all people who would attend that clinic and be recorded with the diagnosis of interest if they had the disease in question. It is important to specify "if they had the disease in question" because clinics serve different populations for different diseases, depending on referral patterns and the reputation of the clinic in specific specialty areas. Unfortunately, without a precisely identified source population, it may be difficult or impossible to select controls in an unbiased fashion.

CONTROL SELECTION

In density case-control studies, the control series is sampled to represent the person-time distribution of exposure in the source population. If the sampling is conducted independently of the exposure, the case-control study can provide a valid estimate of the incidence rate ratio. Each control sampled represents a certain amount of person-time experience. The probability of any given person in the source population being selected as a control should be proportional to his or her person-time contribution to the denominators of the incidence rates in the source population. For example, a person who is at risk of becoming a study case for 5 years should have a five times higher probability of being selected as a control than a person who is at risk for only 1 year.

For each person contributing time to the source population experience, the time that he or she is eligible to be selected as a control is the same time during which he or she is also eligible to become a case if the disease occurs. A person who has already developed the disease or has died is no longer eligible to be selected as a control. This rule corresponds to the treatment of subjects in cohort studies: Every case that is tallied in the numerator of a cohort study contributes to the denominator of the rate until the time that the person becomes a case, when the contribution to the denominator ceases.

One way to implement control sampling according to these guidelines is to choose controls from the unique set of people in the source population who are at risk of becoming a case at the precise time that each case is diagnosed. This set, which changes from one case to the next as people enter and leave the source population, is sometimes referred to as the *risk set* for the case. Risk-set sampling allows the investigator to sample controls so that each control is selected in proportion to his or her time contribution to the person-time at risk.

A conceptually important feature of the selection of controls with density-based sampling is their continuous eligibility to become cases if they develop the disease. Suppose that the study period spans 3 years and that a given person free of disease in year 1 is selected as a control. The same person may develop the disease in year 3, becoming a case. How is such a person treated in the analysis? If the disease is uncommon, it will matter little, because a study is unlikely to have many subjects eligible to be both a case and a control, but the question is nevertheless of some theoretical interest. Because the person in question did develop disease during the study period, many investigators would be tempted to count the person as a case, not as a control. Recall, however, that if a cohort study were being conducted, each person who developed disease would contribute not only to the numerator of the disease rate, but also to the person-time experience counted in the denominator, until the time of disease onset. The control group in density case-control studies is intended to provide estimates of the relative size of the denominators of the incidence rates for the compared groups. Therefore, each case should have been eligible to be a control before the time of disease onset; each control should be eligible to become a case as of the time of selection as a control. A person selected as a control who later develops the disease and is selected as a case should be included in the study both as a control and as a case.

As an extension of the previous point, with density-based sampling, a person selected as a control should remain eligible to be selected again as a control as long as he or she remains at risk for disease in the study population. Although unlikely in typical studies, the same person may appear in the control group two or more times. Note, however, that including the same person at different times does not necessarily lead to exposure (or confounder) information being repeated, because this information may change with time. For example, in a case-control study of viral hepatitis, the investigator may ask about raw shellfish ingested within the previous 6 weeks. Whether a person has consumed raw shellfish during the previous 6 weeks will change with time, and a person included more than once, first as a control and then later as either a control or as a case, may have different exposure information at the different points in time. The same can be true for confounding variables, which may also change with time.

ILLUSTRATION OF DENSITY-BASED CASE-CONTROL DATA

Consider the data for the cohort study in Table 4–7 (see Chapter 4). These data are shown again in Table 5–5 along with a hypothetical control series of 500 women that might have been selected from the two cohorts.

The ratio of the rates for the exposed and unexposed cohorts is $14.6/7.9 = 1.86$. Suppose that instead of conducting a cohort study, the investigators conducted a density case-control study by identifying all 56 breast cancer cases that

Table 5–5 Hypothetical Case-Control Data from a Cohort
Study of Breast Cancer Among Women Treated for
Tuberculosis with X-ray Fluoroscopies and Full Cohort
Data for Comparison

	Radiation Exposure		
	Yes	No	Total
Breast cancer cases	41	15	56
(Person-years)	(28,010)	(19,017)	(47,027)
Control series (people)	298	202	500
Rate (cases/10,000 person-years)	14.6	7.9	11.9

occurred in the two cohorts and a control series of 500 women. The control series should be sampled from the person-time of the source population so that the exposure distribution of the controls sampled mirrors the exposure distribution of the person-time in the source population. Of the 47,027 person-years of experience in the combined exposed and unexposed cohorts, 28,010 (59.6%) are person-years of experience that relate to radiation exposure. If the controls are sampled properly, we would expect that more or less 59.6% of them would be exposed and the remainder unexposed. If we happened to get just the proportion that we would expect to get on the average, we would have 298 exposed controls and 202 unexposed controls, as indicated in Table 5–5.

Table 5–5 shows the case and control series along with the full cohort data for comparison. In an actual case-control study, the data would look like those in Table 5–6. Because there are two rows of data and two columns with four cell frequencies in the table (not counting the totals on the right), this type of table is often referred to as a 2 × 2 table.

From these data, we can calculate the odds ratio to get an estimate of the incidence rate ratio.

$$\text{Odds ratio} = \frac{41 \times 202}{15 \times 298} = 1.85 = \text{Incidence rate ratio}$$

This result differs from the incidence rate ratio from the full cohort data by only a slight rounding error. Ordinarily, we would expect to see additional error because the control group is a sample from the source population, and there may be some difference between the exposure distribution in the control series and the exposure distribution in the source population. In Chapter 9, we see how to take this sampling error into account.

Table 5–6 Case-Control Data Alone from
Table 5–5

	Radiation Exposure		
	Yes	No	Total
Breast cancer cases	41	15	56
Controls	298	202	500

Cumulative Case-Control Studies

Density case-control studies correspond to cohort studies that measure person-time and estimate rates. The effect estimates from density case-control studies are estimates of rate ratios, with each control representing a certain amount of person-time. In cumulative case-control studies or in case-cohort studies, each control represents a certain number of people. These studies correspond to cohort studies that follow a closed population and measure risks, rather than rates. The effect estimate obtained from cumulative case-control studies or from case-cohort studies is a risk ratio rather than a rate ratio.

When sampling controls from a closed source population, an investigator may choose to sample the controls from the entire source population at the start of follow-up or at the end of the follow-up from the noncases that remain after the cases have been identified. If the control sample is drawn from the entire source population at the start of the follow-up, the design is called a *case-cohort study*, which is described later. If the control sample is drawn from the noncases at the end of the follow-up, the design is called a *cumulative case-control study*. Cumulative case-control studies are often conducted at the end of an epidemic period or a specific but time-limited risk period. For example, an investigator may be interested in the effect of specific drug exposures during early pregnancy on the occurrence of birth defects. To conduct a case-control study that addresses this issue, the investigator may identify cases who are born with birth defects. Typically, the control series is sampled from babies born without birth defects. At birth, the period of risk for birth defects is over, so the case and control sampling occurs after the risk period has ended. There is an intuitive appeal to choosing controls from among those babies who did not develop a birth defect, but such babies do not represent the experience of the entire source population. Some babies who were at risk for birth defects may not have survived to be born alive, but even if all had, selecting controls from among those born without birth defects omits the experience of the cases from the population at risk. Because the experience of cases is part of the overall experience of the source population, omitting them from the control series can result in a bias that will overestimate the risk ratio.

In a cumulative case-control study, the risk ratio is estimated from the same measure used in density case-control studies, the odds ratio.

$$\text{Odds ratio} = \frac{ad}{bc}$$

In this equation, a and b are the number of exposed and unexposed cases, respectively, and c and d are the number of exposed and unexposed controls. Because of the sampling approach in a cumulative case-control study, this odds ratio is an estimate of the risk ratio, rather than the rate ratio obtained from density case-control studies. If the disease is rare, the experience of cases will be a small part of the overall experience of the source population, and the odds ratio obtained from cumulative control sampling will be very close to the risk ratio. If the risk for disease is high enough, however, the cumulative case-control study can seriously overestimate the risk ratio.

We can illustrate this phenomenon with a hypothetical example. In Table 5–7, the top section shows hypothetical data from a cohort study of a closed population of 200 people, one half of whom are exposed. The risk of disease is 40% among exposed and 10% among unexposed, for a risk ratio of 4.0. The next section in the table shows the result if a case-control study had been conducted, with all cases included and 50 controls, using cumulative sampling. At the end of follow-up, there were a total of 50 cases, leaving 150 people who did not get the disease. Suppose that 50 controls were sampled from these 150 noncases. The exposure distribution of these controls is shown in the next section of Table 5–7. Although one half of the closed source population was exposed, only 40% of the noncases at the end of follow-up are exposed (there are 60 noncases among those exposed and 90 among those unexposed). The reason for this discrepancy is that exposure is associated with disease, and the disease is common, leaving fewer exposed noncases than unexposed noncases. The estimate of the risk ratio measuring the effect of exposure is obtained from the odds ratio. For the cumulative sampling, the odds ratio = $(40 \times 30)/(10 \times 20) = 6.0$, considerably greater than the correct value for the risk ratio of 4.0. This departure is a bias that results from the sampling method, combined with high risk of disease. If the risks were 4% and 1% among exposed and unexposed, the odds ratio from the same sampling approach would be about 4.1 instead of 6, much closer to the correct value of 4.0 for the risk ratio. As the risk for disease becomes very small, sampling from the noncases at the end of follow-up becomes almost identical to sampling from the entire cohort.

Cumulative sampling results in valid estimates of the risk ratio if the risk of disease is sufficiently low. This condition is described as the *rare disease assumption*. In the past, it has been mistakenly thought to be a necessary assumption to get a valid result for any case-control study, but the rare disease assumption is needed only for cumulative case-control studies. Density case-control studies, for example, provide unbiased estimates of the rate ratio even when the disease is common. When the rare disease assumption is met, it is worth keeping in mind that the risk ratio will approximate the rate ratio, which is to say that in a cumulative case-control study when risks are small, the odds ratio, the risk ratio, and the rate ratio will all be close to the same value.

Case-Cohort Studies

The third basic approach to control sampling is the *case-cohort study*. In this type of study, each control represents a certain number of people in the source

Table 5–7 CUMULATIVE SAMPLING VERSUS CASE-COHORT SAMPLING IN A CASE-CONTROL STUDY

	Exposed	Unexposed	Risk or Odds Ratio
Cases	40	10	
Cohort denominator	100	100	4.0
Controls (cumulative)	20	30	6.0
Controls (case-cohort)	25	25	4.0

population, just as in the cumulative case-control study. As in the cumulative case-control study, the case-cohort study ordinarily provides estimates of risk ratio, rather than rate ratio. In the case-cohort study, however, the controls are sampled from the entire source population rather than from the noncases. Every person in the source population has the same chance of being included in the study as a control, regardless of whether that person becomes a case. The case-cohort design may also be used even if subjects are followed for various amounts of time. With this type of sampling, each control participant represents a fraction of the total number of people in the source population, rather than a fraction of the total person-time. The risk ratio is, as with cumulative case-control studies, estimated from the odds ratio. Because the controls are sampled from the entire source population, however, there is no need for the rare disease assumption in case-cohort studies. As seen in the lower section of Table 5–7, the exposure distribution among controls in a case-cohort study will, on average, reflect the exposure distribution among all persons followed in the source population, even if disease is common.

If the proportion of subjects that is sampled and becomes part of the control series is known, it is possible to estimate the actual size of the cohorts being followed and to calculate separate risks for the exposed and the unexposed cohorts. Usually, this sampling proportion is not known, in which case the actual risks cannot be calculated. As long as the controls are sampled independently of the exposure, however, the odds ratio will still be a valid estimate of the risk ratio, just as the odds ratio in a density case-control study is an estimate of the incidence rate ratio. No rare disease assumption is needed, because the controls are sampled from the entire source population.

One advantage of a case-cohort study over a density case-control study is convenience. Sufficient data to allow risk-set sampling (discussed earlier) may not be available, for example. Moreover, the investigators may intend to study several diseases. In risk-set sampling, each control must be sampled from the risk set (ie, the set of people in the source population who are at risk for disease at that time) for each case. The definition of the risk set changes for each case, because the identity of the risk set is related to the timing of the case. If several diseases are to be studied, each disease will require its own control group to maintain risk-set sampling. Control sampling for a case-cohort study requires only a single sample of people from the roster of people who constitute the cohort. The same control group can used to compare with various case series, just as the same denominators for calculating risks can be used to calculate the risk for various diseases in the cohort. This approach can therefore be considerably more convenient than density sampling.

In a case-cohort study, a person who is selected as a control may also be a case in the study (the same possibility exists in a density case-control study). This possibility may seem bothersome; some epidemiologists take pains to avoid the possibility that a control subject may have even an undetected stage of the disease under study. Nevertheless, there is no theoretical difficulty with a control participant also being a case. The control series in a case-cohort study is a sample of the entire list of people who are in the exposed and unexposed cohorts. If we did not sample at all but included the entire list, we would have a cohort study from which we could directly calculate risks for exposed and unexposed groups. In a cohort study risk calculation, every person in the numerator (ie, every case) is also included in the denominator (ie, is a member of the source population). This situation is analogous to the possibility that a person who is sampled as a control subject in a case-cohort study might be someone who has been included as a case. It may be helpful to consider the timing of control versus case selection. If the control series is seen as a sample of the exposed and unexposed cohorts at the start of their follow-up, the control sampling represents people who were free of disease, because everyone at the start of follow-up in a cohort study is free of disease. It is only later that disease develops in some of these people, who then become cases. These parallels in thinking between case-control and cohort studies help to clarify the principles of control selection and illustrate the importance of viewing case-control studies as cohort studies with sampled denominators. If the same subject is included with the same data as both case and control in a case-cohort study, some refined formulas may be used to analyze the data, taking account of the status of subjects who serve a dual role as case and control. *Modern Epidemiology* offers a more detailed discussion of case-cohort studies.[1]

ILLUSTRATION OF CASE-COHORT DATA

Consider the data in Table 5–1 describing John Snow's natural experiment. Imagine that he had conducted a case-cohort study instead, with a sample of 10,000 controls selected from the source population of the London neighborhoods that he was investigating. If the control series had the same distribution by water company that the entire population in Table 5–1 had, the data might resemble the 2 × 2 table shown in Table 5–8. We would obtain the odds ratio from these hypothetical case-cohort data as follows:

$$\text{Odds ratio} = \frac{4093 \times 3946}{461 \times 6054} = 5.79 = \text{Risk ratio}$$

This result is essentially the same value that Snow obtained from his natural experiment cohort study. In this hypothetical case-cohort study, 10,000 controls were included, instead of the 440,000 people Snow included in the full cohort-study comparison. If Snow had to determine the exposure status of every person in the population, it would have been much easier to conduct the case-cohort study and sample from the source population. As it happened, Snow derived his exposure distribution by estimating the population of water company customers from business records, making it unnecessary to obtain information on each person. He did have to ascertain the exposure status of each case, however.

Table 5–8 HYPOTHETICAL CASE-COHORT DATA FOR
JOHN SNOW'S NATURAL EXPERIMENT

	Water Company	
	Southwark & Vauxhall	Lambeth
Cholera deaths	4,093	461
Controls	6,054	3,946

Sources for Control Series

The ideal method of control selection in a case-control study is to sample controls directly from the source population of cases. If the cases represent all cases or a representative sample of cases within a geographic area, the controls should be sampled from the entire at-risk population of that geographic area. This is a *population-based study*, which means it is based on a geographically defined population. The at-risk subset of the population, which is the source population for cases, is those who met the study inclusion criteria for age, sex, and other factors. This subset also excludes current cases or any other people who were not able to become study cases, such as women with a hysterectomy in a study of endometrial cancer. Control sampling in a population-based study is facilitated if a population registry is available, from which potential controls may be identified, perhaps through random sampling.

Random sampling of controls does not necessarily mean that every person should have an equal probability of being selected to be a control. With density sampling, a person's control selection probability is proportional to the person's time at risk. For example, in a case-control study nested within an occupational cohort, workers on an employee roster have been followed for various lengths of time. Random sampling for a density-based case-control study should reflect the variation in time followed. Random sampling for a case-cohort study in the same setting, however, involves every person on the employee roster having an equal probability of being sampled as a control.

If no registry or roster of the source population is available, other approaches must be found to sample controls from the source population. One approach that has often been used is random-digit dialing. This method is based on the assumption that randomly calling telephone numbers simulates a random sample of the source population. Random-digit dialing offers the advantage of approaching all households in a designated area, even those with unlisted telephone numbers, through a telephone call. The method poses a few challenges, however.

First, the method assumes that every case can be reached by telephone, because the source population being sampled is that part of the total population that is reachable by telephone. If some cases have no telephone, in principle, they should be excluded from a study employing random-digit dialing. The second issue is that random dialing gives every telephone an equal probability of being called, but that is not equivalent to giving every person an equal probability of being called. Households vary in the number of people who reside in them and in the amount of time someone is at home. Third, making contact with a household may require many calls at various times of day and various days of the week. Fourth, it may be challenging to distinguish business from residential telephone numbers, a distinction that affects calculating the proportion of nonresponders. Fifth, the increase in telemarketing in many areas and the availability of caller identification has further compromised response rates to cold calling. Obtaining a control subject meeting specific eligibility characteristics can require dozens of telephone calls. Other problems include answering machines and households with multiple telephone numbers, a rapidly increasing phenomenon. Because telephony is rapidly changing in rich and poor countries, the use of random digit dialing is becoming more complicated, and the possible biases introduced by identifying controls using this method must be carefully considered in each study in which the method is contemplated.

Another method to identify population-based controls when the source population cannot easily be enumerated is sampling residences in some systematic fashion. If a geographic roster of residences is not available, some scheme must be devised to sample residences without enumerating them all. Often, matching is employed as a convenience. After a case is identified, one or more controls who reside in the same neighborhood as that case are identified and recruited into the study. With this type of design, neighborhood must be treated as a matching factor (see Chapter 7).

If the case-control study is not population based, it may be based on a referral population in a hospital or clinic. In these studies, the source population represents a group of people who would be treated in a given clinic or hospital if they developed the disease in question. This population may be hard to identify, because it does not correspond to the residents of a specific geographic area. Any clinic-based study can be restricted to a given geographic area, but the hospitals or clinics that provide the cases for the study often treat only a small proportion of those in the geographic area, making the actual source population unidentifiable. A case-control study is still possible, but the investigator must take into account referral patterns to the hospital or clinic in the sampling of controls. Typically, he or she would draw a control series from patients treated at the same hospitals or clinics as the cases. The source population does not correspond to the population of the geographic area, but only to those who would attend the hospital or clinic if they contracted the disease under study. Other patients treated at the same hospitals or clinics as the cases will constitute a sample, albeit not a random sample, of this source population.

The major problem with any nonrandom sampling of controls is the possibility that they are not selected independently of exposure in the source population. Patients hospitalized with other diseases at the same hospitals, for example, may not have the same exposure distribution as the entire source population, because exposed people are more or less likely than nonexposed people to be hospitalized for the control diseases if they develop them or because the exposure may cause or prevent these control diseases in the first place. Suppose the study aims to evaluate the relation between tobacco smoking and leukemia. If controls are people hospitalized with other conditions, many of them will have been hospitalized for conditions that are caused by smoking. A variety of other cancers, cardiovascular diseases, and respiratory diseases are related to smoking. Thus, a series of people hospitalized for diseases other than leukemia may include more smokers than the source population from which they came. One approach to this problem is to exclude any diagnosis from the control series that is likely to be related to the exposure. For example, in the imagined study of smoking and leukemia, it would be reasonable to exclude from the control series anyone who was hospitalized with a disease thought to be related to smoking. This approach may lead to the exclusion of many diagnostic categories, but even a few remaining diagnostic categories should suffice to find enough control subjects.

It is risky, however, to reduce the control eligibility criteria in a hospital-based case-control study to a single diagnosis. Using a variety of diagnoses has the advantage of diluting any bias that may result from including as the control series only a specific diagnostic group that turns out to be related to the exposure. For the diagnostic categories that constitute exclusion criteria for controls, the exclusion should be based only on the cause of the hospitalization used to identify the study subject, rather than on any previous hospitalization. In the example of a hospital-based case-control study of tobacco smoking and leukemia, a person who was hospitalized because of a traumatic injury and is therefore eligible to be a control should not be excluded if he or she had previously been hospitalized for cardiovascular disease. The reason is that the source population includes people who have had cardiovascular disease, and they must also be included in the control series. In considering whether to exclude potential controls, the investigator must distinguish between the current hospitalization and past hospitalizations.

In some situations, it is impractical or impossible to identify the actual source population for cases. It may still be possible to conduct a valid study, however, by the use of *proxy sampling*. Theoretically, if a control series can be identified that has the same exposure distribution as does the source population for cases, that control series should give the same results as one that draws controls directly from the source population. A control series comprising people who are not in the source population but who serve as valid proxies for those who are in the source population is a reasonable study design.

Consider a case-control study examining the relation between ABO blood type and female breast cancer. Could such a study have a control series comprising the brothers of the (female) cases? The brothers of the cases are not part of the source population. Nevertheless, the distribution of ABO blood type among the brothers should be identical to the distribution of ABO blood type among the source population of women who might have been included as cases, because ABO blood type is not related to sex. Clinic-based studies that use as controls clinic patients with disease diagnoses different from that of the cases may also involve proxy sampling if those control patients would not have come to the same clinic if they had been diagnosed with the disease that the cases have. In studies in which cases who have died are compared with a control series comprising dead people, a comparison sometimes justified by the interest in getting comparable information for cases and controls, the controls cannot be part of the source population. Death precludes the occurrence of any further disease, and dead people therefore are not at risk to become cases. Nevertheless, if a series of dead controls can provide the same exposure distribution as exists in the source population, it may be a reasonable control series to use.

Prospective and Retrospective Case-Control Studies

Case-control studies, like cohort studies, can be prospective or retrospective. In a retrospective case-control study, cases have already occurred when the study begins; there is no waiting for new cases to occur. In a prospective case-control

Is Representativeness Important?

Some textbooks claim that cases should be representative of all persons with the disease and that controls should be representative of the entire non-diseased population. Such advice can be misleading. Cases can be defined in any way that the investigator wishes and need not be representative of all cases. Older cases, female cases, severe cases, or any clinical subset of cases can be studied. These groups are not representative of all cases but are allowable as case definitions. Any type of case that can be used as the disease event in a cohort study also can be used to define the case series in a case-control study.

The case definition implicitly defines the source population for cases, from which the controls should be drawn. It is this source population for the cases that the controls should represent, not the entire nondiseased population.

study, the investigator must wait, just as in a prospective cohort study, for new cases to occur.

Cohort/Case-Control Studies Versus Prospective/Retrospective Studies

Early descriptions of cohort studies often referred to them as prospective studies and to case-control studies as retrospective studies. We now reserve the terms *prospective* and *retrospective* to refer to the timing of the information and events of the study, and we use the term *case-control* to describe studies in which the source population is sampled rather than ascertained in its entirety, as in a cohort study. The early descriptions carried the implication that retrospective studies were less valid than prospective studies, an idea that lingers. It is still commonly thought that case-control studies are less valid than cohort studies. The truth is that validity issues can affect both case-control studies and cohort studies (including randomized trials), whether they are prospective or retrospective. Nevertheless, there is no reason to discount a study simply because it is a case-control study or a retrospective study. Case-control studies represent a high achievement of modern epidemiology, and if conducted well, they can reach the highest standards of validity.

Case-Crossover Studies

Many variants of case-control studies have been described in recent years. One that is compelling in its simplicity and its elegance is the case-crossover study, which is a case-control analog of the crossover study. A *crossover study* is a self-matched cohort study, usually an experimental study, in which two or more interventions are compared, with each study participant receiving each of the interventions at different times. If the crossover study is an experiment, each subject receives the interventions in a randomly assigned sequence, with some time interval between them so that the outcome can be measured after each intervention. A crossover study requires the effect period related to the intervention to be short enough so that it does not persist into the time period during which the next treatment is administered.

The *case-crossover study*, first proposed by Maclure,[14] may be considered a case-control version of the crossover study. Unlike an ordinary case-control study, however, all the subjects in a case-crossover study are cases. The control series, rather than being a different set of people, is represented by information on the exposure distribution drawn from the cases themselves, outside of the time window during which the exposure is hypothesized to cause the disease. Usually, this information is drawn from the experience of cases before they develop disease to address the concern that after getting the disease, a person may modify the exposure, as in someone who cuts back on caffeine after having a myocardial infarction. In some situations, however, when the disease cannot or does not influence subsequent exposure, the experience of cases before and after their disease event may be used. For example, if studying the effect of transient air pollution on asthma attacks, air pollution levels after a case's asthma attack may be used to describe the frequency of air pollution episodes, because the asthma attack cannot affect ambient air pollution levels.

The case-crossover study design can be implemented successfully only for an appropriate study hypothesis. As in a crossover study, in a case-crossover study, the effect of the exposure must be brief, and the disease event ideally will have an abrupt onset. The study hypothesis defines a time window during which the exposure may cause the disease event. The window should be brief in relation to the time between typical successive exposure intervals, so that the effect of exposure will have sufficient time to fade before the next episode of exposure according to the study hypothesis. Each case is classified as exposed or unexposed, depending on whether there was any exposure during the hypothesized time window just before the disease event. Maclure used the example of studying whether sexual intercourse causes myocardial infarction. The period of increased risk after sexual intercourse was hypothesized to be 1 hour. The cases would be a series of people who have had a myocardial infarction. Each case would then be classified as exposed if he or she had sexual intercourse within the hour preceding the myocardial infarction. Otherwise, the case would be classified as unexposed.

This process appears to differ little from what may be done for any case-control study. The key difference is that there is no separate control series; instead, the control information is obtained from the cases themselves. In the example of sexual intercourse and myocardial infarction, the average frequency of sexual intercourse would be ascertained for each case during a period (eg, 1 year) before the myocardial infarction occurred. Under the study hypothesis, after each instance of sexual intercourse, the risk of myocardial infarction during the following hour is elevated, and that hour is considered exposed person-time. All other time would be considered unexposed. If a person had sexual intercourse once per week, 1 hour per week would be considered exposed and the remaining

167 hours would be considered unexposed. Such a calculation can be performed for each case, and from the distribution of these hours within the experience of each case, the incidence rate ratio of myocardial infarction after sexual intercourse in relation to the incidence rate at other times can be estimated. The analysis uses analytic methods based on matching, with each case being self-matched to his or her own experience outside the case time window. Thus, all the information for the study is obtainable from a series of cases.

Only certain types of study questions can be studied with a case-crossover design. The exposure must be something that varies from time to time for a person. The effect of blood type cannot be examined in a case-crossover study, because it does not change. An investigator can study whether coffee drinking triggers an asthma attack within a short time, however, because coffee is consumed intermittently. It is convenient to think of the case-crossover study as evaluating exposures that trigger a short-term effect. The disease also must have an abrupt onset. The causes of multiple sclerosis cannot be considered in a case-crossover study, but whether an automobile driver who is talking on a telephone is at higher risk of having a collision can. The effect of the exposure must be brief. If the exposure had a long effect, it would not be possible to relate the disease to a particular episode of exposure.

CROSS-SECTIONAL VERSUS LONGITUDINAL STUDIES

All of the study types previously described in this chapter can be described as *longitudinal* studies. In epidemiology, a study is considered to be longitudinal if the information obtained pertains to more than one point in time. Implicit in a longitudinal study is the universal premise that the causal action of an exposure comes before the subsequent development of disease as a consequence of that exposure. This concept is integral to the thinking involved in following cohorts over time or in sampling from the person-time at risk based on earlier exposure status. All cohort studies and most case-control studies rely on data in which exposure information refers to an earlier time than that of disease occurrence, making the study longitudinal.

Occasionally, epidemiologists conduct cross-sectional studies, in which all of the information refers to the same point in time. These studies are basically snapshots of the population status with respect to disease or exposure variables, or both, at a specific point in time. A population survey, such as the decennial census in the United States, is a cross-sectional study that attempts to enumerate the population and to assess the prevalence of various characteristics. Surveys are conducted frequently to sample opinions, but they may also be used to measure disease prevalence or even to assess the relation between disease prevalence and possible exposures.

A cross-sectional study cannot measure disease incidence, because risk or rate calculations require information across a time period. Nevertheless, cross-sectional studies can assess disease prevalence. It is possible to use cross-sectional data to conduct a case-control study if the study includes prevalent cases and uses concurrent information about exposure. A case-control study that is based on prevalent cases, rather than new cases, does not necessarily provide information about the causes of disease. Because the cases in such a study are those who have the disease at a given point in time, the study is more heavily weighted with cases of long duration than any series of incident cases would be. A person who died soon after getting disease, for example, would count as an incident case but likely would not be included as a case in a prevalence survey, because the disease duration is so brief.

Sometimes, cross-sectional information is used because it is considered a good proxy for longitudinal data. For example, an investigator may wish to know how much supplemental vitamin E a person consumed 10 years in the past. Because no written record of this exposure is likely to exist, the basic choices are to ask people to recall how much supplemental vitamin E they consumed in the past or to find out how much they consume now. Recall of past use is likely to be hazy, whereas current consumption can be determined accurately. In some situations, accurate current information may be a better proxy for the actual consumption 10 years earlier than the hazy recollections of that past consumption. Current consumption may be cross-sectional, but it would be used as a proxy for exposure in the past. Another example is blood type. Because it remains constant, cross-sectional information on blood type is a perfect proxy for past information about blood type. In this way, cross-sectional studies can sometimes be almost as informative as longitudinal studies with respect to causal hypotheses.

RESPONSE RATES

In a cohort study, if a substantial proportion of subjects cannot be traced to determine the disease outcome, the study validity can be compromised. In a case-control study, if exposure data is missing on a sizable proportion of subjects, it can likewise be a source of concern. The concern stems from the possibility of bias from selectively missing data, which is a form of selection bias (see Chapter 7). The more missing data on outcome there is in a cohort study, or analogously the more missing exposure data there is in a case-control study, the greater the potential for selection bias. For that reason, critics are often skeptical about cohort studies with a high proportion of subjects with unknown disease outcome or about case-control studies with a high proportion of subjects lacking exposure information. These two proportions are sometimes referred to as *response rates*, with the disease outcome corresponding to the response in a cohort study and the exposure information corresponding to the response in a case-control study.

There is no absolute threshold for what a response rate ought to be, but as discussed for tracing subjects in a cohort study, if the response rate or proportion traced is less than 70% to 75%, it may engender some skepticism about the study. Nevertheless, in some settings, a low response rate need not be an important validity concern. Suppose that in a case-control study of risk of acquired immunodeficiency syndrome (AIDS) after transfusion, the exposure information, a history of transfusion, was ascertained from medical records but that only one half of the desired medical records were obtainable for review. Even so, if there is no association between a history of transfusion and the availability of the records for review, an unbiased estimate of the effect of transfusion should be obtainable from the records that are available. Selection bias is a concern when the inter-relation between the study variables in the missing data is different from the corresponding relation in the available data.

In many cohort studies, subjects are recruited as volunteers from a larger population, perhaps from the general population. Recruitment of volunteers is a well-known feature of experimental studies, but it is also common in nonex-perimental cohort studies. The recruitment proportion should not be viewed as a response rate. Even if recruitment is difficult, there may be little reason to be concerned with the validity of the study results. In a randomized experiment, the internal validity of the study flows from the random assignment, which is implemented among those who volunteer to be studied, even if they represent a small proportion of a larger population. In other cohort studies, the partici-pants who are recruited should all be free of disease at the start of follow-up. Regardless of the success or lack of success in recruiting volunteers, there will not be any selection bias from volunteering to be studied unless volunteering is related to both exposure and disease risk. Because disease has not yet occurred in cohort participants, the presence of disease cannot influence volunteering, apart from prodromal effects. The internal comparisons of a cohort study based on a select group of volunteers should ordinarily be free of selection bias stem-ming from volunteering even if recruitment success is poor. The external validity, or generalizability, of the study may be affected by a low recruitment rate, but only if the study participants represent a subset of the population in which the relation between exposure and disease is different from the relation for those who did not volunteer. These considerations have implications for the effort expended to recruit study participants. In some cohort studies, it may be most sensible to have a gentle approach to recruit volunteers as opposed to a hard sell that recruits more reluctant volunteers. If reluctant participants are persuaded to volunteer for the study but later drop out, their missing follow-up data may have a more profound effect on the study's validity than their nonparticipation in the study in the first place. Because dropouts are usually worse for a study than refusals to participate from the beginning, a better strategy is to concen-trate efforts more on follow-up than on recruitment. On the other hand, in case-control studies in which study participants know their exposure status, getting high levels of participation is important, because agreement to be studied may depend on exposure. If study participants do not know their exposure status, because, for example, it is obtainable only from a laboratory test that most peo-ple would not have had, low recruitment into a case-control study is less of a concern.

COMPARISON OF COHORT AND CASE-CONTROL STUDIES

It may be helpful to summarize some of the key characteristics of cohort and case-control studies. The primary difference is that a cohort study involves complete enumeration of the denominator (ie, people or person-time) of the disease mea-sure, whereas case-control studies sample from the denominator. As a result, case-control studies usually provide estimates only of ratio measures of effect, whereas cohort studies provide estimates of disease rates and risks for each cohort, which

Table 5–9 COMPARISON OF THE CHARACTERISTICS OF COHORT
AND CASE-CONTROL STUDIES

Cohort Study	Case-Control Study
Complete source population denominator experience tallied	Sampling from source population
Can calculate incidence rates or risks, and their differences and ratios	Can calculate only the ratio of incidence rates or risks (unless the control sampling fraction is known)
Usually very expensive	Usually less expensive
Convenient for studying many diseases	Convenient for studying many exposures
Can be prospective or retrospective	Can be prospective or retrospective

can then be compared by taking differences or ratios. Case-control studies can be thought of as modified cohort studies, with sampling of the source population being the essential modification.

Consistent with this theme is the idea that many issues that apply to cohort studies apply to case-control studies in the same way. For example, if a person gets a disease, he or she no longer contributes time at risk to the denominator of a rate in a cohort study (assuming that only the first occurrence of disease in a person is being studied). Analogously, in a density case-control study, a person who gets disease is from that point in time forward no longer eligible to be sampled as a control. Another example of the parallels between cohort studies and case-control studies is the classification of studies into prospective and retrospective studies.

Case-control studies are usually more efficient than cohort studies because the cost of the information that they provide is often much lower. With a cohort study, it is often convenient to study many different disease outcomes in relation to a given exposure. With a case-control study, it is often convenient to study many different exposures in relation to a single disease. This contrast, however, is not absolute. In many cohort studies, a variety of exposures can be studied in relation to the diseases of interest. Likewise, in many case-control studies, the case series can be expanded to include more than one disease category, which in effect leads to several parallel case-control studies conducted within the same source population. These characteristics are summarized in Table 5–9.

QUESTIONS

1. During the second half of the 20th century, there was a sharp increase in hysterectomy in the United States. Concurrent with that trend, there was an epidemic of endometrial cancer that has been attributed to widespread use of replacement estrogens among menopausal women. The epidemic of endometrial cancer was not immediately evident, however, in data on endometrial cancer rates compiled from cancer registries. Devise a hypothesis based on considerations of the population at risk for endometrial cancer that can explain why the epidemic went unnoticed.

2. What is the purpose of randomization in an experiment? How is the same goal achieved in nonexperimental studies?

3. When cancer incidence rates are calculated for the population covered by a cancer registry, the usual approach is to take the number of new cases of cancer and divide by the person-time contributed by the population covered by the registry. Person-time is calculated as the size of the population from census data multiplied by the time period. This calculation leads to an underestimate of the incidence rate in the population at risk. Explain.

4. In the calculations of rates for the data in Figure 5–2, the rate in the exposed group declined after taking the induction period into account. If exposure does cause disease, would you expect that the rate in exposed people would increase, decrease, or stay the same after taking into account an appropriate induction period?

5. If a person already has disease, can that person be selected as a control in a case-control study of that disease?

6. If a person has already been selected as a control in a case-control study and then later during the study period develops the disease that is being studied, should the person be kept in the study as (1) a case, (2) a control, (3) both, or (4) neither?

7. In case-cohort sampling, a single control group can be compared with various case groups in a set of case-control comparisons, because the control sampling depends on the identity of the cohorts and has nothing to do with the cases. Analogously, the denominators of risk for a set of several different diseases occurring in the cohort will be the same. Risk-set sampling, in contrast, requires that the investigator identify the risk set for each case; the sample of controls will be different for each disease studied. If the analogy holds, this observation implies that the denominators of incidence rates will differ when calculating the rates for different diseases in the same cohort. Is that true? If not, why not? If so, why should the denominators for the risks not change no matter what disease is studied, whereas the denominators for the rates change from studying one disease to another?

8. Explain why it would not be possible to study the effect of cigarette smoking on lung cancer in a case-crossover study but why it would be possible to study the effect of cigarette smoking on sudden death from arrhythmia using that design.

9. Cumulative case-control studies are conducted by sampling the controls from people who remain free of disease after the period of risk for disease (eg, an epidemic period) has ended. With this sampling strategy, demonstrate why the odds ratio will tend to be an overestimate of the risk ratio.

10. Often, the time at which disease is diagnosed is used as the time of disease onset. Many diseases, such as cancer, rheumatoid arthritis, and schizophrenia, may be present in an undiagnosed form for a considerable time before the diagnosis. Suppose you are conducting a case-control study of a cancer. If it were possible, would it be preferable to exclude people with undetected cancer from the control series?

REFERENCES

1. Rothman KJ, Greenland S, Lash TL. *Modern Epidemiology.* 3rd ed. Philadelphia, PA: Lippincott Williams & Wilkins; 2008.
2. Porta M. *A Dictionary of Epidemiology.* 5th ed. New York, NY: Oxford University Press; 2008.
3. Snow J. *On the Mode of Communication of Cholera.* 2nd ed. London, England: John Churchill; 1860. (Facsimile of 1936 reprinted edition by Hafner, New York, 1965.)
4. Kinloch-de Loes S, Hirschel BJ, Hoen B, et al. Controlled trial of zidovudine in primary human immunodeficiency virus infection. *N Engl J Med.* 1995;333: 408–413.
5. Francis TF, Korns RF, Voight RB, et al. An evaluation of the 1954 poliomyelitis vaccine trials. *Am J Public Health.* 1955;45(suppl):1–63.
6. Bang AT, Bang RA, Baitule SB, Reddy MH, Deshmukh MD. Effect of home-based neonatal care and management of sepsis on neonatal mortality: field trial in rural India. *Lancet.* 1999;354:1955–1961.
7. Milunsky A, Jick H, Jick SS, et al. Multivitamin/folic acid supplementation in early pregnancy reduces the prevalence of neural tube defects. *JAMA.* 1989;262: 2847–2852.
8. Rothman KJ, Moore LL, Singer MR, Nguyen US, Mannino S, Milunsky A. Teratogenicity of high vitamin A intake. *N Engl J Med.* 1995;333:1369–1373.
9. Dawber TR, Moore FE, Mann GV. Coronary heart disease in the Framingham study. *Am J Public Health.* 1957;47:4–24.
10. Richardson DB, MacLehose RF, Langholz B, Cole SR. Hierarchical latency models for dose-time-response associations. *Am J Epidemiol.* 2011;173:695–702.
11. Morrison AS, Kirshner J, Molho A. Epidemics in Renaissance Florence. *Am J Public Health.* 1985;75:528–535.
12. Huybrechts KF, Mikkelsen EM, Christensen T, et al. A successful implementation of e-epidemiology: evidence from the Danish pregnancy planning study "Snart-Gravid." *Eur J Epidemiol.* 2010;25:297–304.
13. Labarthe D, Adam E, Noller KL, et al. Design and preliminary observations of National Cooperative Diethylstilbestrol Adenosis (DESAD) Project. *Obstet Gynecol.* 1978;4:453–458.
14. Maclure M. The case-crossover design: a method for studying transient effects on the risk of acute events. *Am J Epidemiol.* 1991;133:144–153.

6

Infectious Disease Epidemiology

Symbiosis refers to the interactive relation between different species. It encompasses a broad range of patterns ranging from *mutualism* at one end of the spectrum, in which both species benefit, to *parasitism* at the other end, in which one species, the parasite, obtains nutriment from the other, the host, while offering little or nothing in return. Parasitism is a ubiquitous feature of life. Virtually every animal and plant is either a parasite or host to a parasite during part or all of its life cycle. Parasites tend to reproduce more quickly than their hosts and to evolve rapidly in response to host defenses, perpetuating a continual struggle that determines the boundary between disease and health and life or death. An infectious parasite is typically much smaller than its host, living within or on the host, on which it depends for its sustenance. Agents that infect humans include a range of microorganisms, including viruses, bacteria, fungi, and protozoa, as well as some larger animals such as helminths. In this chapter, we refer to the microscopic agents as *pathogens* and reserve the term *parasite* for larger animals.

Evolution has fostered the development of defenses against infection. The skin is an effective, if passive, barrier against most bacteria and viral infections. Surface responses that help resist infection include sweating and desquamation, cilia movement in the respiratory tract, and production of mucus along interior epithelial surfaces. Mucous membranes have antibacterial properties; stomach acid, saliva, and tears help to resist infection. In the gut, entrenched but friendly bacteria compete with pathogens, limiting opportunities for the pathogens to establish themselves. For pathogens that manage to penetrate skin or mucous membranes, the immune system provides two more levels of defense. The first comes from the *innate immune system*. Injury to cells triggers a nonspecific inflammatory reaction, which is a cascade of events involving chemical and cellular responses to the local injury. The inflammatory reaction recruits a variety of blood cells, including mast cells, phagocytes, neutrophils, and others that play various roles in the host response. The innate immune system also activates the *adaptive immune system*, which allows a specific response to infectious agents. This system produces antibodies that are designed to attach to specific sites on the pathogen or its toxins, neutralizing the threat. Specialized B-cell lymphocytes work in conjunction with helper T cells to produce antibodies. These cells also record the antigenic pattern that stimulated their response, enabling a faster and more effective response if the antigen is encountered again. This antigenic memory is what is commonly referred to as *immunity* to an infectious agent. Immunity occurs naturally after an infection, but it can also be stimulated by vaccination, which is intended to provoke an immunogenic reaction without causing an initial pathogenic infection. Immunity can vary in duration from a relatively short period to lifetime protection.

The sophistication of host defenses implies that humans have always had to reckon with infectious disease. The balance between host and pathogen, however, is readily tipped by changing social conditions. For example, human invasions or migrations sometimes brought immunologically naïve populations into contact with diseases to which they had not previously been exposed. Urbanization during the Middle Ages brought on the conditions that fostered spread of the plague. Europeans brought with them to the New World a host of infections, such as smallpox, measles, typhus, and cholera, which had catastrophic consequences for natives of the Western Hemisphere. Europeans had adapted to these agents, but the newly exposed natives of the Americas had no natural defenses. Conversely, some speculate that syphilis was prevalent in the Americas but unknown in Europe until after Columbus' first voyage to the New World.

The public-health burden from infectious disease began to diminish after the acceptance of the germ theory and the arrival of greatly improved sanitation and hygiene. Wealthy nations saw much faster progress than poorer ones, because implementing the needed public-health programs was expensive. The advent of antibacterials was another crucial development in fighting infection. This tool was also more available to wealthy nations. Nevertheless, sanitation and hygiene had the more powerful effect, as can be seen in Figure 6–1. This graph depicts the steady decline in mortality from infectious disease in the United States over the course of the 20th century. The figure also indicates the spike in deaths during 1919, the year with the majority of cases of pandemic H1N1 influenza that

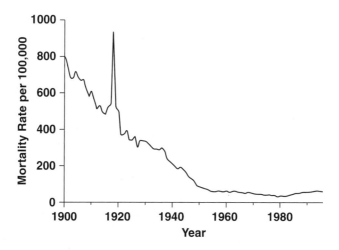

Figure 6–1 Crude death rate from infectious disease in the United States between 1900 and 1996.

Adapted from Armstrong et al.[2]

swept the world beginning in 1918 and continuing into 1919. This epidemic may have accounted for more human deaths than any catastrophe humanity has faced, apart from bubonic plague, the notorious Black Death that swept Europe in the 14th century. (In light of this graph, it is understandable that the 2009 outbreak of H1N1 was initially a cause for great concern[1] and fortunate that it turned out to be much less deadly than the 1918 version.) Antibiotics did not come into widespread use in medicine until the mid–20th century, when most of the decline in mortality rates from infectious disease had already occurred.

WHAT MAKES A PANDEMIC?

In Chapter 4, an epidemic was defined as an unusually high occurrence of disease. A *pandemic* is defined in the *Dictionary of Epidemiology*[2] as "an epidemic occurring worldwide or over a very wide area, crossing boundaries of several countries and usually affecting a large number of people." The World Health Organization (WHO) had a more specific description that it had used for *pandemic influenza:* "An influenza pandemic occurs when a new influenza virus appears against which the human population has no immunity, resulting in several, simultaneous epidemics worldwide with enormous numbers of deaths and illness." Just before WHO announced that the H1N1 influenza of 2009 (swine flu) had become pandemic, it changed its description of pandemic by dropping the phrase "with enormous numbers of deaths and illness." This new description of pandemic was more consistent with the definition quoted from the *Dictionary of Epidemiology.*[2] It also allowed the WHO to declare a pandemic for a disease that did not have extraordinary mortality and morbidity. The announcement of the pandemic in 2009 led to criticism that the declaration was motivated by ties between the WHO and the pharmaceutical industry, a claim that the WHO denied.[3–5]

TYPES OF TRANSMISSION

The host population constitutes the *reservoir* for the pathogen; this is the biologic space that serves as the primary habitat for the pathogen. Reservoirs are usually a collection of discrete organisms, which creates a problem for the pathogen, because to survive beyond the life of a particular host, it must find a way to spread to another host within its reservoir. First, it usually needs to reproduce within the host. Most pathogens reproduce extracellularly within the host, but a virus is unusual in that it can reproduce only after penetrating a host cell. While within a host cell, it is protected from the immune system, but it can be intercepted and deactivated by antibodies before entry into a cell. The specific immune response, which is a key defense against viral pathogens, typically does not occur rapidly enough to avert disease on the initial infection. It can take days for the antibody response to build, so those who lack previous contact are generally susceptible to infection from a virus. After an initial infection, the antibody response is typically rapid enough to prevent subsequent disease or at least to mitigate it, leading to immunity.

To move from one host to another, pathogens have evolved a variety of mechanisms. Pathogens whose infection leads to early death of the host have a more pressing problem, because they may not long survive the death of the host. This problem exerts an evolutionary pressure for the pathogen to spread more efficiently or to become more benign, at least to the extent that it allows the host to survive long enough for the pathogen to be transmitted to a new host.

Table 6–1 lists a variety of mechanisms that pathogens have evolved to move from one human host to another. The most direct of these involve *person-to-person transmission*. Diseases that spread from one person to another, such as measles, are described as *communicable* or *contagious*. The only reservoir for measles virus is humans. It spreads from one infected person to another largely through coughing or sneezing, which produces a cloud of infected droplets. These droplets can be inhaled directly by a susceptible person or spread indirectly after landing on a contaminated surface, where the virus will remain viable for a couple of hours.

Some agents have both human and animal reservoirs, and they spread from person to person by means of a transmitting animal, which is called *vector-borne* transmission. Technically, when pathogens are spread through vectors, the vector represents an intermediate host for the pathogen that is necessary to its life cycle and its transmission. Human malaria is an infection with the *Plasmodium* protozoa, which is transmitted from human to human by certain species of the *Anopheles* mosquito, the vector of malaria transmission. A mosquito that bites an infected person acquires a blood meal that contains infected *Plasmodium* gametocytes, and it can transmit the infection to other people during subsequent blood meals. In rare cases, malaria can spread from person to person without the *Anopheles* vector (eg, through contaminated blood, from a pregnant mother to a fetus), but most transmission occurs through the mosquito vector. Many other infectious diseases, such as yellow fever, Chagas disease, Lyme disease, plague, West Nile encephalitis, and dengue fever are spread by animal vectors. In all these examples, the vectors are arthropods. (Viruses that are transmitted through arthropod vectors are called *arboviruses*, which is short for arthropod-borne viruses.)

Table 6–1 MAJOR ROUTES OF TRANSMISSION FOR INFECTIOUS DISEASE

Transmission	Route	Examples
Direct transmission	Airborne	Anthrax, chicken pox, common cold, influenza, measles, mumps, rubella, tuberculosis, whooping cough
	Direct contact	Athlete's foot, impetigo, warts
	Fecal-oral	Cholera, hepatitis A, rotavirus, salmonella
	Maternal-fetal	Hepatitis B, syphilis
	Sexual	Chlamydia, gonorrhea, hepatitis B, herpes, syphilis, human papillomavirus (HPV)
Indirect transmission	Intermediate host	Tapeworm (from consuming inadequately cooked pork)
	Vector-borne	Bubonic plague, malaria, typhus, West Nile encephalitis, yellow fever

Diseases that spread from animal reservoirs to humans are called *zoonoses*. Zoonoses may be vector-borne, as with equine encephalitis or plague, or may spread from the animal reservoir directly to humans, as with toxoplasmosis (for which the primary reservoir is cats) and Ebola virus (for which the primary reservoir is thought to be bats). Influenza virus infects humans, birds, and pigs and frequently jumps from one species to another. Rabies is a zoonotic virus that infects all warm-blooded animals. The case-fatality rate from untreated rabies is close to 100%, but despite killing its hosts, the virus is an old one that has spread throughout the world. Like some other pathogens, it causes changes in behavior in infected hosts that are conducive to its transmission. In the case of rabies, it affects the brain directly and leads to hyperexcitability, spasms, and aggressive behavior that can help the parasite spread through bite wounds from infected hosts. Because the disease is transmitted to humans from animal bites but rarely is transmitted from a human host, humans are considered an incidental or "dead-end" host for rabies.

Giardia is a protozoan parasite, a zoonosis that infects many species. It spreads through contaminated water or by oral-fecal transmission. It takes the form of dormant cysts that get excreted in feces and can survive for weeks or months in warm water, from which it may be ingested by a susceptible host. Cholera is another infection that spreads by oral-fecal transmission; its spread through contaminated water was the focus of Snow's landmark investigations in London (see Chapters 4 and 5).

In Chapter 4, two types of epidemic outbreaks were described, *point source* and *propagated*. Person-to-person transmission of a pathogen can manifest as either type of outbreak. The famous outbreak of cholera in Golden Square that Snow investigated was a point-source epidemic, transmitted from one infected person to the population that partook of water from the Broad Street pump. In a propagated epidemic, infection may begin from a single source, but it spreads through propagation in the population, transmitted from many infected people to uninfected people who come in contact with them.

HERD IMMUNITY AND BASIC REPRODUCTIVE NUMBER

For an infection that depends on person-to-person transmission, the relative proportions of immune and susceptible persons in a population can determine whether the infection will take hold in the community or die out quickly. If a substantial proportion of the population is immune from previous experience with the pathogen or from vaccination, an infected person will be less likely to spread the infection to another susceptible person because many of the contacts who might have provided an opportunity for person-to-person transmission will be immune and therefore not susceptible to infection. If enough are immune, the prevalence of the infection will decrease with time and the outbreak will wane until it is extinguished. This situation is described as *herd immunity*. When it exists, susceptible people in the population are protected indirectly by the immunity of the people with whom they interact. The immunity of potential contacts limits the interactions that can expose a susceptible person to infection. Thus, vaccination campaigns protect those who get vaccinated and also confer protection on the unvaccinated.

A key concept in assessing whether an outbreak that is spread by person-to-person transmission will ignite or die out is the *basic reproductive number*, usually written as R_0. It is the average number of secondary cases that occur from a single index case in a susceptible population in which no interventions are being taken. If the basic reproductive number is less than 1, each case will on average lead to less than one additional case, and the outbreak will die out, unless fueled by external re-infections. The rate at which disease disappears from the population depends on how much below 1 the basic reproductive number is and on the interval between successive generations of infection. If the basic reproductive number is above 1, each case in the early stage of an outbreak produces more than one new secondary case, and the epidemic grows. The speed at which it grows depends on the magnitude of the basic reproductive number for that disease and the time between successive infections.

The reproductive number reflects the biologic potential of the infectious agent and the social intercourse that leads to situations in which transmission might occur. For example, if infected persons are too sick to move about while they are infectious, there may be few contacts and a low reproductive number. The basic reproductive number varies from population to population, because the number of potential contacts differs by population. For the same reason, it also varies by subgroups within a population. The overall basic reproductive number is an average over these subgroups. Even if the basic reproductive number is low, transmission probabilities may vary considerably from person to person, and some social networks within a population may form a subset in which an epidemic spreads rapidly even if the overall basic reproductive number for the total population is low, perhaps even below 1.[6] A few "superspreaders" such as needle-sharers transmitting a blood-borne infection can suffice to spark an outbreak. Table 6–2 gives some examples of the basic reproductive number for various human diseases that are spread by person-to-person transmission.

Table 6–2 Basic Reproductive Number for Various Diseases Spread by Person-to-Person Transmission

Disease	Primary Mode of Transmission	Basic Reproductive Number
Measles	Airborne	15
Pertussis	Airborne droplet	15
Diphtheria	Saliva	6
Smallpox	Social contact	6
Polio	Fecal-oral route	6
Rubella	Airborne droplet	6
Mumps	Airborne droplet	5
HIV/AIDS	Sexual contact	3
SARS	Airborne droplet	3
Ebola	Bodily fluids	2
1918 influenza (H1N1)	Airborne droplet	2
2009 influenza (H1N1) flu	Airborne droplet	1.5

Abbreviations: AIDS, acute immunodeficiency syndrome; HIV, human immunodeficiency virus; SARS, severe acute respiratory syndrome.

The basic reproductive number indicates the potential for spread of an outbreak in a population of susceptibles. In practice, given some immunity (which may come from vaccinations, recovery from the infection during the outbreak, or previous exposure to the same or a similar agent) and given attempts to reduce person-to-person contact after an outbreak begins, the reproductive number that characterizes an outbreak as it develops will be lower than the basic reproductive number. The *effective reproductive number*, R_t, is the value of the reproductive number that takes into account the mix of immunity and social interaction at any point in time as an outbreak progresses. The effective reproductive number changes with time, usually decreasing as immunity spreads among those who have recovered from their infection. While the effective reproductive number remains above 1, an epidemic spreads, but the effective reproductive number eventually decreases to 1 or below as the proportion of susceptible people remaining in the population diminishes or as control measures are implemented. In the long run, R_t will fall below 1, and the epidemic will sputter out, or it will maintain an *endemic equilibrium* at an R_t of 1. In the equilibrium state, the prevalence of infection remains level over time as new susceptibles are added to the population to balance those who acquire immunity. In such an endemic equilibrium, $R_t = 1 = R_0 \times p_s$, where p_s is the proportion of the population susceptible to infection at equilibrium. Therefore, in an equilibrium state one can estimate the basic reproductive number, R_0 as $1/p_s$.

A basic strategy to reduce transmission and contain an outbreak of a disease spread by person-to-person transmission is isolation of infected persons. By reducing contacts of infectious persons, isolation can limit the spread of an infection, and if applied on a broad enough scale, it can lower the effective reproductive number. A related strategy that has been used since antiquity is *quarantine* (see Chapter 2). The intent of quarantine is to restrict contacts among people who are not yet ill but who have come into contact with infected persons. Like isolation, quarantine can lower the effective reproductive number. The combination of isolating infected patients and quarantining contacts together can be effective in cutting short an outbreak.

This strategy of isolation and quarantine worked well against severe acute respiratory syndrome (SARS), a viral disease that nearly became a pandemic in 2003. The disease rapidly spread from its index location in China to 37 countries, infecting more than 8000 people, with a case-fatality rate of almost 10%. Within months of the first appearance of SARS, the possibility of a calamitous pandemic with a high case-fatality rate seemed like a strong possibility. In Toronto, where it seemed that the spread of SARS was nearly out of control, Canadian officials quarantined more than 23,000 people who had been in contact with SARS cases, about 100 persons for every identified case of SARS. The movement of those under quarantine was restricted until 10 days after their last patient contact. Such stringent methods ultimately contained the epidemic.

SARS was a new disease in 2003, and no vaccine was available. If vaccine is available, a vaccination campaign can contain an outbreak. The basic strategy is to lower the reproductive number from the basic value to an effective reproductive number < 1, providing sufficient herd immunity to stop the outbreak. In a population in which some people are vaccinated, the effective reproductive number depends on vaccine efficacy and the vaccination coverage of the population. If V_e

---

Glossary of Key Terms in Infectious Disease Epidemiology

Communicable: capable of person-to-person transmission.

Generation time: the time interval between one person getting infected and another person getting infected from the first.

Herd immunity: a prevalence of susceptibles in a population low enough so that transmission cannot be sustained.

Immunity: resistance to infection.

Incubation period: the time interval between getting infected and developing symptoms.

Reproductive number: the average number of infected persons resulting from contact with a single infected person. The basic reproductive number is the average number of infections that would be caused by one infected person when everyone else is susceptible. The effective reproductive number is the average number of infections resulting from one infected person given that not everyone is susceptible.

Reservoir: the host population for an infectious agent.

Secondary cases: cases of infection that occur from contact with a primary case.

Secondary attack rate: risk of infection among susceptibles exposed to an infected source.

Susceptibility: at risk of contracting disease (lack of immunity).

Transmission probability: probability of transmission from an infected person to a susceptible person during a contact.

Vector: an animal that transmits disease from an infected person to an uninfected person.

Virulence: the degree to which a pathogen can cause disease and death.

---

is vaccine efficacy and V_c is vaccine coverage, the proportional reduction in the basic reproductive number will be $(1 - V_e \times V_c)$. The effective reproductive number, R_t, will be $R_0 (1 - V_e \times V_c)$. From this relation, it can be shown that to lower R_t so that it is less than 1, V_c must exceed the following quantity:

$$V_c > \frac{1 - \frac{1}{R_0}}{V_e} \qquad [6\text{--}1]$$

When R_0 is large, high coverage and high efficacy are required for vaccination to succeed in curtailing the epidemic. If R_0 is 10 and the vaccine efficacy is 95%, the vaccine coverage must be greater than $(1 - 1/10)/0.95 = 95\%$ to reduce the effective reproductive number below 1. Measles, with a basic reproductive number of 15, requires more than 93% coverage with a vaccine of 100% efficacy to stop an epidemic. For a vaccine with the same high efficacy aimed at preventing infection of a disease for which R_0 is 2, the vaccine coverage need only exceed $(1 - 1/2)/0.95 = 53\%$ to reduce the effective reproductive number below 1. From the inequality in Equation 6–1, we observe that if the vaccine efficacy is less than

$1 - 1/R_0$, even 100% coverage of the population will not be sufficient to lower the effective reproductive number below 1. In this situation, herd immunity cannot be achieved from the vaccine. Although the vaccine would still be valuable in lowering the risk of infection among those who were vaccinated, there would be enough secondary infections to keep the epidemic growing, perhaps until natural immunity lowered the effective reproductive number further.

THE REED-FROST EPIDEMIC MODEL

In 1928, Lowell Reed and Wade Hampton Frost developed a simple deterministic mathematical model to simulate the spread of an outbreak through a susceptible population. The model assumes that the epidemic began with one or few infected people and progressed through a succession of time periods, which correspond to the *generation time*, defined as the time between acquiring an infection and transmitting it. Within each of these time periods, the basic Reed-Frost model assumes that (1) there is random mixing, with contact between infected people and susceptible people within the population during each time period; (2) there is a uniform, fixed probability that a contact between an infected person and a susceptible person would result in transmission; (3) an infection is always followed by immunity; (4) the population is isolated from other populations; and (5) these conditions remain constant with time. Despite these mostly unrealistic assumptions, the model serves as a reasonable teaching tool about the course of an outbreak.

The Reed-Frost model uses the following formula:

$$C_{t+1} = S_t\left(1-(1-p)^{C_t}\right)$$

In this equation, C_t is the number of infected people at time t, C_{t+1} is the number of infected people at time $t + 1$, S_t is the number of susceptible people at time t, and p is the probability that within one time period an infected person will transmit the infection to a susceptible person with whom there is contact. If $S_t \times p$ is above 1, the epidemic grows, and when $S_t \times p$ declines below 1, the epidemic abates.

Figure 6–2 shows the application of a Reed-Frost model to a population of 100 people, all of whom are susceptible except for a single initially infected person. In the upper diagram, the probability of effective contact is set at 4%. Because one person is infected initially, with a 4% probability of transmission on contact, four will be infected after one generation time. This corresponds to an R_0 of 4, a high value that produces an explosive outbreak and infects most of the population within a few generation times. In the lower diagram, the probability of effective contact is set at 1.5%, corresponding to a lower R_0 of 1.5, which leads to a more gradual epidemic that ultimately infects only about 60% of the population.

The Reed-Frost and many other mathematical models of the spread of infection make unrealistic assumptions. For example, the assumption that there is random mixing with contact between infected and susceptible people may be extremely unrealistic, because subgroups of any community form affinities that may well be

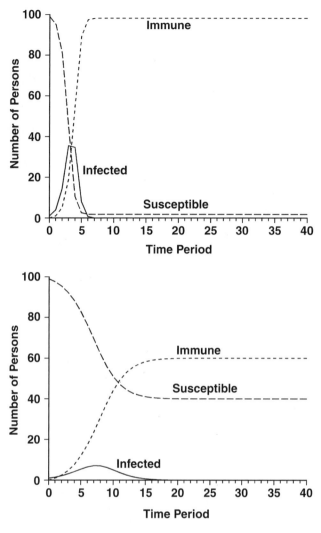

Figure 6-2   Reed-Frost projection of epidemic curve for infected, susceptible, and immune subpopulations among 100 people with one initial infected person and an effective contact probability of 4% (high R_0 in upper panel) and 1.5% (low R_0 in bottom panel). The time scale is measured in generation times.

related to susceptibility. Such was the case in an extended outbreak of measles in Quebec, where more than 95% of the population was vaccinated, but pockets of those who objected to vaccination on religious grounds had numerous contacts with one another and created conditions in which the epidemic could spread over an extended period.[7]

INFECTIOUS DISEASE EPIDEMIOLOGY INVESTIGATIONS

Several types of epidemiologic studies are unique to the investigation of infectious disease or figure more prominently than in other areas. Four types of studies are worthy of mention: contact-tracing studies, outbreak investigations, seroprevalence surveys, and vaccine trials.

1. *Contact-tracing studies.* In the early stage of an epidemic, it may be possible to interrupt person-to-person transmission enough to bring the reproductive number, R_v below the critical threshold value of 1. The most effective approach is to isolate cases to prevent further contacts and to identify any previous contacts so they may be treated or quarantined. This "shoe-leather" approach to stemming an outbreak has been effective in preventing the spread of many sexually transmitted diseases, such as syphilis, chlamydia, and gonorrhea, and it has been effective in containing outbreaks of airborne-spread disease, such as diphtheria and SARS.

2. *Outbreak investigations.* When a local epidemic occurs, epidemiologists are typically tasked with documenting the outbreak and then investigating its origin and propagation. The first job is not trivial. Many apparent disease clusters represent nothing more than a chance aggregation of cases, and they may include cases whose disease does not meet rigorous criteria for diagnosis but have been included as a result of their proximity in time or place to other apparent cases. For epidemics of infectious diseases that are indisputable and represent immediate public-health problems, epidemiologists will be called on to assess the origin of the epidemic and its means of spread. Often, these investigations can also be characterized as shoe-leather epidemiology, calling for detective work that follows leads about infective or contaminated sources and that requires knocking on doors and traveling to factories, farms, food-processing plants, and other spots where an epidemic may have originated. In other cases, these investigations involve more classic study designs, cohort or case-control studies aimed at determining which hypothesis of several can account for an outbreak. Some of these research studies will be prosaic, perhaps doing little more than pinning the blame for a diarrhea outbreak at the church supper on the potato salad. Others may become scientific milestones, elucidating a new disease, as did early studies of acute immunodeficiency syndrome (AIDS), toxic shock syndrome, and SARS.

3. *Seroprevalence surveys.* Seroprevalence surveys are like any other prevalence study, aiming to estimate the prevalence of a characteristic in a population. Like other prevalence surveys, they usually rely on sampling methods to estimate the population prevalence and require a representative sample for the prevalence estimates to be valid. The characteristic of interest is immunity to a specific antigen, which requires obtaining a blood sample to measure antibody response. Getting blood samples from representative cross sections of a population can be challenging. It often is easier to collect samples in the context of delivering health care, although patient populations may differ in the immune status from the general population. Seroprevalence data are invaluable for assessing the vulnerability of a population to existing infectious agents, for finding subgroups that are susceptible to outbreaks, and for setting priorities for vaccination campaigns. Seroprevalence studies may be an important component of surveillance activities that are conducted to monitor the health of a population

with respect to potential infectious diseases. Surveillance for epidemic diseases is a crucial public function that is usually the responsibility of one or more government agencies tasked with monitoring the health of a population.

4. *Vaccine trials.* A randomized trial of a preventive measure is called a *field trial* (see Chapter 5). Trials of therapies (ie, clinical trials) are usually easier to conduct than field trials. One reason is that if the outcome that the preventive measure is intended to prevent is rare, the study must be large, which can be prohibitively expensive. The Salk Vaccine trial, with hundreds of thousands of elementary school children as study subjects, was the largest formal human experiment ever conducted. The aim was to prevent paralytic poliomyelitis. Although infection with the poliomyelitis virus was common, the complication of muscle paralysis was rare, requiring an extremely large study. Some vaccine trials can be successful even if small, because they are aimed at preventing common outcomes. Vaccine trials for influenza, for example, can be relatively small if the population studied is susceptible to the strain of the virus that circulates, because a large proportion of a susceptible population will succumb to influenza during an epidemic. As vaccines become established for diseases that represent continuing threats, it may be difficult to study new versions of vaccines in randomized studies. If vaccination provides lengthy immunity, those who need vaccination may be only a small proportion of a population, such as immigrants or newborns. If herd immunity exists, investigators may have to look outside a population to find enough people who are susceptible to an infective agent and in whom an outbreak might occur. Furthermore, if a new vaccine is being compared with an older vaccine, the study will have to be large enough to measure what may be a small difference in efficacy between the two vaccines.

OUTLOOK FOR INFECTIOUS DISEASE EPIDEMIOLOGY

For a brief time at the dawn of the antibiotic era, it seemed that humans might have found the ultimate defense against infection from bacteria. During the same era, continued progress in the development of vaccines gave rise to hope that viral illness also might be tamed and in some cases eradicated, as was the case for smallpox. With these successes, it looked like infectious disease might become a historical problem. Unfortunately, the high reproductive rate of microorganisms and their ability to mutate have enabled them to evade many of our technologically driven defenses. Widespread and possibly some unnecessary use of antibiotics has produced antibiotic-resistant bacteria. Increasing urbanization and intercontinental travel have added to the risks of communicating infectious illnesses. Social and medical practices that change rapidly have opened new routes of transmission for infectious agents to spread, as illustrated by the spread of human immunodeficiency virus (HIV) through needle sharing, blood banks, and increased sexual contacts. Even good sanitation and hygiene, the most important weapon in the struggle against infectious disease, is unavailable to an appallingly large proportion of the world's population, and where present, it is easily disrupted by natural disaster or economic instability.

Infectious disease epidemiology is a frontier that has observed two remarkable triumphs that go beyond the good news conveyed by Figure 6–1. One is the eradication from the planet of an age-old human scourge, smallpox. By a combination of vaccination, contact tracing, and other containment methods employing a rapid response to contain any new outbreak, the spread of smallpox was gradually constricted until, in 1977, the last case was reported. With no animal reservoir, smallpox cannot recur in humans, apart from the risk of deliberate spread from biologic samples stored for research purposes. The second triumph is the near-elimination of a second disease, poliomyelitis, currently the focus of a global eradication campaign. In 2009, there were fewer than 1600 cases of poliomyelitis recorded. Control of smallpox and poliomyelitis are major achievements of epidemiology and public health. There is hope that other diseases can also be eradicated. Malaria is one candidate, but eradication has proved challenging. An effective malaria vaccine has been elusive because the life cycle of the multistage *Plasmodium* parasites that cause malaria is complex, the parasite is spread by mosquito, and some forms of *Plasmodium* have a primate reservoir other than humans.[8]

Our vulnerability to infectious agents remains high. Nevertheless, these successes indicate that the prospect of eradication of some infectious diseases and better control of others is a realistic, if ambitious, goal. This combination of vulnerability on some fronts and the hope of success on others ensures that infectious disease epidemiology will remain an important subdiscipline for epidemiologists in the 21st century and beyond.

QUESTIONS

1. Give reasons why crowding can foster the spread of infection.

2. Figure 6–1 displays crude death rates over time. The age distribution of the population was changing over the time scale shown, gradually shifting toward an older age distribution. If age had been controlled so that the curve reflected the change in death rates among people with the same age distribution, would the curve drop more steeply or less steeply than what is shown in Figure 6–1? Comment on the apparent rise in the crude death rate in the past 15 years covered by the graph.

3. Explain the relation between quarantine and the effective reproductive number.

4. The Reed-Frost model is a simplified model of transmission that assumes the population is closed. Suppose that with each generation time there is some migration into and out of the population. Under what conditions would that mixing hasten the transmission of disease, and under what conditions would it slow the transmission?

5. Varicella infection (chicken pox) results in long-term immunity to the virus that causes it, but infected people can experience a recrudescence of their infection, known as *shingles*, years or decades after their initial infection. How does the virus persist in the body over such a long period despite an immune system that is primed to deactivate the virus with specific antibodies?

6. Despite evidence of person-to-person spread, contact tracing was not widely used to control the spread of HIV in the early stages of the epidemic. Give pro and con arguments regarding the desirability of contact tracing to contain the transmission of HIV.

REFERENCES

1. Yang Y, Sugimoto JD, Halloran ME, et al. The transmissibility and control of pandemic influenza A (H1N1) virus. *Science.* 2009;326:729–733.
2. Porta M. *A Dictionary of Epidemiology.* 5th ed. New York, NY: Oxford University Press; 2008.
3. Doshi P. Calibrated response to emerging infections. *BMJ.* 2009;339:b3471.
4. Godlee F. Conflicts of interest and pandemic flu. *BMJ.* 2010;340:c2947.
5. Chan M: WHO Director-General replies to the BMJ. *BMJ.* 2010;340:c3463.
6. Dallaire F, De Serres G, Tremblay FW, Markowski F, Tipples G. Long-lasting measles outbreak affecting several unrelated networks of unvaccinated persons. *J Infect Dis.* 2009;200:1602–1605.
7. Armstrong GL, Conn LA, Pinner RW. Trends in infectious disease mortality in the United States during the 20th century. *JAMA.* 1999;281:61–66.
8. Plowe CV, Alonso P, Hoffman SL. The potential role of vaccines in the elimination of *Falciparum malaria* and the eventual eradication of malaria. *J Infect Dis.* 2009;200:1646–1649

SUGGESTED READING

Halloran ME, Struchiner CJ. Study designs for dependent happenings. *Epidemiology.* 1991;2:331–338.
Heymann DL, ed. *Control of Communicable Diseases Manual.* Washington, DC: American Public Health Association; 2008.

7

Dealing with Biases

Two broad types of error afflict epidemiologic studies: random error and systematic error. In designing a study, an epidemiologist attempts to reduce both sources of error. In interpreting a study, a reader should be aware of both types of error and how they have been addressed.

What is meant by error in a study? In Chapter 5, I said that an epidemiologic study could be viewed as an attempt to obtain an epidemiologic measure. The object of measurement may be a rate or a risk, but it typically is a measure of effect, such as an incidence rate ratio. Suppose a study is conducted to attempt to measure the ratio of the incidence rate of Alzheimer's disease among those who are physically active compared with those who are physically inactive. We can imagine that there is a correct value for the incidence rate ratio. A given study will produce an estimate of this correct value. If the study estimates a value of the incidence rate ratio that is close to the correct value, we would consider the study to be accurate, which means that it has little error. Conversely, a study estimate that differs considerably from the correct value is inaccurate. Unfortunately, we can never know the correct value for the rate ratio of Alzheimer's disease among physically active people compared with the physically inactive or for any other measure that we try to estimate; all we can know is the value of the estimates from a study. Because the correct values are unknown, we cannot determine the actual amount of error in any given study. Nevertheless, epidemiologists can still take steps in the design and analysis of studies to reduce errors. We also can look for features in the design and analysis of a study that may contribute to or prevent errors.

This chapter focuses on systematic error; random error is discussed in Chapter 8, which deals with statistical issues in epidemiologic research. Another term for systematic error is *bias*. Bias can refer to an attitude on the part of the investigator, but it is also used to describe any systematic error in a study. A study can be biased because of the way in which the subjects have been selected, the way the study variables are measured, or some confounding factor that is not completely controlled.

There is a simple way to distinguish random errors from systematic errors. Imagine that a given study could be increased in size until it was infinitely large.

Some errors would be reduced to zero if a study became infinitely large; these are the random errors. Other errors are not affected by increasing the size of the study. Errors that remain even in an infinitely large study are the systematic errors, also described as biases (Fig. 7–1). As study size increases and as random error concomitantly decreases, the relative role of systematic error becomes greater. In a sufficiently large study, virtually all errors of concern are systematic errors.

To see the difference between systematic errors and random errors, consider the following example. Suppose your task is to determine the average height of women in the city of Centerville, which has a population of 500,000 women. To conduct this work, you are supplied with an official measuring tape. You may decide to measure the height of 100 women sampled randomly from the population of all women in the city. You can use the average of the 100 measurements as an estimate of the average height of women in Centerville. What sources of error affect your estimate? A measuring tape will give different readings depending on how it is held, how it is read, the time of day the measurement is taken, and who is taking the measurement. Some of these errors, such as how the measuring tape is held during a given measurement, may be random; some of these errors sometimes lead to a reading that is too high and sometimes to a reading that is too low, but on average, readings do not tend to be too high or too low. If the sample of 100 were increased to 1000 or to 10,000 women, the effect of these random errors would become less important because the greater number of measurements would ensure that the discrepancy between the average measured height for women in the sample and the height of all women in Centerville would be close to zero. Other errors, however, would not be affected by increasing the number of women measured. Suppose that the official tape used in the measurements was a cloth tape that had been laundered before the project began. Unknown to anyone, the laundering shrank the tape. Consequently, the height

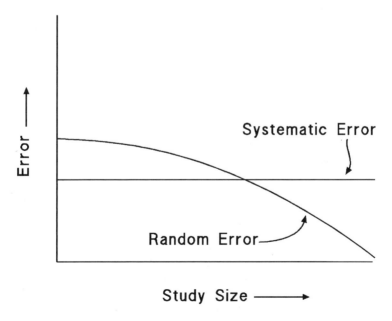

Figure 7–1   The relation of systematic error and random error to study size.

estimates derived from using the shrunken tape would tend to be high by an amount that depends on the amount of shrinkage. This systematic error cannot be reduced by taking more measurements with the same shrunken tape. Similarly, any defect in the measuring technique, such as a tendency to hold the tape crookedly, may also lead to measurements that are systematically wrong and would not be offset by increasing the number of subjects.

SOURCES OF BIAS IN EPIDEMIOLOGIC STUDIES

Error can creep into epidemiologic studies from myriad directions. Although many types of specific biases have been described, it is helpful to classify bias into three broad categories: selection bias, information bias, and confounding.

Selection Bias

Selection bias is a systematic error in a study that stems from the procedures used to select subjects and from factors that influence study participation. It comes about when the association between exposure and disease differs for those who participate and those who do not participate in the study. Because the association between exposure and disease among nonparticipants is unknown, the presence of selection bias must usually be inferred, rather than observed.

Suppose that a new screening test was devised to detect colon cancer and that this test was offered to a community in a pilot evaluation. Later, the efficacy of the test was assessed by comparing the incidence rate of colon cancer among those who volunteered to be tested with the incidence rate among community residents who were not tested. We would suspect that such a comparison would suffer from a selection bias. At issue is whether we could expect any difference in colon cancer incidence between these two groups regardless of whether the screening test had any effect. There likely would be a difference, because people who volunteer for cancer screening usually are more health conscious than those who do not volunteer, and people who are more health conscious may have a diet that lowers the risk of colon cancer. If so, those who volunteer for screening might be expected to have a lower rate of colon cancer for reasons that do not result from the screening. This difference would be superimposed on any effect of the screening and would represent a bias in assessing the screening effect.

Another possibility is that some of those who volunteer for screening may volunteer because they are especially worried about their colon cancer risk. They may, for example, have a family history of colon cancer. Some volunteers may be at lower risk than nonvolunteers, and other volunteers may be at a higher risk than nonvolunteers. These biases would tend to counteract one another, but because neither one is easy to quantify, the net bias would be unknown. Concern about selection bias has been the main reason why the efficacy of many screening procedures is evaluated by randomized trials. Although a randomized trial is much more cumbersome and expensive than a cohort study, the randomization ensures that the groups studied are reasonably comparable if the study is reasonably large.

The selection bias in the previous example is a bias arising from self-selection, because the study subjects selected themselves to be screened. Selection bias can also arise from choices made more directly by the investigator. For example, many studies of workers' health have compared the death rate among workers in a specific job with that among the general population. This comparison is biased because the general population contains many people who cannot work because of ill health. Consequently, overall death rates for workers are often substantially lower than death rates for the general population, and any direct comparison of the two groups is biased. This selection bias is often referred to as the *healthy worker effect*. One way to avert the bias is to compare the workers in a specific job with workers in other jobs that differ in their occupational exposures or hazards. If all subjects involved in the comparison are workers, the investigator can avoid bias from the healthy worker effect.

Table 7–1 shows how the healthy worker effect comes about. If the mortality rate of an exposed group of workers at a specific plant is compared with that of the general population (the Total column in Table 7–1), their overall mortality rate appears much lower; in this hypothetical example, their overall mortality rate is 5/7, or 71% of the rate in the general population. The general population, however, comprises two groups: a majority that is healthy enough to work and a minority that is too ill to work. The latter group is included among the nonworkers in Table 7–1, and results in the nonworkers having a higher mortality rate than the remainder of the general population that comprises current workers. In this hypothetical example, workers in the general population have the same mortality rate as the exposed workers at the study plant, but because the nonworkers in the general population have a rate that is five times as great as that of workers, the overall rate in the general population is considerably greater than that of the exposed workers. In a study that compared the mortality rate of the exposed workers with that of the general population, the exposed workers would have a lower mortality rate as a result of this selection bias.

The data in Table 7–1 are hypothetical data chosen to illustrate the healthy worker selection bias. Some actual data that show an effect of selection bias come from studies of influenza vaccine efficacy among the elderly. One such study combined cohort data from several health plans over many years, thereby including 713,872 person-seasons of experience. The investigators found that those who were vaccinated had a 48% decrease in overall mortality during influenza season.[1] Other evidence, however, indicates that perhaps 5% and at most 10% of deaths among the elderly during influenza season are attributable to influenza.[2] How can

Table 7–1 HEALTHY WORKER EFFECT[a]

	Exposed Workers	General Population		
		Workers	Nonworkers	Total
Deaths	50	4500	2500	7000
Person-time	1,000	90,000	10,000	100,000
Mortality rate (cases/yr)	0.05	0.05	0.25	0.07

[a]The healthy worker effect is an example of a selection bias that underestimates the mortality related to occupational exposures, as illustrated by these hypothetical rates for workers and the general population.

a vaccine, even one that is completely effective in preventing influenza, prevent one half of all deaths among those vaccinated if influenza itself accounts for at most 10% of those deaths? In simple terms, it cannot. The huge decrease in over-all mortality must reflect a selection bias. The unvaccinated group in this study is likely to include most of the elderly patients who are at the brink of death, because for them vaccination is most likely not seen as a priority. Evidence to support this hypothesis about selection bias comes from a study that examined the effect of influenza vaccine on mortality in the elderly during three periods each year: before influenza arrived, during influenza season, and after the influenza season.[3] The findings are summarized in Figure 7–2. During the influenza period, the investigators found about the same vaccine efficacy as had been reported by others, with almost 50% of all deaths being "prevented." They also found, how-ever, that the effect estimate indicating protection from the vaccine for all causes of death appeared even greater during the period each winter before the influenza virus arrived, when the vaccine could not have had any effect and all the apparent effect must stem from bias. Smaller biases were evident after the influenza season, when the vaccine efficacy should also theoretically be zero. The biases observed before and during the influenza season would also be operating during the influ-enza season. The selection factors responsible for the bias appear to be strongest at the outset of the study period, just after the vaccinations are administered, and they then weaken with the passage of time, as can be expected if the effect is the result of vaccine not being offered to those with a high risk of near-term death. A similar trend, also indicating strong selection bias, was evident for the outcome of hospitalization for pneumonia or influenza. These data indicate that selection bias among the elderly getting vaccinated for influenza is much stronger than any possible effect of the vaccine. These findings leave open the question of the actual magnitude of the vaccine effect on death in the elderly.

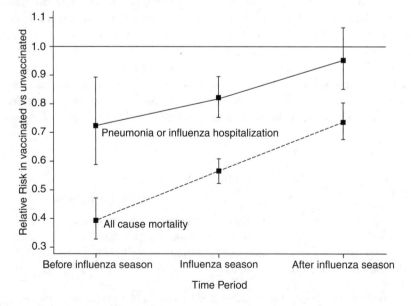

Figure 7–2 The relation of systematic error and random error to study size. (Reproduced with permission from Jackson et al.[3])

MATCHING IN CASE-CONTROL STUDIES

Another prominent form of selection bias comes from a design feature of some case-control studies. When *matching* is used to select controls in case-control studies, ostensibly to prevent confounding, matching usually paradoxically results in selection bias. In Chapter 5, the point was made that to get a valid effect estimate in a case-control study, the controls must be sampled independently of the exposure. Matching in case-control studies typically violates this assumption. With matching, controls are selected because they have one or more characteristics that match the corresponding characteristics of a case in the study. Commonly used matching factors are age, sex, and geographic location, but they may also include many other factors that may be specific to a given study. The motivation for matching usually is to prevent confounding, and the matching factors therefore are usually potential confounding factors. As described later in this chapter, confounding factors are associated with both exposure and disease. By matching controls to cases on possible confounding factors, the investigator selects controls according to factors that are related to exposure, depending on the extent that the exposure is associated with the matching factors. Because of the matching, the exposure distribution in the control series may not reflect the exposure distribution of the source population for cases. Instead, the exposure distribution among matched controls will tend toward the exposure distribution of the cases. If the exposure were perfectly correlated with one of the matching factors, controls would then have exactly the same exposure distribution as the cases, which would appear to indicate no effect of exposure, regardless of the actual effect that the exposure has.

Suppose 10% of a community is exposed to an agent that multiplies the risk of disease tenfold. Let us hypothesize that males have a five times greater risk for the disease than females, and 90% of males are exposed, compared with only 10% of females. If we have 100,000 males and 100,000 females in the population, the data for this community describing the risk during 1 year is summarized in Table 7–2. Because males and exposed people are at higher risk, and most males are exposed, most cases occur in exposed males.

Because males have a much greater risk of disease than females and because the preponderance of exposed people are males, whereas most unexposed people are females, the imbalance of males between exposed and unexposed subgroups will confound the effect of exposure. Although the effect of exposure is to increase the risk of disease tenfold, if we calculated the risk among all exposed, 4600/100,000,

Table 7–2 HYPOTHETICAL DATA SHOWING RISK FOR A DISEASE DURING 1 YEAR BY EXPOSURE STATUS AND SEX

	Sex[a]	Population	Data Risk	No. of Cases
Exposed	Male	90,000	5.00%	4500
	Female	10,000	1.00%	100
Unexposed	Male	10,000	0.50%	50
	Female	90,000	0.10%	90

[a]Being male is associated with exposure and is a risk factor for disease.

and compared it with the risk among all unexposed, 140/100,000, we would obtain a risk ratio estimate of 32.9, rather than the value of 10 that corresponds to the actual effect of exposure.

Can matching prevent confounding? We could try conducting a cohort study within this population and match the unexposed subjects to the exposed subjects by sex. We could take a random 10% sample of the total exposed population as the exposed cohort and match 10,000 unexposed people to this group of 10,000 exposed people so that each person in a matched pair has the same sex. The summary data after this matching is given in Table 7–3.

After matching by sex, there is no longer an imbalance of males between exposed and unexposed. The crude data for the study represented in Table 7–3 produce an estimate of risk among exposed of 460/10,000 and among unexposed of 46/10,000, for a risk ratio of 10. Matching has prevented the confounding by male sex.

The situation is not so pretty, however, if a case-control study is conducted with the aim of using matching to prevent confounding by male sex. Suppose we include in such a study all the cases occurring during 1 year in the community. From Table 7–2, we have a total of 4740 cases. We can then select a control group of 4740 people from the community, matched by sex, in an attempt to prevent confounding. Ideally, the controls should be selected from the entire population at risk to be cases, which in this setting is the entire population of the community, rather than just the noncases (see Chapter 5). Of the 4740 cases, 4550 are males and 190 are females. The 4740 controls, after matching by sex, include 4550 male controls and 190 female controls. Because 90% of males are exposed and 10% of females are exposed, we would expect, on average, that there would be $0.9 \times 4550 = 4095$ exposed male controls and $0.1 \times 190 = 19$ exposed female controls, for a total of $4095 + 19 = 4114$ exposed controls. The summary data for this case-control study is given in Table 7–4.

Unlike the cohort study, matching in the case-control study does not give the correct risk ratio of 10. The estimate also differs from that of the confounded relation, RR = 32.9, which was seen for the total population. The RR estimate of 5.0 that is obtained is an underestimate of the correct value, rather than an overestimate. What happened? This result stems from selection bias. Choosing controls based on their sex leads to a control series that is mostly male, and that has an exposure distribution that has been shifted toward that of the cases, leading to an underestimate of the effect. The matching has substituted one bias for

Table 7–3 HYPOTHETICAL COHORT STUDY[a]

	Sex	Population	Data Risk	No. of Cases
Exposed	Male	9,000	5.00%	450
	Female	1,000	1.00%	10
Unexposed	Male	9,000	0.50%	45
	Female	1,000	0.10%	1

[a]Based on a 10% sample of exposed from the population in Table 7–2 and 10,000 unexposed people matched by sex.

Table 7–4 HYPOTHETICAL CASE-CONTROL STUDY
BASED ON ALL CASES IN THE STUDY POPULATION
AND ONE CONTROL PER CASE MATCHED BY SEX

	Exposed	Unexposed	Total
Cases	4,600	140	4,740
Controls	4,114	626	4,740

another. As is explained in Chapter 5, the key design element in a case-control study is that controls must be selected independently of exposure. If they are not, selection bias results. Matching controls to cases for a variable that is correlated with exposure introduces selection bias because it violates the design element that controls must be selected independently of exposure.

In Table 7–5, the case-control data are shown separately for males and females. Among males and among females, the case-control data give the correct estimate of $RR = 10$. This analysis illustrates that in case-control studies the selection bias introduced by the matching can be removed by appropriate analytic methods, such as stratifying the data by the matching factor or factors. Regression models that condition on the matching factors can also be used to remove the selection bias.

As explained in Chapter 10, stratifying the data into male and female groups can suffice to control confounding by sex, even without matching by sex in subject selection. Because matching by sex introduces a bias that also requires control of sex in the data analysis to be removed, what does matching by sex in subject selection achieve? The answer is very little and perhaps nothing. One argument for matching in a case-control study is that the data analysis becomes more efficient in a technical sense. The distribution of controls over the two strata in Table 7–5 is identical to that of the cases as a result of the matching. Having controls distributed across strata identically to cases ordinarily makes for a statistically efficient stratified analysis. Without matching, one half of controls would have been female, and there would have been more than 2000 female controls to compare with only 190 female cases, whereas male cases would have outnumbered male controls. Although matching in a case-control study does not appear to improve validity (by preventing confounding), it may improve the efficiency of a stratified analysis that is employed to remove the confounding.

Unfortunately, the argument for efficiency gain from matching in case-control studies is not clear-cut. One problem is that analytic control of the matched variable may not have even been necessary without the matching. If the matched variable is related to exposure, matching on it will introduce selection bias. But if it is not related to disease, it is not a confounding factor and can be ignored. Matching

Table 7–5 CASE-CONTROL DATA FROM TABLE 7–4,
STRATIFIED BY SEX

	Males		Females	
	Exposed	Unexposed	Exposed	Unexposed
Cases	4,500	50	100	90
Controls	4,095	455	19	171
	RR = 10		RR = 10	

for such a variable introduces the need to control it in the analysis, which typically cannot improve efficiency compared with not needing to control for that factor in the first place. Another problem is that matching on some variables or a set of variables may lead to small numbers within strata. In the illustration, we matched on sex and combined all matched pairs that were male into a male stratum and all female pairs into a female stratum. If matching is implemented for many variables, however, it may produce unique combinations of values for each matched set, leading to strata for the stratified analysis that will each have a single case with one or more matched controls. With such small numbers in the strata, there is a reasonably high likelihood that the case and all the matched controls within a set will have the same value for exposure: all exposed or all unexposed. When exposure does not vary within a stratum, the stratum does not contribute information to the analysis. Effectively, any subjects in such a stratum, which is described as a *concordant set,* are lost to the analysis, leading to a loss of efficiency.

Given these potential problems, is matching worthwhile in case-control studies? Sometimes it is, but often it is not. Matching can be expensive, and in case-control studies, it does not improve validity. Efficiency gains are possible but not guaranteed and may not be worth the added cost. In some settings, efficiency may be lost rather than gained because of concordant sets. For these reasons, matching usually is best avoided in case-control studies, except for some specific exceptions. One exception is *convenience matching.* There may be circumstances in which some types of matching may simply be a convenient way to identify controls. *Risk-set sampling* is an example of a type of matching often done for convenience (see Chapter 5); it involves matching on time as a means of selecting controls proportional to their person-time contribution to the source population of cases. With convenience matching, the matching factor may not be related to exposure, and the matching may not introduce any selection bias. In that event, it can be ignored in the analysis. On the other hand, if the time variable in risk-set sampling is related to exposure, it must be controlled in the analysis, as is the case for any matching factor in a case-control study that is related to exposure. For example, consider a case-control study of mobile telephone use and brain cancer that matched risk sets on time of occurrence of the brain cancer. If mobile telephone use changed appreciably over the time scale in which the cases were identified, it might be necessary to retain the matched sets in the analysis, even if the only matching factor were calendar time. Ordinarily, the need to take the matching into account in the analysis is evaluated by comparing the results of an analysis that does take the matching into account with an analysis that ignores the matching. If the results are close, the matching need not be considered further in the analysis.

Another motivation for matching in case-control studies may be to control for variables that would be impossible to control in the analysis without matching. For example, suppose an investigator wishes to control for early-childhood environmental and genetic influences by controlling for family, specifically by using sibling controls. The only practical way to ensure that sibling controls can be used is to select them by matching on sibship during subject ascertainment. Apart from such exceptions, however, the drawbacks of matching typically may outweigh any advantages. If the investigator does decide to match in a case-control study, it may be worth considering using a high matching ratio (the number of controls matched to each case). A high matching ratio will reduce the probability that any matched set would have completely concordant exposures and reduce the number of matched sets that would be lost to the analysis.

Information Bias

Systematic error in a study can arise because the information collected about or from study subjects is erroneous. Such information is often referred to as *misclassified* if the variable is measured on a categorical scale and the error leads to a person being placed in an incorrect category. For example, a heavy smoker who is categorized as a light smoker is misclassified. Misclassification of subjects can be *differential* or *nondifferential*. Nondifferential misclassification is a misclassification that is unrelated to other study variables. In contrast, with differential misclassification, the misclassification differs according to the value of other study variables. The two key variables to consider with regard to misclassification are exposure and disease.

A common type of information bias is *recall bias*, which occurs in case-control studies in which a subject is interviewed to obtain exposure information after disease has occurred. For example, case-control studies of babies born with birth defects sometimes obtain interview information from mothers after the birth. Mothers who have given birth to a baby with a serious birth defect are thought to be able to recall accurately many exposures during early pregnancy, such as taking nonprescription drugs or experiencing a fever, because the adverse pregnancy outcome serves as a stimulus for the mother to consider potential causes of the birth defect. Mothers of normal babies, however, have had no comparable stimulus to search their memories and may consequently fail to recall exposures such as nonprescription drugs or fevers. The discrepancy in recall gives rise to a particular version of recall bias known as *maternal recall bias*. This problem is distinct from the more general problem of remembering and reporting exposures, which affects all people to some extent and tends to be a nondifferential rather than a differential misclassification.

How can recall bias be prevented? One approach is to frame the questions to aid accurate recall. Improving accuracy of recall reduces recall bias, because it limits the inaccurate recall among controls. Another approach is to use an entirely different control group that will not be subject to the incomplete recall. For example, mothers of babies born with birth defects other than the one under study may provide recall of earlier exposures comparable with that of case mothers. Another approach to avoiding recall bias is to conduct a study that does not use interview information but instead uses information from medical records that was recorded before the birth outcome was known.

Recall bias is a differential misclassification because the exposure information is misclassified differentially for those with or without disease. Although it occurs only in case-control studies, there is an analogous type of differential misclassification that occurs in follow-up studies, in which unexposed people are underdiagnosed for disease more than exposed people. Suppose an investigator conducts a cohort study to assess the effect of tobacco smoking on the occurrence of emphysema. Suppose also that the study asks about medical diagnoses but does not involve any examinations to check the diagnoses. It may happen that emphysema, a diagnosis that is often missed, is more likely to be diagnosed in smokers than in nonsmokers. Both the smokers and their physicians may be inclined to search more thoroughly for respiratory disease because they are concerned about the effects of smoking. As a result, the diagnosis of emphysema may be missed more frequently among nonsmokers, leading to a differential misclassification of disease. Even if smoking did not lead to emphysema, smokers would appear to have a greater incidence rate of emphysema than nonsmokers because of the greater likelihood that a case of emphysema would remain undiagnosed in a nonsmoker. This bias could be avoided by conducting examinations for emphysema as part of the study itself, thereby avoiding the biased follow-up.

The previous biases are examples of differential misclassification, when the exposure is misclassified differentially according to a person's disease status or disease is misclassified differentially according to a person's exposure status. Differential misclassification can exaggerate or underestimate an effect. A more pervasive type of misclassification, which affects every epidemiologic study to some extent, is nondifferential misclassification. With nondifferential misclassification, exposure or disease (or both) is misclassified, but the misclassification does not depend on a person's status for the other variable. For example, suppose that the study hypothesis concerns the relation between consumption of red wine and the development of emphysema; assume for this example that consumption of red wine is not related to smoking. Unlike the situation for smoking, there is little reason to suppose that those who drink more or less red wine will have a greater or a lesser tendency to be diagnosed with emphysema if they have it. As a result, although some people with emphysema will not have it diagnosed, the proportion of people who do not have their emphysema diagnosed would be expected to be the same for those who do and who do not drink red wine. The underdiagnosis represents some misclassification of emphysema, but because the tendency for underdiagnosis is the same for exposed and unexposed people, the misclassification of disease is nondifferential with respect to exposure. Similarly, if an exposure is misclassified in a way that does not depend on disease status, the exposure misclassification is nondifferential with respect to disease.

Nondifferential misclassification leads to more predictable biases than does differential misclassification. Misclassification of a dichotomous exposure that is nondifferential with respect to disease tends to produce estimates of the effect that are "diluted" or closer to the null or no-effect value than the actual effect. If there is no effect to begin with, nondifferential misclassification of the exposure will not bias the effect estimate.

The simplest case to consider is nondifferential misclassification of an exposure that is measured on a dichotomous scale: exposed versus nonexposed. Suppose that an investigator conducts a case-control study to assess the relation between eating a high-fat diet and subsequent heart attack. Everyone in the study is classified according to some arbitrary cutoff value of dietary fat intake as having a high-fat diet or not. This classification cannot be perfectly accurate because it is almost impossible to avoid some measurement error. In the case of measuring the fat content of a person's diet, there is likely to be substantial error, and some people who do not have a high-fat diet may be classified as having one and vice versa. If these misclassifications are not related to whether a person gets a heart attack, the misclassification is nondifferential with respect to disease.

The effect of nondifferential misclassification of a dichotomous exposure is illustrated in Table 7–6. On the left are hypothetical data that presume no misclassification with respect to a high-fat diet. The incidence rate ratio (calculated from the odds ratio) is 5.0, indicating a substantially greater mortality rate among those eating a high-fat diet. The center columns show the result if 20% of those who actually do not eat a high-fat diet were inaccurately classified as eating a high-fat diet. This level of misclassification is higher than ordinarily expected, even for an exposure as difficult to measure as diet, but it still involves only a small proportion of the subjects. By moving 20% of those from the No column to the Yes column, the resulting data give a rate ratio of 2.4, less than one half as great as the value with the correct data. In terms of the effect part of the risk ratio, the excess risk ratio of 4.0 ($= 5.0 - 1$) has been reduced to 1.4 ($= 2.4 - 1$), which means that about two thirds of the effect has been obscured. Notice that we have transferred both 20% of cases and 20% of controls. Nondifferential misclassification of exposure implies that these percentages of misclassified subjects among cases and controls will be equal. If the proportions of cases and controls that were misclassified differed from one another, the misclassification would be differential with respect to disease.

The third set of columns in Table 7–6 adds further nondifferential misclassification: 20% of cases and controls who ate a high-fat diet are misclassified as not having a high-fat diet. This misclassification is added to the misclassification in the other direction, with the result as shown in the right part of the table. With this additional misclassification, the rate ratio has declined to 2.0, even closer to the null value of 1.0, nullifying three fourths of the effect seen in the correctly classified data.

Nondifferential misclassification of a dichotomous exposure will always bias an effect, if there is one, toward the null value. If the exposure is not dichotomous, there may be bias toward the null value, but there may also be bias away from the null value, depending on the categories to which individuals get misclassified.

Table 7–6 Nondifferential Misclassification in a Hypothetical Case-Control Study

	Correct Classification		Nondifferential Misclassification			
			20% of No → Yes		20% of No → Yes 20% of Yes → No	
	High-Fat Diet		High-Fat Diet		High-Fat Diet	
	No	Yes	No	Yes	No	Yes
Myocardial infarction cases	450	250	360	340	410	290
Controls	900	100	720	280	740	260
	RR = 5.0		RR = 2.4		RR = 2.0	

Nondifferential misclassification between two exposure categories usually makes the effect estimates for those two categories converge toward one another.[4]

Confounding

Confounding is a central issue for epidemiologic study design. A simple definition of confounding is the *confusion of effects*. This definition implies that the effect of the exposure is mixed with the effect of another variable, leading to a bias. Consider a classic example: the relation between birth order and the occurrence of Down syndrome. Figure 7–3 shows data on birth order and Down syndrome from the work of Stark and Mantel.[5]

These data show a striking trend in prevalence of Down syndrome with increasing birth order, which can be described as the effect of birth order on the occurrence of Down syndrome. The effect of birth order, however, is a blend of whatever effect birth order has by itself and the effect of another variable that is closely correlated with birth order: the age of the mother. Figure 7–4 gives the relation between mother's age and occurrence of Down syndrome from the same data. It indicates a much stronger relation between mother's age and Down syndrome. In Figure 7–3, the prevalence increased from about 0.6/1000 at the first birth to 1.7/1000 for birth order of 5 or greater, a respectably strong trend. In Figure 7–4, however, the prevalence increases from 0.2/1000 at the youngest category of mother's age to 8.5/1000 at the highest category of mother's age, more than a 40-fold increase. (The vertical scale changes from Figure 7–3 to Figure 7–4.)

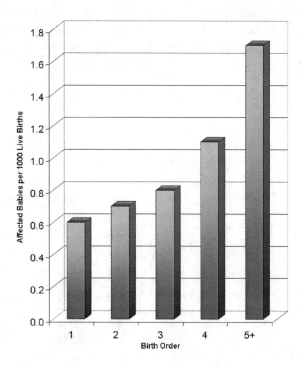

Figure 7–3 Prevalence of Down syndrome at birth by birth order. (Data from Stark and Mantel.[2])

CONFOUNDING BY INDICATION

Pharmacoepidemiologists study the epidemiology of intended and unintended drug effects, often by using nonexperimental studies. In these studies, the essential comparisons involve a contrast of outcomes for individuals who have taken a specific drug with those who have not taken the drug. Without a randomized trial, it can be challenging to design a study that yields a valid comparison of drug takers with nontakers. The main challenge comes from a phenomenon that epidemiologists refer to as *confounding by indication*. The problem arises from the fact that those who take a drug usually differ from those who do not according to the medical indication for which the drug was prescribed. Even if the comparison group represents patients with the same disease who received a different therapy or none at all, there typically are differences in disease severity or other risk factors between populations who receive different treatments. These differences introduce a bias in the comparison that is called confounding by indication, which is described further in Chapter 13.

Because birth order and the age of the mother are highly correlated, we can expect that the mothers who are giving birth to their fifth baby are, as a group, considerably older than mothers who are giving birth to their first baby. Therefore the comparison of high-birth-order babies with lower-birth-order babies is to some extent a comparison of babies born to older mothers with babies born to younger mothers. Thus, the birth-order comparison in Figure 7–3 mixes the effect of mother's age with the effect of birth order. The extent of the mixing depends on the extent to which mother's age is related to birth order. This mixing of effects is called *confounding*; the birth order effect depicted in Figure 7–3 is confounded by the effect of mother's age.

Is the effect of mother's age in Figure 7–4 also confounded by the effect of birth order? This is a reasonable question; the answer depends on whether birth order has any effect at all on its own. Because the effect in Figure 7–4 for mother's age is so much stronger than the effect in Figure 7–3 for birth order, we know that birth order cannot fully explain the maternal age effect, whereas it remains a possibility that maternal age fully accounts for the apparent effect of birth order. A good way to resolve the extent to which one variable's effect explains the apparent effect of the other is to examine both effects simultaneously. Figure 7–5 presents the prevalences of Down syndrome at birth by both birth order and mother's age simultaneously.

Figure 7–5 shows that within each category of birth order, looking from the front to the back, there is the same striking trend in prevalence of Down syndrome with increasing maternal age. In contrast, within each category of maternal age, looking from left to right, there is no discernible trend with birth order. Thus, the apparent trend with birth order in Figure 7–3 is entirely explained by confounding by maternal age. There is no confounding in the other direction: Birth order does not confound the maternal age association, because birth order has no effect. We call the apparent effect of birth order in Figure 7–3 the *crude*

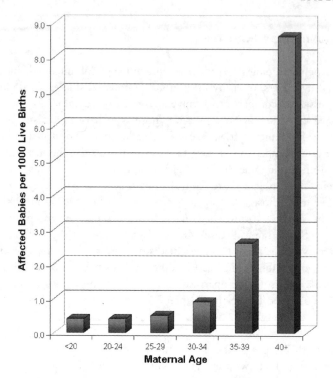

Figure 7–4 Prevalence of Down syndrome at birth by mother's age.

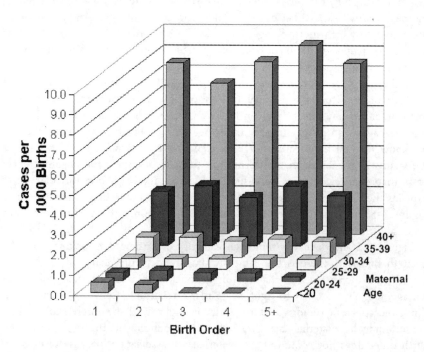

Figure 7–5 Prevalence of Down syndrome at birth by birth order and mother's age.

effect of birth order. In Figure 7–5, we can see that within categories of maternal age there is no birth order effect, and the crude effect in this instance is entirely a result of confounding.

Although the maternal age effect in Figure 7–4 is not confounded by birth order, which appears to have no effect on its own, it is confounded by other factors. We can be sure of that because age is just a marker of time. There must be biologic events that occur during a woman's aging process that lead to the sharp increase in occurrence of Down syndrome among the offspring of older mothers. Mother's age is thus a proxy for unidentified events that more directly account for the occurrence of Down syndrome. When these events are identified, we may ultimately find that mother's age has no effect after we take into account the biologic changes that are correlated with age. In this sense, we can say that the apparent effect of mother's age is presumably confounded by unknown factors.

The research process of learning about and controlling for confounding can be thought of as a walk through a maze toward a central goal. The path through the maze eventually permits the scientist to penetrate deeper levels of understanding. In this example, the apparent relation between Down syndrome and birth order can be explained entirely by the effect of mother's age, but that effect ultimately will be explained by other factors that have not yet been identified. As the layers of confounding are left behind, we gradually approach a deeper causal understanding of the underlying biology. Unlike a maze, however, this journey toward the goal of biologic understanding does not have a clear end point, because there is always room to understand the biology in a deeper way.

Confounding previously was defined as the confusion of or mixing of effects. Strictly speaking, the exposure variable may or may not have an effect; in the Down syndrome example, birth order did not have an effect. The confounding variable, however, must have an effect on the outcome to be confounding. Theoretically, a confounding variable should be a cause of the disease, but in practice, it may be only a proxy or a marker for a cause. That is the case for mother's age, which by itself does not cause Down syndrome but serves as a marker for unknown biologic events that accumulate with time. Whether an actual cause or just a marker for a cause, a confounder is a predictor of disease occurrence.

Nevertheless, not every predictor of disease occurrence is a confounding factor. For confounding to occur, a predictor of disease occurrence must also be imbalanced across exposure categories. Suppose that age is a risk factor for a given disease (as it usually is). Age would not be confounding unless the age distributions of people in the various exposure categories differed, as they did for smoking and nonsmoking women in Table 1–2. If every exposure category contains people whose age distribution is the same as that for people in other exposure categories, the comparison of disease rates across exposure categories is not distorted by age differences. On the other hand, if age is imbalanced across exposure categories, the comparison of one exposure category with another involves the comparison of people whose age distributions differ. Under those circumstances, the effect of exposure will be confounded with the effect of age to an extent that depends on the strength of the relation between age and the disease and on the extent of the age imbalance across exposure categories.

Table 7–7 DEATHS AMONG PATIENTS WHO
RECEIVED TOLBUTAMIDE AND PLACEBO IN THE
UNIVERSITY GROUP DIABETES PROGRAM IN 1970

	Tolbutamide	Placebo
Deaths	30	21
Surviving	174	184
Total	204	205
Mortality proportion	0.147	0.102

Consider another example. In 1970, the University Group Diabetes Program published the results of a randomized trial designed to assess how well three treatments for diabetes prevented fatal complications.[6] Table 7–7 presents the crude data comparing one of the treatments, the drug tolbutamide, with placebo, with respect to total mortality over a period that averaged 7 years.

The proportion of subjects who died was greater in the tolbutamide group than in the placebo group, a surprising result that spurred a long and bitter controversy and brought tremendous scrutiny to these study results. If we measure the effect of treatment as the difference in proportion of those who died in the tolbutamide and placebo groups, we estimate an adverse effect of tolbutamide of $0.147 - 0.102 = 0.045$. This result translates to an estimate that subjects who receive tolbutamide face an additional risk of 4.5% of dying over 7 years compared with subjects receiving placebo.

Although this study was a randomized experiment, the random assignment in this case led to imbalances between the tolbutamide and placebo groups with respect to age. Randomization is intended to balance potential confounding factors between the compared groups, but it cannot guarantee such a balance. In this case, the tolbutamide group comprised subjects who were older on average than the placebo group. Because age is strongly related to the risk of death, this imbalance in age introduced confounding. In the Down syndrome example, we removed the confounding by examining the effect of birth order within categories of mother's age. This process is called *stratification*. We can also stratify the data from the University Group Diabetes Program by age (Table 7–8).

Table 7–8 shows that of the 204 subjects who received tolbutamide in the study, 98 (48%) were 55 years old or older; in contrast, only 85 of 205 placebo subjects (41%) were age 55 or older. This difference may not appear striking,

Table 7–8 DEATHS AMONG SUBJECTS WHO RECEIVED TOLBUTAMIDE
AND PLACEBO IN THE UNIVERSITY GROUP DIABETES PROGRAM IN 1970,
STRATIFIED BY AGE

	Age < 55		Age 55>	
	Tolbutamide	Placebo	Tolbutamide	Placebo
Dead	8	5	22	16
Surviving	98	115	76	69
Total	106	120	98	85
Mortality proportion	0.076	0.042	0.224	0.188
Difference in proportion	0.034		0.036	

but the difference in the risk of dying during the 7 years is strikingly greater for those age 55 or older than for younger subjects. With age so strongly related to the risk of death, the difference in the age distribution is potentially worrisome. Did it lead to confounding by age? To answer that, we can look at the difference in the proportion who died, comparing tolbutamide with placebo, in each of the two age groups. In both groups, there is an approximately 3.5% greater risk of death over the 7 years for the tolbutamide group than for the placebo group. (The data show a difference of 3.4% for the younger group and 3.6% for the older group. As a summary measure, we can average these two values and call the overall difference 3.5%. Technically, we would want to take an average that weighted each of the age categories according to the amount of data in that category.) When age was ignored, we found a difference of 4.5%. The value of 4.5% that we obtained from the crude data is confounded and gives an overestimate of the adverse effect of tolbutamide. The value of 3.5% obtained after the age stratification may not be completely unconfounded by age. Because we used only two age categories, it is possible that age differences remain within the age categories in Table 7–8. Nevertheless, even with this simple age stratification, the estimate of effect is lower than the estimate from the crude data. The crude data overestimate the adverse effect of tolbutamide by almost 30% (4.5% is almost 30% greater than 3.5%). The topic of stratification is discussed further in Chapter 10.

PROPERTIES OF A CONFOUNDING FACTOR

Confounding can be thought of as a mixing of effects. A confounding factor therefore must have an effect, and it must be imbalanced between the exposure groups that are being compared. These conditions imply that a confounding factor must have two associations:

- A confounder must be associated with the disease (either as a cause or as a proxy for a cause, but not as an effect of the disease).
- A confounder must be associated with the exposure.

There is also a third requirement. A factor that is an effect of the exposure and is an intermediate step in the causal pathway from exposure to disease will have the previously described properties, but causal intermediates are not confounders; they are part of the effect that we wish to study. For example, if a diet high in saturated fat leads to higher levels of low-density lipoproteins (LDL) in the blood, and a high LDL level leads to atherosclerosis, a high LDL level will be associated with both diet and atherosclerosis. Nevertheless a high LDL level does not confound the relation between diet and atherosclerosis; it is part of the exposure's effect and should not be considered confounding. Any effect of the exposure, whether it is part of the causal pathway to the disease or not, is not a confounder. Thus, the third property of a confounder is the following:

- A confounder must not be an effect of the exposure.

The University Group Diabetes Program illustrates that even randomization cannot prevent confounding in all instances. In this case, it led to an age imbalance, which caused a moderate amount of confounding. The confounding in the Down syndrome example was greater, in large part because the association between mother's age and birth order is stronger than the association between age and tolbutamide that the randomization produced in the University Group Diabetes Program.

Notice that confounding can cause a bias in either direction. It can cause an overestimate of the effect, as the confounder mother's age did for birth order and Down syndrome and the confounder age did for tolbutamide and death, or it can cause an underestimate of an effect, as the confounder age did for smoking and death in the example in Chapter 1. The bias introduced by confounding occasionally can be strong enough to reverse the apparent direction of an effect,[7] as illustrated in Chapter 1 when comparing the death rates in Panama and Sweden.

CONTROL OF CONFOUNDING

Confounding is a systematic error that investigators aim to prevent or to remove from a study. There are three methods that are used to prevent confounding. One of them, *randomization*, or the random assignment of subjects to experimental groups, can be used only in experiments. The second method, *restriction*, involves selecting subjects for a study who all have the same value or almost the same value for a variable that would otherwise be a confounding variable. Restriction can be used in any epidemiologic study, regardless of whether it is an experiment or not. The third approach is *matching*, which is an effective way to prevent confounding in cohort studies, but as discussed earlier, causes a selection bias in case-control studies. Because no method prevents confounding completely, these design methods may be best viewed as methods to limit confounding.

In experiments, in which the investigator assigns the exposure to study subjects, randomization confers powerful benefits. With a sufficiently large study population, randomization produces two or more study groups with almost the same distribution of characteristics. This similarity for all variables implies that the compared groups will be similar for risk factors that predict the outcome of interest and that these risk predictors therefore will not confound. Randomization cannot guarantee the absence of confounding; a random process can still lead to confounding imbalances, such as the age imbalance that occurred in the University Group Diabetes Program experiment and shown in Tables 7–7 and 7–8. The likelihood of a large imbalance, however, becomes small as the number of subjects who are randomized increases. Perhaps the most important benefit of randomization is that it prevents confounding for unidentified factors as well as for factors that are already known to be of concern. Even unknown risk factors will not confound a randomized experiment of sufficient size.

Restriction, unlike randomization, cannot control for unknown confounding factors, but it is more certain to prevent confounding for those factors for which it is employed. For example, in a study of alcohol drinking and cancer of the throat, smoking may be considered a likely confounding variable. Smoking is a cause of throat cancer, and people who drink alcohol smoke more than people who do not drink alcohol. If the study were confined to nonsmokers, smoking

IS CONFOUNDING IN A RANDOMIZED EXPERIMENT A BIAS?

Earlier in this chapter, I proposed that if an error in a study would decrease if the study were larger, then that error is a random error, whereas an error that would not decrease if the study were larger is a systematic error. Confounding is usually considered a systematic error, but confounding in an experiment is an exception. In all types of epidemiologic studies, confounding arises from imbalances in risk factors for the outcome across the exposure categories. Uniquely in randomized experiments, however, these imbalances are determined by random assignment. As a result of the law of large numbers, the larger the experiment, the more closely the randomly assigned groups will resemble one another in their distributions of risk factors. Because the amount of confounding depends on the size of the experiment, confounding in an experiment is an example of random error rather than systematic error. For systematic errors, replicating the study replicates the error, but for confounding in an experiment, replicating the study (with a new random assignment) will not replicate the same confounding because there will be an entirely new set of assignments to the study groups. Despite being an example of random error rather than systematic error, confounding in an experiment can be controlled using the same methods to control confounding in nonexperimental studies.

In this discussion, a large experiment does not necessarily mean one with many participants; rather, it is one that has a large number of random assignments. For example, a study may involve the random assignment of a community intervention to eight cities that contain millions of people. With only eight random assignments, however, it is not large enough to prevent substantial confounding.

could not be confounding. Similarly, if age is thought to be a likely confounding factor in a study, confounding by age can be prevented by enrolling subjects who are all the same age. If everyone in a study has the same value for a variable, that factor can no longer vary in the study setting; it becomes a constant. For confounding to occur, a confounding factor must be associated with exposure, but if a factor is constant, it cannot be associated with anything. Restriction is an effective way to prevent confounding in any study.

Restriction is used in experiments in addition to randomization to be certain that confounding for certain factors does not occur. It is also used by laboratory scientists conducting animal experiments to prevent confounding and enhance the validity of their studies. Typically, a researcher conducting an experiment with mice seeks only mice bred from the same laboratory and that have the same genotype, the same age, and sometimes the same sex.

It may appear puzzling that restriction is not used more often in epidemiologic research. One explanation is that many researchers have been taught that an epidemiologic study, whether an experiment or a nonexperimental study, should comprise study subjects whose characteristics are representative of the target population for whom the study results are intended. The goal of *representativeness* appears to work contrary to the method of restriction, which provides a study population that is homogeneous and therefore not similar to most target populations of interest. Elevating the importance of representativeness is a fallacy that has plagued epidemiologic studies for decades. As explained in Chapter 3, the notion that representativeness is a worthwhile goal presumably stems from the arena of survey research, in which a sample of a larger population is surveyed to avoid the expense and trouble of surveying the entire population. The statistical inference that such sampling allows is only superficially similar to the scientific inference that is the goal of epidemiologic research. For scientific inference, the goal is not to infer a conclusion that would apply to a specific target population but rather to infer an abstract theory that is not tied to a specific population. It is possible to make such a scientific inference more readily without confounding; restriction enhances the ability to make a scientific inference, as those who work with laboratory animals know.

What about the concern that restriction makes it difficult to know whether a studied relation applies to people with characteristics different from those in a study population? For example, suppose that an investigator uses restriction to study the effect of drinking wine on cardiovascular disease risk among people who are 60 years old. Would the study results apply to people who are 45-years old? The answer is maybe; without outside knowledge, it is not possible to say whether the study results apply to people who are 45 years old. This uncertainty leaves open the possibility of an erroneous or incomplete conclusion, but such is the nature of science. It is nevertheless wrong to think that the theorization needed to apply the results of a study to people with different characteristics could be replaced by mechanical sampling. If an investigator suspects that the effect of wine consumption on cardiovascular risk is different for 60-year-olds and 45-year-olds, he or she would want to select a group of 45-year-olds to study in addition to 60-year-olds. The number of the study subjects and their age distribution should not reflect the age distribution in some target population; why let the demographics of a locale dictate the age distribution of subjects that are chosen for study? Instead, the investigator can choose to study subjects of whatever age seems interesting and in numbers that suit the study design rather than reflect the numbers of people in a target population at those ages. Scientifically, there is no specific target population. There is instead a scientific theory about wine, cardiovascular disease risk, and perhaps age. The theory is the real target of inference. A valid study is the best route to a correct inference, and restriction, rather than representativeness, is the more desirable means to achieve the correct inference.

Matching should be distinguished from restriction. With restriction, all subjects are confined to a single value or narrow range of values for one or more factors that are suspected of being possible confounding factors. Matching imposes no constraint on the index subjects, those who are the target of the matching. The other subjects are selected to conform to the index series for whatever matching factors are employed. Suppose one is conducting a cohort study and wishes to control for age by matching. Generally, when matching in a cohort study, the index series is the exposed series, and the goal of matching is to assemble an unexposed series that has the same age distribution as the exposed subjects. There are two ways to accomplish this goal. One approach is to describe the age distribution of exposed subjects and then select unexposed subjects to replicate that age distribution. That approach is called *frequency matching*. The other approach is to take the exposed subjects one by one and to find for each of them an unexposed subject that has a matching age. The investigator also can select two or three or any fixed number of unexposed subjects to match with each exposed subject. This approach is called *individual matching*. Whether frequency matching or individual matching is used, the result is that for the matched factor, the exposed and unexposed cohorts will have the same distribution, and therefore that factor will not be confounding. To the extent that the matching is loose rather than tight, such as matching within 5 years of age rather than match to the exact year of age, there may still be minor differences in the age distribution. The tighter the match, the more effective the elimination of age confounding. For variables that are categorical, such as sex, defining a tight match is not an issue.

Matching is very effective in preventing confounding, but there are a few cautions to consider. The greatest caution, described earlier in this chapter, is that it does not work to prevent bias in case-control studies. In cohort studies, it does work well, and it can lead to results that are unbiased by the matching factors, provided that the cohort is followed for a short enough time for the matching to be maintained. Because matching is accomplished for people, not person-time, as people are lost to follow-up for various reasons, the initially equal distributions across cohorts for matching factors may become different if exposed people and unexposed people are lost to the study at different rates.

Matching can be an expensive process. To match an unexposed cohort to a sizable exposed cohort can be costly and consequently has seldom been attempted. The main exception is when all potential subjects and their data are already stored in a data warehouse or database. In that case, matching an unexposed cohort is no more costly than implementing a computer program to find the matching subjects, and matching becomes considerably more cost-effective. There is a drawback to using matching within a database, however. If the data are already available in a database, matching will result in excluding some subjects from the study. Some excluded subjects will be possible matches that were not used because there were closer matches that were chosen instead; others may be outliers that are unmatchable. This loss of subjects may lessen the appeal of matching compared with alternative methods that can be employed in the data analysis that retain all possible subjects. On the other hand, the exclusion of unmatchable subjects may enhance the validity of the study and be preferable to including them; this point is discussed further in Chapter 12.

Control of confounding in the data analysis requires that the study data include adequate information about the confounding factor or factors. Two methods can be used to deal with confounding in the data analysis. One is stratification, a technique that was illustrated in Table 7–8 and in Chapter 1. It is discussed in greater detail in Chapter 10. The other approach is by using regression models, an analytic technique that is described in Chapter 12.

QUESTIONS

1. Suppose a case-control study could be expanded to be infinitely large. Which sources of error would be eliminated by such a study, and which would not? Suppose that a randomized trial could be infinitely large. Which sources of error would remain in such a trial?

2. Will a larger study have less bias than a smaller study? Why or why not?

3. When recall bias occurs, patients who have been afflicted with a medical problem, such as a heart attack, give responses about possible causes of that problem that differ from those given by nonafflicted subjects. Whose responses are thought to be more accurate?

4. Suppose that in analyzing the data from an epidemiologic study, a computer coding error led to the exposed group being classified as unexposed and the unexposed group being classified as exposed. What specific effect would this error have on the reported results? Is this a bias? If so, what type? If not, what type of error is it?

5. Explain the difference between a confounding factor and a potential confounding factor. In what situations might a potential confounding factor not end up being a confounding factor?

6. The incidence rate of cardiovascular disease increases with increasing age. Does that mean that age always confounds studies of cardiovascular disease in the same direction? Why or why not?

7. The effectiveness of randomization in controlling confounding depends on the size of the experiment. Consider an experiment to study the effect of nutritional education of schoolchildren on their serum cholesterol levels. Suppose that the study involved randomly assigning 10 classrooms with 30 children each to receive a new curriculum and assigning another 10 classrooms with 30 children each to receive the old curriculum. Should this be considered a study that compares two groups with 300 in each group or 10 in each group from the viewpoint of the effectiveness of controlling confounding by randomization?

8. Confounding by indication arises because those who take a given drug differ for medical reasons from those who do not take the drug. Is this problem truly confounding, or is it more appropriately described as a selection bias?

9. Those who favor representative studies claim that one should not generalize a study to a population whose characteristics differ from those of the study population. A study of smoking and lung cancer in men would tell nothing about the relation between smoking and lung cancer in women. Give the counterarguments. (Hint: if the study were conducted in London, would the results apply to those who lived in Paris?)

REFERENCES

1. Nichol KL, Nordin JD, Nelson DB, Mullooly JP, Hak E. Effectiveness of influenza vaccine in the community-dwelling elderly. *N Engl J Med.* 2007;357:1373–1381.

2. Simonsen L, Reichert TA, Viboud C, Blackwelder WC, Taylor RJ, Miller MA. Impact of influenza vaccination on seasonal mortality in the US elderly population. *Arch Intern Med.* 2005;165:265–272.

3. Jackson LA, Jackson ML, Nelson JC, Neuzil KM, Weiss NS. Evidence of bias in estimates of influenza vaccine effectiveness in seniors. *Int J Epidemiol.* 2006;35:337–344.

4. Rothman KJ, Greenland S, Lash TL. *Modern Epidemiology.* 3rd ed. Philadelphia, PA: Lippincott Williams & Wilkins; 2008.

5. Stark CR, Mantel N. Effects of maternal age and birth order on the risk of mongolism and leukemia. *J Nat Cancer Inst.* 1966;37:687–698.

6. University Group Diabetes Program. A study of the effects of hypoglycemic agents on vascular complications in patients with adult onset diabetes. *Diabetes.* 1970;19(suppl 2):747–830.

7. Reintjes R, de Boer A, van Pelt W, Mintjes-de Groot J. Simpson's paradox: an example from hospital epidemiology. *Epidemiology.* 2000;11:81–83.

8

Random Error and the Role

of Statistics

Statistics plays two main roles in the analysis of epidemiologic data: first, to measure variability in the data in an effort to assess the role of chance, and second, to estimate effects after correcting for biases such as confounding. This chapter concentrates on the assessment of variability. The use of statistical approaches to control confounding is discussed in Chapters 10 and 12.

An epidemiologic study can be viewed as an exercise in measurement. As in any measurement, the goal is to obtain an accurate result, with as little error as possible. Systematic error and random error can distort the measurement process. Chapter 7 describes the primary categories of systematic error. The error that remains after systematic error is eliminated is *random error*. Random error is nothing more than variability in the data that cannot be readily explained. Sometimes, random error stems from a random process, but it may not. In randomized trials, some of the variability in the data reflects the random assignment of subjects to the study groups. In most epidemiologic studies, however, there is no random assignment to study groups. For example, in a cohort study that compares the outcome of pregnancy among women who drink heavily chlorinated water with the outcome among women who drink bottled water, it is not chance but the decision making or circumstances of the women themselves that determines the cohort in which the women are grouped. The individual assignments to categories of water chlorination are not random; nevertheless, some of the variability in the outcome is considered to be random error. Much of this variation may reflect hidden biases and presumably can be accounted for by factors other than drinking water that affect the outcome of pregnancy. These factors may not have been measured among these women or perhaps not even discovered.

ESTIMATION

If an epidemiologic study is thought of as an exercise in measurement, the result of the study should be an estimate of an epidemiologic quantity. Ideally, the analysis of data and the reporting of results should report the magnitude of that epidemiologic quantity and portray the degree of precision with which it is measured. For example, a case-control study may be undertaken to estimate the incidence rate ratio (RR) between use of cellular telephones and the occurrence of brain cancer. The report on the results of the study should present a clear estimate of the RR, such as $RR = 2.5$. When an estimate is presented as a single value, we refer to it as a *point estimate*. In this example, the point estimate of 2.5 quantifies the estimated strength of the relation between the use of cellular telephones and the occurrence of brain cancer. To indicate the precision of the point estimate, we use a *confidence interval,* which is a range of values around the point estimate. A wide confidence interval indicates low precision, and a narrow interval indicates high precision.

CHANCE

In ordinary language, the word *chance* has a dual meaning. One meaning refers to the outcome of a random process, implying an outcome that could not be predicted under any circumstances; the other refers to outcomes that cannot be predicted easily but are not necessarily random phenomena. For example, if you unexpectedly encounter your cousin on the beach at Cape Cod, you may describe it as a chance encounter. Nevertheless, there were presumably causal mechanisms that can explain why you and your cousin were on the beach at Cape Cod at that time. It may be a coincidence that the two causal mechanisms led to both of you being there together, but randomness does not necessarily play a role in explaining the encounter.

Flipping a coin is usually considered to be a randomizing event, one that is completely unpredictable. Nevertheless, the flip of a coin can be predicted with sufficient information about the initial conditions and the forces applied to the coin. The reason we consider it a randomizing event is that most of us do not have the necessary information nor the means to figure out from it what the outcome of the flip would be. Some individuals, however, have practiced flipping coins enough to predict the outcome of a given toss almost perfectly. For the rest of us, the flip of a coin appears random, despite the fact that the underlying process is not actually random. As we practice flipping or learn more about the sources of error in a body of data, we can reduce errors that may appear random at first. Physicists tell us that we will never be able to explain all components of error, but for the problems that epidemiologists address, it is reasonable to assume that much of the random error that we observe in data could be explained with better information.

POINT ESTIMATES, CONFIDENCE INTERVALS, AND *P* VALUES

We use confidence intervals because a point estimate, being a single value, cannot express the statistical variation, or random error, that underlies the estimate.

If a study is large, the estimation process can be comparatively precise, and there may be little random error in the estimation. A small study, however, has less precision, which means that the estimate is subject to more random error. A confidence interval indicates the amount of random error in the estimate. A given confidence interval is tied to an arbitrarily set level of confidence. Commonly, the level of confidence is set at 95% or 90%, although any level in the interval of 0% to 100% is possible. The confidence interval is defined statistically as follows: If the level of confidence is set to 95%, it means that if the data collection and analysis could be replicated many times and the study were free of bias, the confidence interval would include within it the correct value of the measure 95% of the time. This definition presumes that the only thing that would differ in these hypothetical replications of the study would be the statistical, or chance, element in the data. It also presumes that the variability in the data can be described adequately by a statistical model and that biases such as confounding are nonexistent or completely controlled. These unrealistic conditions are typically not met even in carefully designed and conducted randomized trials. In nonexperimental epidemiologic studies, the formal definition of a confidence interval is a fiction that at best provides a rough estimate of the statistical variability in a set of data. It is better not to consider a confidence interval to be a literal measure of statistical variability but rather a general guide to the amount of random error in the data.

The confidence interval is calculated from the same equations that are used to generate another commonly reported statistical measure, the *P value*, which is the statistic used for statistical hypothesis testing. The *P* value is calculated in relation to a specific hypothesis, usually the *null hypothesis*, which states that there is no relation between exposure and disease. For the *RR* measure, the null hypothesis is $RR = 1.0$. The *P* value represents the probability, assuming that the null hypothesis is true and the study is free of bias, that the data obtained in the study would demonstrate an association as far from the null hypothesis or farther than what was actually obtained. For example, suppose that a case-control study gives, as an estimate of the relative risk, $RR = 2.5$. The *P* value answers this question: What is the probability, if the true $RR = 1.0$, that a given study may give a result as far as this or farther from 1.0? The *P* value is the probability, conditional on the null hypothesis, of observing as strong an association as was observed or a stronger one.

P values can be calculated using statistical models that correspond to the type of data that have been collected (see Chapter 9). In practice, the variability of collected data is unlikely to conform precisely to any given statistical model. For example, most statistical models assume that the observations are independent of one another. Many epidemiologic studies, however, are based on observations that are not independent. Data also may be influenced by systematic errors that increase variation beyond that expected from a simple statistical model. Because the theoretical requirements are seldom met, a *P* value usually cannot be taken as a meaningful probability value. Instead, it can be viewed as something less technical: a measure of relative consistency between the null hypothesis and the data in hand. A large *P* value indicates that the data are highly consistent with the null hypothesis, and a low *P* value indicates that the data are not very consistent with the null hypothesis. More specifically, if a *P* value were as small as .01, it would mean that the data were not very consistent with the null hypothesis, but a *P* value as large as .5 would indicate that the data were reasonably consistent with the null hypothesis. Neither of these P values should be interpreted as a strict probability. Neither tells us whether the null hypothesis is correct or not. The ultimate judgment about the correctness of the null hypothesis will depend on the existence of other data and the relative plausibility of the null hypothesis and its alternatives.

WHAT IS THE PROBABILITY THAT THE NULL HYPOTHESIS IS CORRECT?

Some people interpret a P value as a probability statement about the correctness of the null hypothesis, but that interpretation cannot be defended. First, the null hypothesis, like any hypothesis, should be regarded as true or false but not as having a probability of being true. A probability would not be assigned to the truth of any hypothesis except in a subjective sense, as in describing betting odds. Even in framing a subjective interpretation or in assigning betting odds, the P value should not be considered to be equivalent to the probability that the null hypothesis is correct.

It is true that the P value is a probability measure. When the data are very discrepant with the null hypothesis, the P value is small, and when the data are concordant with the null hypothesis, the P value is large. Nonetheless, the P value is not the probability that the null hypothesis is correct. It is calculated only after assuming that the null hypothesis is correct, and it refers to the probability that the association observed in the data, divided by its standard error, would deviate from the null value as much as it did or more. It can thus be viewed as a measure of consistency between the data and the null hypothesis, but it does not address whether the null hypothesis is correct. Suppose you buy a ticket for a lottery. Under the null hypothesis that the drawing is random, your chance of winning is slim. If you win, the P value evaluating the null hypothesis (that you won by chance) is tiny, because your winning is not a likely outcome in a random lottery with many tickets sold. Nevertheless, someone must win. If you did win, does that constitute evidence that the lottery was not random? Should you reject the null hypothesis because you calculated a very low P value? The answer is that even with a very low P value, the tenability of the null hypothesis depends on what alternative theories you have. One woman who twice won the New Jersey state lottery said she would stop buying lottery tickets to be fair to others. The more reasonable interpretation is that her two wins were chance events. The point is that the null hypothesis may be the most reasonable hypothesis for the data even if the P value is low. Similarly, the null hypothesis may be implausible or just incorrect even if the P value is high.

STATISTICAL HYPOTHESIS TESTING VERSUS ESTIMATION

Often, a P value is used to determine the presence or absence of *statistical significance*. Statistical significance is a term that appears laden with meaning, although it tells nothing more than whether the P value is less than some arbitrary value, almost always .05. The term *statistically significant* and the statement "$P < .05$" (or whatever level is taken as the threshold for statistical significance) are equivalent. Neither is a good description of the information in the data.

Statistical hypothesis testing is a term used to describe the process of deciding whether to reject or not to reject a specific hypothesis, usually the null hypothesis. Statistical hypothesis testing is predicated on statistical significance as determined from the P value. Typically, if an analysis gives a result that is statistically significant, the null hypothesis is rejected as false. If a result is not statistically significant, it means that the null hypothesis cannot be rejected. It does not mean that the null hypothesis is correct. No data analysis can determine definitively whether the null hypothesis or any hypothesis is true or false. Nevertheless, it is unfortunately often the case that a statistical significance test is interpreted to mean that the null hypothesis is false or true according to whether the statistical test of the relation between exposure and disease is or is not statistically significant. In practice, a statistical test, accompanied by its declaration of "significant" or "not significant," is often mistakenly used as a forced decision on the truth of the null hypothesis.

A declaration of statistical significance offers less information than the P value, because the P value is a number, whereas statistical significance is just a dichotomous description. There is no reason that the numeric P value must be degraded into this less-informative dichotomy. Even the more quantitative P value has a problem, however, because it confounds two important aspects of the data, the strength of the relation between exposure and disease and the precision with which that relation is measured. To have a clear interpretation of data, it is important to be able to separate the information on strength of relation and precision, which is the job that estimation does for us.

P-VALUE (CONFIDENCE INTERVAL) FUNCTIONS

To illustrate how estimation does a better job of expressing strength of relation and precision, we describe a curve that is often called a *P-value function* but is also referred to as a *confidence interval function*. The P-value function enlarges on the concept of the P value. The P value is a statistic that can be viewed as a measure of the compatibility between the data in hand and the null hypothesis. We can enlarge on this concept by imagining that instead of testing just the null hypothesis, we also calculate a P value for a range of other hypotheses. Consider the rate ratio measure, which can range from 0 to infinity and equals 1.0 if the null hypothesis is correct. The ordinary P value is a measure of the consistency between the data and the hypothesis that $RR = 1.0$. Mathematically, however, we are not constrained to test only the hypothesis that $RR = 1.0$. For any set of data, we can in principle calculate a P value that measures the compatibility between those data and any value of RR. We can even calculate an infinite number of P values that test every possible value of RR. If we did so and plotted the results, we end up with the P-value function. An example of a P-value function is given in Figure 8–1, which is based on the data in Table 8–1 describing a case-control study of drug exposure during pregnancy and congenital heart disease.[1]

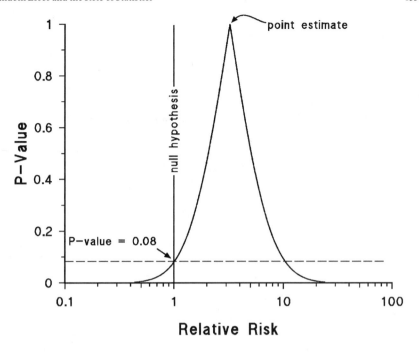

Figure 8–1 *P-value* function for the case-control data in Table 8–1.

The curve in Figure 8–1, which resembles a tepee, plots the P value that tests the compatibility of the data in Table 8–1 with every possible value of RR. When RR = 1.0, the curve gives the P value testing the hypothesis that RR = 1.0; this is the usual P value testing the null hypothesis. For the data depicted in Figure 8–1, the ordinary P value is .08. This value would be described by many observers as not significant, because the P value is greater than .05. To many people, *not significant* implies that there is no relation between exposure and disease in the data. It is a fallacy, however, to infer a lack of association from a P value. The curve also gives the P values testing every other possible value of the RR, thus indicating the degree of compatibility between the data and every possible value of RR. The full P-value function in Figure 8–1 makes it clear that there is a strong association in

Table 8–1 CASE-CONTROL DATA FOR
CONGENITAL HEART DISEASE AND
CHLORDIAZEPOXIDE USE IN EARLY
PREGNANCY

	Chlordiazepoxide Use		
	Yes	No	Total
Cases	4	386	390
Controls	4	1250	1254
Total	8	1636	1644

$$OR = (4 \times 1250)/(4 \times 386) = 3.2$$

Data from Rothman et al.[1]

the data, despite the ordinary P value being greater than .05. Where the curve reaches its maximum (for which $P = 1.0$), the value of RR at that point is the value most compatible with the observed data. This RR value is called the *point estimate*. In Figure 8–1, the point estimate is $RR = 3.2$. As the RR departs from the point estimate in either direction, the corresponding P values decline, indicating less compatibility between the data and these relative risk hypotheses. The curve provides a quantitative overview of the statistical relation between exposure and disease. It indicates the best single value for the RR based on the data, and it gives a visual appreciation for the degree of precision of the estimate, which is indicated by the narrowness or the breadth of the tepee.

For those who rely on statistical significance for their interpretation of data, the ordinary P value (testing the hypothesis that $RR = 1.0$) of .08 in Figure 8–1 may be taken to imply that there is no relation between exposure and disease. But that interpretation is already contradicted by the point estimate, which indicates that the best estimate is more than a threefold increase in risk among those who are exposed. Moreover, the P-value function shows that values of RR that are reasonably compatible with the data extend over a wide range, from roughly $RR = 1$ to $RR = 10$. The P value for $RR = 1$ is identical to the P value for $RR = 10.5$, so there is no reason to prefer the interpretation of $RR = 1$ over the interpretation that $RR = 10.5$. A better estimate than either of these is $RR = 3.2$, the point estimate. The main lesson here is how misleading it can be to try to base an inference on a test of statistical significance, or, for that matter, on a P value.

The lesson is reinforced when we consider another P-value function that describes a set of hypothetical data given in Table 8–2. These hypothetical data lead to a narrow P-value function that reaches a peak slightly above the null value, $RR = 1$. Figure 8–2 contrasts the P-value function for the data in Table 8–2 with the P-value function given earlier for the data in Table 8–1. The narrowness of the second P-value function reflects the larger size of the second set of data. Large size translates to better precision, for which the visual counterpart is the narrow P-value function.

There is a striking contrast in messages from these two P-value functions. The first function suggests that the data are imprecise but reflect an association that is strong; the data are readily compatible with a wide range of effects, from very little or nothing to more than a 10-fold increase in risk. The first set of data thus raises the possibility that the exposure is a strong risk factor. Although the data do not permit a precise estimate of effect, the range of effect values consistent with the data includes mostly strong effects that would warrant concern about the exposure. This concern comes from data that give a "nonsignificant" result for a test of the null hypothesis. In contrast, the other set of data, from Table 8–2, gives a precise estimate of an effect that is close to the null. The data are not very compatible with a strong effect and, indeed, may be interpreted as reassuring about the absence of a strong effect. Despite this reassurance, the P value testing the null hypothesis is .04; a test of the null hypothesis would give a "statistically significant" result, rejecting the null hypothesis. In both cases, reliance on the significance test would be misleading and conducive to an incorrect interpretation. In the first case, the association is "not significant," but the study is properly interpreted as raising concern about the effect of the exposure. In the second case, the study provides reassurance about the absence of a strong effect, but the

Table 8–2 Hypothetical Case-Control Data

	Exposure		
	Yes	**No**	**Total**
Cases	1,090	14,910	16,000
Controls	1,000	15,000	16,000
Total	2,090	29,910	32,000

$$OR = (1{,}090 \times 15{,}000)/(1{,}000 \times 14{,}910) = 1.1$$

significance test gives a result that is "significant," rejecting the null hypothesis. This perverse behavior of the significance test should serve as a warning against using significance tests to interpret data.

Although it may superficially seem like a sophisticated application of quantitative methods, significance testing is only a qualitative proposition. The end result is a declaration of "significant" or "not significant" that provides no quantitative clue about the size of the effect. Contrast that approach with the *P*-value function, which is a quantitative visual message about the estimated size of the effect. The message comes in two parts, one relating to the strength of the effect and the other to precision. Strength is conveyed by the location of the curve along the horizontal axis and precision by the amount of spread of the function around the point estimate.

Because the *P* value is only one number, it cannot convey two separate quantitative messages. To get the message about both strength of effect and precision,

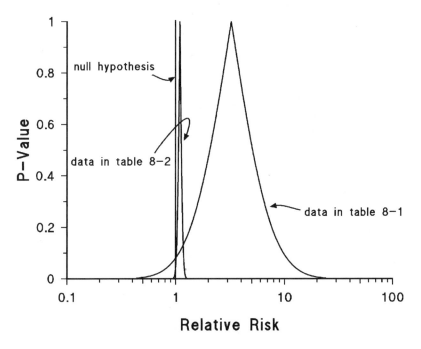

Figure 8–2   *P*-value function for the data in Table 8–1 and the hypothetical case-control data in Table 8–2.

at least two numbers are required. Perhaps the most straightforward way to get both messages is from the upper and lower confidence limits, the two numbers that form the boundaries to a confidence interval. The P-value function is closely related to the set of all confidence intervals for a given estimate. This relation is depicted in Figure 8–3, which shows three different confidence intervals for the data in Figure 8–1. These three confidence intervals differ only in the arbitrary level of confidence that determines the width of the interval. In Figure 8–3, the 95% confidence interval can be read from the curve along the horizontal line where $P = .05$ and the 90% and 80% intervals along the lines where $P = .1$ and .2, respectively. The different confidence intervals in Figure 8–3 reflect the same degree of precision but differ in their width only because the level of confidence for each is arbitrarily different. The three confidence intervals depicted in Figure 8–3 are described as *nested* confidence intervals. The P-value function is a graph of all possible nested confidence intervals for a given estimate, reflecting all possible levels of confidence between 0% and 100%. It is this ability to find all possible confidence intervals from a P-value function that leads to its description as either a P-value function or a confidence interval function.

It is common to see confidence intervals reported for an epidemiologic measure, but it is uncommon to see a full P-value function or confidence interval function. Fortunately, it is not necessary to calculate and display a full P-value function to infer the two quantitative messages, strength of relation and precision, for an estimate. A single confidence interval is sufficient, because the upper and lower confidence bounds from a single interval are sufficient to determine the entire P-value function. If we know the lower and upper limit to the confidence interval, we know the location of the P-value function along the horizontal axis

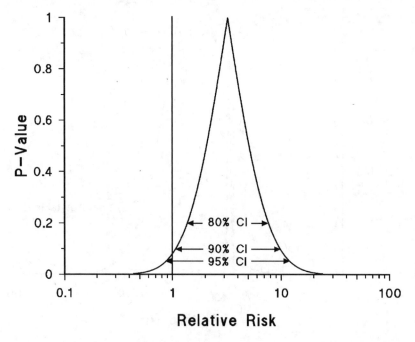

Figure 8–3   *P*-value function for the data from Table 8–1, showing how nested confidence intervals can be read from the curve.

and the spread of the function. Thus, from a single confidence interval, we can construct an entire P-value function. We do not need to go through the labor of calculating this function if we can visualize the two messages that it can convey directly from the confidence interval.

Regrettably, confidence intervals are too often not interpreted with the image of the corresponding P-value function in mind. A confidence interval can unfortunately be used as a surrogate test of statistical significance: a confidence interval that contains the null value within it corresponds to a significance test that is "not significant," and a confidence interval that excludes the null value corresponds to a significance test that is "significant." The allure of significance testing is so strong that many people use a confidence interval merely to determine "significance" and thereby ignore the potentially useful quantitative information that the confidence interval provides.

Example: Is Flutamide Effective in Treating Prostate Cancer?

In a randomized trial of flutamide, which is used to treat prostate cancer, Eisenberger et al.[2] reported that patients who received flutamide fared no better than those who received placebo. Their interpretation that flutamide was ineffective contradicted the results of 10 previous studies, which collectively had pointed to a modest benefit. The 10 previous studies, on aggregate, indicated about an 11% survival advantage for patients receiving flutamide [odds ratio $(OR) = 0.89$]. The actual data reported by Eisenberger et al. are given in Table 8–3. From these data, we can calculate an OR of 0.87, almost the same result (slightly better) as was obtained in the 10 earlier studies. (We usually calculate odds ratios only for case-control data; for data such as these from an experiment, we normally calculate risk ratios or mortality rate ratios. The meta-analysis of the first 10 experiments on flutamide, however, reported only the OR, so we use that measure also for consistency.) Why did Eisenberger et al.[2] interpret their data to indicate no effect when the data indicated about the same beneficial effect as the 10 previous studies? They based their conclusion solely on a test of statistical significance, which gave a result of $P = .14$. By focusing on statistical significance testing, they ignored the small beneficial effect in their data and came to an incorrect interpretation.

Table 8–3 SUMMARY OF SURVIVAL DATA
FROM THE STUDY OF FLUTAMIDE AND
PROSTATE CANCER

	Flutamide	Placebo
Died	468	480
Survived	229	205
Total	697	685

$OR = 0.87$
95% CI: 0.70–1.10

Data from Eisenberger et al.[2]

The original 10 studies on flutamide were published in a review that summarized the results.[3] It is helpful to examine the P-value function from these 10
studies and to compare it with the P-value function after adding the study of
Eisenberger et al.[2] to the earlier studies (Fig. 8–4).[4] The only change apparent
from adding the data of Eisenberger et al.[2] is a slightly improved precision of the
estimated benefit of flutamide in reducing the risk of dying from prostate cancer.

Example: Is St. John's Wort Effective in Relieving
Major Depression?

Extracts of St. John's Wort (*Hypericum perforatum*), a small, flowering weed, have
long been used as a folk remedy. It is a popular herbal treatment for depression.
Shelton et al.[5] reported the results of a randomized trial of 200 patients with major
depression who were randomly assigned to receive either St. John's Wort or placebo. Of 98 who received St. John's Wort, 26 responded positively, whereas 19 of
the 102 who received placebo responded positively. Among those whose depression was relatively less severe at entry into the study (a group that the investigators thought might be more likely to show an effect of St. John's Wort), the

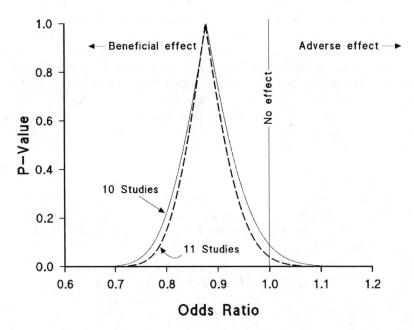

Figure 8–4 P-value functions for the first 10 studies of flutamide and prostate cancer
survival *(solid line)*[3] and for the first 11 studies *(dashed line)* after adding the study by
Eisenberger et al.[2] The study by Eisenberger et al. did not shift the overall findings
toward the null value but instead shifted the overall findings a minuscule step away
from the null value. Nevertheless, because of an inappropriate reliance on statistical
significance testing, the data were incorrectly interpreted as refuting earlier studies and
indicating no effect of flutamide, despite the fact that the findings replicated previous
results. (Reproduced with permission from Rothman et al.[4])

Table 8–4 REMISSIONS AMONG PATIENTS
WITH LESS SEVERE DEPRESSION

	St. John's Wort	Placebo
Remission	12	5
No remission	47	45
Total	59	50

RR = 2.0

90% CI: 0.90–4.6

Data from Shelton et al.[5]

proportion of patients who had remission of disease was twice as great among the 59 patients who received St. John's Wort as among the 50 who received a placebo (Table 8–4).

In Table 8–4, *risk ratio* refers to the "risk" of having a remission in symptoms, which is an improvement, so any increase above 1.0 indicates a beneficial effect of St. John's Wort; the RR of 2.0 indicates that the probability of a remission was twice as great for those receiving St. John's Wort. Despite these and other encouraging findings in the data, the investigators based their interpretation on a lack of statistical significance and concluded that St. John's Wort was not effective. A look at the P-value function that corresponds to the data in Table 8–4 is instructive (Fig. 8–5).

Figure 8–5 shows that the data regarding remissions among the less severely affected patients hardly support the theory that St. John's Wort is ineffective. The data for other outcomes were also generally favorable for St. John's Wort but, for

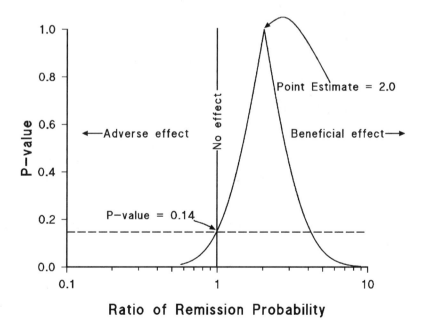

Figure 8–5 *P*-value function for the effect of St. John's Wort on remission from major depression among relatively less severely affected patients. (Data from Shelton et al.[5])

almost all comparisons, not statistically significant. Instead of concluding, as they should have, that these data are readily compatible with moderate and even strong beneficial effects of St. John's Wort, the investigators drew the wrong conclusion, based on the lack of statistical significance in the data. Although the P value from this study is not statistically significant, the P value for the null hypothesis has the same magnitude as the P value testing the hypothesis that the $RR = 4.1$ (on the graph, the dashed line intersects the P-value function at $RR = 1.0$ and $RR = 4.1$). Although the investigators interpreted the data as supporting the hypothesis that $RR = 1.0$, the data are equally compatible with values of 1.0 or 4.1. Furthermore, it is not necessary to construct the P-value function in Figure 8–5 to reach this interpretation. An investigator need look no farther than the confidence interval given in Table 8–4 to appreciate the location and the spread of the underlying P-value function.

SIMPLE APPROACHES TO CALCULATING CONFIDENCE INTERVALS

The following chapters present basic methods for analyzing epidemiologic data. The focus is on estimating epidemiologic measures of effect, such as risk and rate ratios and, in cohort studies, risk and rate differences as well. The overall strategy in a data analysis is to obtain a good point estimate of the epidemiologic measure that we seek and an appropriate confidence interval.

Confidence intervals are usually calculated on the presumption that the estimate comes from the statistical distribution called a *normal distribution*, the usual bell-shaped curve. Estimates based on the normal distribution are always reasonable with enough data. When data are sparse, it may be necessary to use more specialized formulas for small numbers (usually called *exact methods*), but such situations are the exception rather than the rule. A given normal distribution is described with regard to its mean, or center point, and its spread, or *standard deviation* (*standard error* is an equivalent term for the standard deviation in the applications discussed here).

In estimating the confidence interval for an incidence rate difference (RD), we can use basic formulas to calculate an estimate of the standard deviation (SD) of the RD from the data, and from the SD, we can calculate a confidence interval around the point estimate. To calculate a 95% confidence interval, we would add and subtract $1.96 \times SD$ to the point estimate to get the 95% confidence limits. The value 1.96 is a constant multiplier for the SD that determines an interval encompassing 95% of the normal distribution. For a different level of confidence for the interval, we would use a different multiplier. For example, the multiplier 1.645 corresponds to 90% confidence.

We have the following formula for a 90% confidence interval for the rate difference:

$$RD_L, RD_U = RD \pm 1.645 \times SD \qquad [8\text{–}1]$$

In Equation 8–1, RD_L refers to the lower confidence limit, obtained using the minus sign, and RD_U refers to the upper confidence limit, obtained by using the

---

STATISTICAL SIGNIFICANCE TESTING VERSUS ESTIMATION

Statistical significance testing is so ingrained that it is almost ubiquitous. Even those who acknowledge the impropriety of basing a conclusion on the results of a statistical significance test often fall into the bad habit of equating a lack of significance with a lack of effect and the presence of significance with "proof" of an effect. Significance testing evaluates only one theory that is an alternative to causation to explain the data, the theory that chance accounts for the findings. Nonchance alternative theories, such as confounding, selection bias, and bias from measurement error, are all more important to consider. For example, if an investigator finds a nonsignificant result and consequently does not explore it further, he or she may be ignoring an important and even strong association that has been underestimated because of confounding or nondifferential misclassification. To evaluate these issues, it is crucial to take a quantitative view of the data and their interpretation. That is, it is essential to think in terms of estimation rather than testing.

Significance testing is qualitative, not quantitative. When P values are calculated, they are often reported using inequalities, such as $P < .05$, rather than equalities, such as $P = .023$. Nothing is gained by converting the continuous P-value measure into a dichotomy, but even the numeric P value is far inferior to an estimate of effect, such as that obtained from a confidence interval. Estimation using confidence intervals allows the investigator to quantify separately the strength of a relation and the precision of an estimate and to reach a more reasonable interpretation. The key issue in interpreting a confidence interval is not to take the limits of the interval too literally. Instead of sharp demarcation boundaries, they should be considered gray zones. Ideally, a confidence interval should be viewed as a tool to conjure up an image of the full P-value function, a smooth curve with no boundary on the estimate. In most instances, there is no need for any test of statistical significance to be calculated, reported, or relied on, and we are much better off without them.

---

plus sign. We use the point estimate of RD as the center point for the interval. If 95% confidence limits had been desired, the value 1.96 could be substituted for 1.645. The values for the RD point estimate and for the SD would be calculated from the data, as is demonstrated in subsequent chapters.

Equation 8–1 is the same general form that would be used to calculate risk differences or rate differences. We modify this equation slightly, however, when we estimate risk or rate ratios. The reason is that for small or moderate amounts of data, the distribution of ratio measures is asymmetrically skewed toward large values. To counteract the skewness, it is customary to set the confidence limits on the log scale (ie, after a logarithmic transformation). For the RR, we can use the following equation to determine a 90% confidence interval.

$$\ln(RR_{L}), \ln(RR_{U}) = \ln(RR) \pm 1.645 \times SD(\ln(RR))$$

The term ln() refers to the natural logarithm transformation. A natural logarithm is a logarithm using the base $e \approx 2.7183$. Because this equation gives confidence limits on the log scale, the limits need to be converted back to the RR scale after they are calculated, by reversing the transformation, which involves taking antilogarithms. The whole process can be summarized by Equation 8–2 (for a 90% confidence interval):

$$RR_L, RR_U = e^{(\ln(RR)\pm1.645\times SD(\ln(RR)))} \qquad [8-2]$$

In the next chapter, we apply these equations to the analysis of simple epidemiologic data.

QUESTIONS

1. Why should confidence intervals and P values have a different interpretation in a case-control study or a cohort study than a randomized experiment? What is the effect of the difference on the interpretation?

2. Which has more interpretive value, a confidence interval, a P value, or a statement about statistical significance? Explain.

3. In what way is a P value inherently confounded?

4. What are the two main messages that should come with a statistical estimate? How are these two messages conveyed by a P-value function?

5. Suppose that a study showed that former professional football players experienced a rate ratio for coronary heart disease of 3.0 compared with science teachers of the same age and sex, with a 90% confidence interval of 1.0 to 9.0. Sketch the P-value function. What is your interpretation of this finding, presuming that there is no confounding or other obvious bias that distorts the results?

6. One argument sometimes offered in favor of statistical significance testing is that it is often necessary to come to a yes-or-no decision about the effect of a given exposure or therapy. Significance testing has the apparent benefit of providing a dichotomous interpretation that could be used to make a yes-or-no decision. Comment on the validity of the argument that a decision is sometimes needed based on a research study. What would be the pros and cons of using statistical significance to judge whether an exposure or a therapy has an effect?

7. Are confidence intervals always symmetric around the point estimate? Why or why not?

8. What is the problem with using a confidence interval to determine whether or not the null value lies within the interval?

9. Consider two study designs, A and B, that are identical apart from the study size. Study A is planned to be much larger than study B. If both studies are conducted, which of the following statements is correct? (1) The 90% confidence interval for the rate ratio from study A has a greater probability of including the true rate ratio value than the 90% confidence interval from study B. (2) The 90% confidence interval for the rate ratio from study A has a smaller probability of including the true rate ratio value than the 90% confidence interval from study B. (3) The 90% confidence intervals for the rates ratio from study A and study B have equal probabilities of including the true rate ratio value. Before answering, be sure to take into account the fact that no study is without some bias.

REFERENCES

1. Rothman KJ, Fyler DC, Goldblatt A, et al. Exogenous hormones and other drug exposures of children with congenital heart disease. *Am J Epidemiol.* 1979;109:433–439.
2. Eisenberger MA, Blumenstein BA, Crawford ED, et al. Bilateral orchiectomy with or without flutamide for metastatic prostate cancer. *N Engl J Med.* 1998;339:1036–1042.
3. Prostate Cancer Trialists' Collaborative Group. Maximum androgen blockade in advanced prostate cancer: an overview of 22 randomised trials with 3283 deaths in 5710 patients. *Lancet.* 1995;346:265–269.
4. Rothman KJ, Johnson ES, Sugano DS. Is flutamide effective in patients with bilateral orchiectomy? *Lancet.* 1999;353:1184.
5. Shelton RC, Keller MB, Gelenberg A, et al. Effectiveness of St John's wort in major depression: a randomized controlled trial. *JAMA.* 2001;285:1978–1986.

9

Analyzing Simple Epidemiologic Data

This chapter provides the statistical tools to analyze simple epidemiologic data, such as crude data from a study with no confounding. Because our emphasis is on estimation rather than statistical significance testing, we concentrate on formulas for obtaining confidence intervals for basic epidemiologic measures, although we also include formulas to derive P values.

The equations presented in this chapter give only approximate results and are valid only for data with sufficiently large numbers. More accurate estimates can be obtained by using what is called *exact* methods. It is difficult to determine a precise threshold of data above which we can say that the approximate results are good enough and below which we would say that exact calculations are needed. Fortunately, even for studies with modest numbers, the interpretation of results rarely changes when exact rather than approximate results are used to estimate confidence intervals. For those who inappropriately place emphasis on whether a confidence interval contains the null value (thereby converting the confidence interval into a statistical test), it may appear to matter if the limit changes its value slightly with a different equation and the limit is near the null value—a situation equivalent to being on the borderline of statistical significance. As explained in the previous chapter, however, placing emphasis on the exact location of a confidence interval, equivalent to placing emphasis on statistical significance, is an inappropriate and potentially misleading way to interpret data. With proper interpretation, which ignores the precise location of a confidence limit and instead considers the general width and location of an interval, the difference between results from approximate and exact formulas becomes much less important.

CONFIDENCE INTERVALS FOR MEASURES OF DISEASE FREQUENCY

Risk Data and Prevalence Data

Suppose we observe that 20 people of 100 become ill with influenza during the winter season. We would estimate the risk, R, of influenza to be 20/100, or 0.2.

To obtain a confidence interval, we need to apply a statistical model. For risk data or prevalence data, the model usually applied is the binomial model. To use the model to obtain a confidence interval, it helps to have some simple notation. We can use a to represent cases and N to represent people at risk. Using this notation, our estimate of risk is the number of cases divided by the total number of people at risk: $R = a/N$. We can obtain a confidence interval from the following equation:

$$R_L, R_U = R \pm Z \cdot SE(R) \qquad [9-1]$$

In Equation 9–1, the minus sign is used to obtain the lower confidence limit and the plus sign is used to obtain the upper confidence limit. Z is a fixed value, taken from the standard normal distribution, that determines the confidence level. If Z is set at 1.645, the result is a 90% confidence interval; if it is set at 1.96, the result is a 95% confidence interval. $SE(R)$ is the *standard error* of R. The standard error is a measure of the statistical variability of the estimate. Under the binomial model, the standard error of R would be

$$SE(R) = \sqrt{\frac{a(N-a)}{N^3}}$$

Example: Confidence Limits for a Risk or Prevalence

Using the following equation with the example of 20 cases of influenza among 100 people, we can calculate a 90% confidence interval for the risk as follows. The lower bound would be

$$R_L = R - Z \cdot SE(R) = 0.20 - 1.645 \cdot \sqrt{\frac{20 \cdot 80}{100^3}} = 0.13$$

The upper bound could be obtained by substituting a plus sign for the minus sign in the calculation. Making this substitution gives a value 0.27 for the upper bound. With 20 influenza cases in a population of 100 at risk, the 90% confidence interval for the risk estimate of 0.2 is 0.13 to 0.27.

Incidence Rate Data

For incidence rate data, we use a to represent cases and PT to represent person-time. Although the notation is similar to that for risk data, these data differ conceptually and statistically from the binomial model used to describe risk data. For binomial data, the number of cases cannot exceed the total number of people at risk. In contrast, for rate data, the denominator does not relate to a specific number of people but rather to a time total. We do not know from the value of the person-time denominator, PT, how many people might have contributed time.

For statistical purposes, we invoke a model for incidence rate data that allows the number of cases to vary without any upper limit. It is the Poisson model.

We take a/PT as the estimate of the disease rate, and we calculate a confidence interval for the rate using Equation 9–1 with the following standard error:

$$SE(R) = \sqrt{\frac{a}{PT^2}}$$

Do Rates Always Describe Population Samples?

Some theoreticians propose that if a rate or risk is measured in an entire population, there is no point to calculating a confidence interval, because a confidence interval is intended to convey only the imprecision that comes from taking a sample from a population. According to this reasoning, if the entire population is measured instead of a sample, there is no sampling error to worry about and therefore no confidence interval to compute. There is another side to this argument, however. Others hold that even if the rate or risk is measured in an entire population, that population represents only a sample of people from a hypothetical superpopulation. In other words, the study population, even if enumerated completely without any sampling, represents merely a biologic sample of a larger set of people; therefore, a confidence interval is justified.

The validity of each argument may depend on the context. If one is measuring voter preference, it is the actual population in which one is interested, and the first argument is reasonable. For biologic phenomena, however, what happens in an actual population may be of less interest than the biologic norm that describes the superpopulation. Therefore, for biologic phenomena the second argument is more compelling.

Example: Confidence Limits for an Incidence Rate

Consider as an example a cancer incidence rate estimated from a registry that reports 8 cases of astrocytoma among 85,000 person-years at risk. The rate is 8/85,000 person-years, or 9.4 cases/100,000 person-years. A lower 90% confidence limit for the rate would be estimated as

$$R_L = R - Z \cdot SE(R) = \frac{8}{85,000 \text{ person-years}} - 1.645 \cdot \sqrt{\frac{8}{(85,000 \text{ person-years})^2}}$$

$$= 3.9/100,000 \text{ person-years}$$

Using the plus sign instead of the minus sign in the equation gives 14.9/100,000 person-years for the upper bound.

CONFIDENCE INTERVALS FOR MEASURES OF EFFECT

Studies that measure the effect of an exposure involve the comparison of two or more groups. Cohort studies may be conducted using a fixed follow-up period for each person. These studies allow direct calculation of risks, which may then be compared. Alternatively, cohort studies may allow for different follow-up times for each person, giving rise to data from which incidence rates may be estimated and compared. Case-control studies also come in more than one variety, depending on how the controls are sampled. Usually, the analysis of case-control studies is based on a single underlying statistical model that describes the statistical behavior of the odds ratio. Prevalence data, obtained from surveys or cross-sectional studies, usually may be treated as risk data for statistical analysis because, like risk data, they are expressed as proportions. Similarly, case-fatality rates, which are more aptly described as data on risk of death among those with a given disease, may usually be treated as risk data.

Cohort Studies with Risk Data or Prevalence Data

Consider a cohort study of a dichotomous exposure, classified into exposed and unexposed. If the study followed all subjects for a fixed period of time and there were no important competing risks and no confounding, we could display the essential data as follows:

	Exposed	**Unexposed**
Cases	a	b
People at risk	N_1	N_0

From this table, it is easy to estimate the risk difference, RD, and the risk ratio, RR:

$$RD = \frac{a}{N_1} - \frac{b}{N_0}$$

and

$$RR = \frac{a}{N_1} \Big/ \frac{b}{N_0}$$

To apply Equation 8–1 and 8–2 to get confidence intervals for the risk difference and the risk ratio, we need formulas for the standard error of the RD and the $\ln(RR)$:

$$SE(RD) = \sqrt{\frac{a(N_1 - a)}{N_1^{\,3}} + \frac{b(N_0 - b)}{N_0^{\,3}}} \qquad [9\text{--}2]$$

and

$$SE(\ln(RR)) = \sqrt{\frac{1}{a} - \frac{1}{N_1} + \frac{1}{b} - \frac{1}{N_0}} \qquad [9\text{--}3]$$

Example: Confidence Limits for Risk Difference and Risk Ratio

As an example of risk data, consider Table 9–1, which describes recurrence risks among women with breast cancer treated either with tamoxifen or with a combination of tamoxifen and radiotherapy. From the data in Table 9–1, we can calculate a risk of recurrence of $321/686 = 0.47$ among women treated with tamoxifen and radiotherapy and a risk of $411/689 = 0.60$ among women treated with tamoxifen alone. The risk difference is $0.47 - 0.60 = -0.13$, with the minus sign indicating that the treatment group receiving both tamoxifen and radiotherapy had the lower risk. To obtain a 90% confidence interval for this estimate of risk difference, we use Equation 8–1 and 9–2 as follows:

$$RD_L = -0.13 - 1.645 \cdot \sqrt{\frac{321 \cdot 365}{686^3} + \frac{411 \cdot 278}{689^3}}$$

$$= -0.13 - 1.645 \cdot 0.027 = -0.17$$

$$RD_U = -0.13 + 1.645 \cdot \sqrt{\frac{321 \cdot 365}{686^3} + \frac{411 \cdot 278}{689^3}}$$

$$= -0.13 + 1.645 \cdot 0.027 = -0.08$$

This calculation gives 90% confidence limits around −0.13 of −0.17 and −0.08. The 90% confidence interval for the risk difference ranges from a risk that is 17% lower in absolute terms to a risk that is 8% lower in absolute terms for women receiving the combined tamoxifen and radiotherapy treatment.

We can also compute the risk ratio and its confidence interval from the same data. The risk ratio is $(321/686)/(411/689) = 0.78$, indicating that the group receiving combined treatment faces a risk of recurrence that is 22% lower $(1 - 0.78)$ relative to the risk of recurrence among women receiving tamoxifen alone. The 90% lower confidence bound for the risk ratio is calculated as follows:

$$RR_L = e^{\ln(0.78) - 1.645 \cdot \sqrt{\frac{1}{321} - \frac{1}{686} + \frac{1}{411} - \frac{1}{689}}}$$

$$= e^{-0.24 - 1.645 \cdot 0.051} = e^{-0.327} = 0.72$$

Substituting a plus sign for the minus sign before the Z multiplier of 1.645 gives 0.85 for the upper limit. The 90% confidence interval for the risk ratio estimate of

Table 9–1 RISK OF RECURRENCE OF BREAST CANCER IN
A RANDOMIZED TRIAL OF WOMEN TREATED WITH TAMOXIFEN
AND RADIOTHERAPY OR TAMOXIFEN ALONE

	Tamoxifen and Radiotherapy	Tamoxifen Only
Women with recurrence	321	411
Total women treated	686	689

Data from Feychting et al.[1]

0.78 is 0.72 to 0.85, which is equivalent to saying that the benefit of combined treatment ranges from a 28% lower risk to a 15% lower risk, measured in relative terms. (It is common when describing a reduced risk to convert the risk ratio to a relative decrease in risk by subtracting the risk ratio from unity; a lower limit for the risk ratio equal to 0.72 indicates a 28% lower risk because $1 - 0.72 = 0.28$, or 28%.) Keep in mind that these percentages indicate a risk measured in relation to the risk among those receiving tamoxifen alone: the 28% lower limit refers to a risk that is 28% lower than the risk among those receiving tamoxifen alone.

CONFIDENCE INTERVALS VERSUS CONFIDENCE LIMITS

A *confidence interval* is a range of values about a point estimate that indicates the degree of statistical precision that describes the estimate. The level of confidence is set arbitrarily, but for any given level of confidence, the width of the interval expresses the precision of the measurement. A wider interval implies less precision, and a narrower interval implies more precision. The upper and lower boundaries of the interval are the *confidence limits*.

Cohort Studies with Incidence Rate Data

For cohort studies that measure incidence rates, we use the following notation:

	Exposed	Unexposed
Cases	a	b
People-time at risk	PT_1	PT_0

The incidence rate among exposed is a/PT_1, and that among unexposed is b/PT_0. To obtain confidence intervals for the incidence rate difference (*ID*), $a/PT_1 - b/PT_0$, and the incidence rate ratio (*IR*), $(a/PT_1)/(b/PT_0)$, we use the following equations for the standard error of the rate difference and the logarithm of the incidence rate ratio:

$$SE(ID) = \sqrt{\frac{a}{PT_1^2} + \frac{b}{PT_0^2}} \qquad [9\text{--}4]$$

$$SE(\ln(IR)) = \sqrt{\frac{1}{a} + \frac{1}{b}} \qquad [9\text{--}5]$$

Example: Confidence Limits for Incidence Rate Difference and Incidence Rate Ratio

The data in Table 9–2 are taken from a study by Feychting et al.[1] that compared cancer occurrence among the blind with occurrence among those who were not blind but had severe visual impairment. The study hypothesis was that a high

Table 9–2 INCIDENCE RATE OF CANCER AMONG A BLIND
POPULATION AND A POPULATION THAT IS VISUALLY
SEVERELY IMPAIRED BUT NOT BLIND

	Totally Blind	Visually Severely Impaired but Not Blind
Cancer cases	136	1,709
Person-years	22,050	127,650

Data from Petitti et al.[2]

circulating level of melatonin protects against cancer. Melatonin production is greater among the blind because visual detection of light suppresses melatonin production by the pineal gland.

From these data, we can calculate a cancer rate of 136/22,050 person-years = 6.2/1000 person-years among the blind, compared with 1709/127,650 person-years = 13.4/1000 person-years among those who were visually impaired but not blind. The incidence rate difference (ID) is (6.2 − 13.4)/1000 person-years = −7.2/1000 person-years. The minus sign indicates that the rate is lower among the group with total blindness, which is here considered to be the exposed group. To get a 90% confidence interval for this estimate of rate difference, we use Equations 8–1 in combination with Equation 9–4, as follows.

$$ID_L = \frac{-7.2}{1{,}000 \text{ pyrs}} - 1.645 \cdot \sqrt{\frac{136}{22{,}050^2} + \frac{1{,}709}{127{,}650^2}}$$

$$= \frac{-7.2}{1{,}000 \text{ pyrs}} - 1.645 \cdot \frac{0.62}{1{,}000 \text{ pyrs}} = \frac{-8.2}{1{,}000 \text{ pyrs}}$$

$$ID_U = \frac{-7.2}{1{,}000 \text{ pyrs}} + 1.645 \cdot \sqrt{\frac{136}{22{,}050^2} + \frac{1{,}709}{127{,}650^2}}$$

$$= \frac{-7.2}{1{,}000 \text{ pyrs}} + 1.645 \cdot \frac{0.62}{1{,}000 \text{ pyrs}} = \frac{-6.2}{1{,}000 \text{ pyrs}}$$

This calculation gives 90% confidence limits around the rate difference, −7.2/1000 person-years, of −8.2/1000 person-years and −6.2/1000 person-years.

The incidence rate ratio for the data in Table 9–2 is (136/22,050)/ (1709/127,650) = 0.46, indicating a rate among the blind that is less than one half that among the comparison group. The lower limit of the 90% confidence interval for this rate ratio is calculated as follows:

$$IR_L = e^{\ln(0.46) - 1.645 \cdot \sqrt{\frac{1}{136} + \frac{1}{1{,}709}}}$$

$$= e^{-0.775 - 1.645 \cdot 0.089} = e^{-0.922} = 0.40$$

A corresponding calculation for the upper limit gives $IR_U = 0.53$, for a 90% confidence interval around the incidence rate ratio of 0.46 of 0.40 to 0.53.

Case-Control Studies

This and later chapters deal with methods for the analysis of a density case-control study or a cumulative case-control study. The analysis of case-cohort studies and case-crossover studies is slightly different and is left for more advanced texts. For the data display from a case-control study, we use the following notation:

	Exposed	Unexposed
Cases	a	b
Controls	c	d

The primary estimate of effect that we can derive from these data is the incidence rate ratio or risk ratio, depending on how controls were sampled. In either case, the effect measure is estimated from the odds ratio (OR), ad/bc. We obtain an approximate confidence interval for the odds ratio using the following equation for the standard error of the logarithm of the odds ratio:

$$SE(\ln(OR)) = \sqrt{\frac{1}{a} + \frac{1}{b} + \frac{1}{c} + \frac{1}{d}} \qquad [9\text{-}6]$$

Example: Confidence Limits for the Odds Ratio

Consider as an example the data in Table 9–3 on amphetamine use and stroke in young women, from the study by Petitti et al.[2] For these case-control data, we can calculate an odds ratio (OR) of $(10)(1{,}016)/[(5)(337)] = 6.0$. An approximate 90% confidence interval for this odds ratio can be calculated from the standard error Equation 9–6 in combination with Equation 8–1:

$$OR_L = e^{\ln(6.0) - 1.645 \cdot \sqrt{\frac{1}{10} + \frac{1}{337} + \frac{1}{5} + \frac{1}{1{,}016}}}$$

$$= e^{1.797 - 1.645 \cdot 0.551} = e^{1.797 - 0.907} = e^{0.890} = 2.4$$

Using a plus sign instead of the minus sign in front of the Z multiplier of 1.645, we get $OR_U = 14.9$. The point estimate of 6.0 for the odds ratio is the geometric mean between the lower limit and the upper limit of the confidence interval. This relation applies whenever we set confidence intervals on the log scale, which we do for all approximate intervals for ratio measures. The limits are symmetrically placed about the point estimate on the log scale, but the upper bound appears

Table 9–3 FREQUENCY OF RECENT AMPHETAMINE USE
AMONG STROKE CASES AND CONTROLS AMONG WOMEN
BETWEEN 15 AND 44 YEARS OLD

	Amphetamine Users	No Amphetamine Use
Stroke cases	10	337
Controls	5	1,016

Adapted from Petitti et al.[2]

farther from the point estimate on the untransformed ratio scale. This asymmetry on the untransformed scale for a ratio measure is especially apparent in this example because the OR estimate is large.

CALCULATION OF P VALUES

Although the investigator is better off relying on estimation rather than tests of statistical significance for inference, for completeness, we give the basic formulas from which traditional P values can be derived that test the null hypothesis that exposure is not related to disease.

Risk Data

For risk data, we use the following expansion of the notation used earlier in the chapter:

	Exposed	Unexposed	Total
Cases	a	b	M_1
Noncases	c	d	M_0
People at risk	N_1	N_0	T

The P value testing the null hypothesis that exposure is not related to disease can be obtained from the following equation for χ:

$$\chi = \frac{a - \dfrac{N_1 M_1}{T}}{\sqrt{\dfrac{N_1 N_0 M_1 M_0}{T^2(T-1)}}} \qquad [9\text{--}7]$$

For the data in Table 9–1, Equation 9–7 gives χ as follows:

$$\chi = \frac{321 - \dfrac{686 \cdot 732}{1375}}{\sqrt{\dfrac{686 \cdot 689 \cdot 732 \cdot 643}{1375^2 \cdot 1374}}} = \frac{321 - 365.20}{\sqrt{85.64}} = -4.78$$

The P value that corresponds to this χ statistic must be obtained from tables of the standard normal distribution (see Appendix). For a χ of −4.78 (minus sign indicates only that the exposed group had a lower risk than the unexposed group), the P value is very small (roughly 0.0000009). The Appendix tabulates values of χ only from −3.99 to +3.99.

Incidence Rate Data

For incidence rate data, we use the following notation, which is an expanded version of the table we used earlier:

	Exposed	Unexposed	Total
Cases	a	b	M
Person-time	PT_1	PT_0	T

for which we can use the following equation to calculate χ:

$$\chi = \frac{a - \dfrac{PT_1}{T} M}{\sqrt{M \dfrac{PT_1}{T} \dfrac{PT_0}{T}}} \qquad [9\text{--}8]$$

Applying this equation to the data of Table 9–2 gives the following result for χ:

$$\chi = \frac{136 - \dfrac{22{,}050 \cdot 1845}{149{,}700}}{\sqrt{1845 \cdot \dfrac{22{,}050}{149{,}700} \dfrac{127{,}650}{149{,}700}}} = \frac{136 - 271.76}{\sqrt{231.73}} = -8.92$$

This χ is so large in absolute value that the P value cannot be readily calculated. The P value corresponding to a χ of -8.92 is much smaller than 10^{-20}, implying that the data are not readily consistent with a chance explanation.

Case-Control Data

For case-control data, we can apply Equation 9–7 to the data in Table 9–3.

$$\chi = \frac{10 - \dfrac{15 \cdot 347}{1368}}{\sqrt{\dfrac{15 \cdot 1353 \cdot 347 \cdot 1021}{1368^2 \cdot 1367}}} = \frac{10 - 3.80}{\sqrt{2.81}} = 3.70$$

From the appendix table, we see that this result corresponds to a P value of 0.00022.

QUESTIONS

1. With person-time data, the numerators of rates are considered Poisson random variables, and the denominators are treated as if they were constants, not subject to variability. Nevertheless, the person-time must be measured and is therefore subject to measurement error. Why are the denominators treated as constants if they are subject to measurement error? What would be the effect on the confidence interval of taking this measurement error into account instead of ignoring it?

2. The approximate formulas for confidence intervals described in this chapter do not work well with small numbers. Suppose 20 people are followed, and 1 develops a disease of interest, giving a risk estimate of $1/20 = 0.05$.

The binomial model would give a 90% confidence interval for the risk from −0.03 to 0.13. The lower limit implies a negative risk, which does not make sense. The lower limit should never go below zero, and the upper limit should never go above 1. These risk estimates, based on only one case, are too small for these approximate formulas. Instead, exact formulas based on the binomial distribution can be used. Would you expect a confidence interval for risk calculated from an exact formula to be symmetric around the point estimate (0.05), as the approximate confidence interval is?

3. There is another approximation for obtaining the confidence interval for a binomial proportion that comes closer to the exact method. It is an expression that was proposed in 1927 by Wilson[3]:

$$\frac{N}{N+Z^2}\left[\frac{a}{N}+\frac{Z^2}{2N}\pm Z\sqrt{\frac{a(N-a)}{N^3}+\frac{Z^2}{4N^2}}\right]$$

In this formula, a is the number of cases (numerator), N is the number at risk (denominator), and Z is the multiplier from the standard normal distribution that corresponds to the confidence level. The $\pm$ sign gives the lower bound when the minus sign is used and the upper bound when the plus sign is used. Even with only 1 case among 20 people, this formula gives results very close to the exact confidence interval, and its accuracy only improves with larger numbers. What is the 90% confidence interval for the risk estimate of 1/20 using Wilson's equation? If Wilson's equation is so accurate, why do you suppose that it has not been adopted more widely as the usual approach to getting confidence limits for a binomial variable?

4. Why are the estimation equations to obtain confidence intervals the same for prevalence data and for risk data (see Equations 9–2 and 9–3)?

5. Why do the estimation equations for confidence intervals differ for risk data and case-control data (see Equations 9–3 and 9–6), whereas the formula for obtaining a χ statistic to test the null hypothesis is the same for risk data and case-control data (see Equation 9–7)?

6. Does it lend a false sense of precision to present a 90% confidence interval instead of a 95% confidence interval?

7. Calculate a 90% confidence interval and a 95% confidence interval for the odds ratio from the following crude case-control data relating to the effect of exposure to magnetic fields on risk of acute leukemia in children[4]:

	Median Nighttime Exposure		
	≥2 μT	<2 μT	Total
Cases	9	167	176
Controls	5	409	414
Total	14	576	590

REFERENCES

1. Feychting M, Osterlund B, Ahlbom A. Reduced cancer incidence among the blind. *Epidemiology.* 1998;9:490–494.
2. Petitti DB, Sidney S, Quesenberry C, Bernstein A. Stroke and cocaine or amphetamine use. *Epidemiology.* 1999;9:596–600.
3. Wilson EB. Probable inference. The law of succession and statistical inference. *J Am Stat Assoc.* 1927;22:209–212.
4. Michaelis J, Schütz, Meinert R, et al. Combined risk estimates for two German population-based case-control studies on residential magnetic fields and childhood acute leukemia. *Epidemiology.* 1997;9:92=94.

10

Controlling Confounding by Stratifying Data

In an earlier chapter, we saw that the apparent effect of birth order on the prevalence at birth of Down syndrome (see Fig. 7–3 in Chapter 7) is attributable to confounding. As demonstrated in Figure 7–4, maternal age has an extremely strong relation to the prevalence of Down syndrome. Figure 7–5, which classifies the Down syndrome data simultaneously by birth order and maternal age, shows that there is a maternal-age effect at every level of birth order, but no clear birth order effect at any level of maternal age. The birth order effect in the crude data is confounded by maternal age, which is correlated with birth order.

Figure 7–5 is a graphic demonstration of *stratification*. Stratification is used here to mean the cross-tabulation of data; usually, in this context, stratification refers to cross-tabulation of data on exposure and disease by categories of one or more other variables that are potential confounding variables. Another example of stratification was discussed in Chapter 1, which introduced the concept of confounding. Stratification is an effective and straightforward means to control confounding. In this chapter, we explore stratification in greater detail and present formulas to derive an unconfounded estimate of an effect from stratified data.

AN EXAMPLE OF CONFOUNDING

Consider another example of confounding. The data in Table 10–1 are mortality rates for male and female patients with trigeminal neuralgia, a recurrent paroxysmal pain of the face.

The rate ratio of 1.10 indicates a slightly greater mortality rate for males than for females in these crude data. (The male group may be thought of as the exposed group and the female group as the unexposed group to make this example analogous to other settings in which the exposure variable is a specific agent.) This estimate of the association between being male and death among trigeminal neuralgia

Table 10–1 Mortality Rates Among Patients with Trigeminal Neuralgia Categorized by Sex[1]

	Males	Females
Deaths	90	131
Person-years (pyr)	2465	3946
Mortality rate	36.5/1000 pyr	33.2/1000 pyr
Rate ratio		1.10
90% CI		0.88–1.38

Data from Rothman and Monson.[1]

patients is confounded. Table 10–2 shows the data stratified into two age strata, which are split at age 65. The age stratification reveals several interesting things about the data. First, as might have been predicted, patients in the older age group have much higher death rates than those in the younger age group. The striking increase in risk of death with age is typical of any population of older adults, even adults in the general population. Second, the stratification shows a difference in the age distribution of the person-time of male and female patients; the male person-time is mainly found in the younger than 65 years category, whereas the female person-time is predominantly found in the 65 years or older category. Thus, the female experience is older than the male experience. This age difference lowers the overall death rate for males relative to females, because to some extent comparing the death rate among males with that of females is a comparison of young with old. Third, in the crude data the rate ratio (male/female) was 1.10, but in the two age categories, it was 1.57 and 1.49, respectively. This discrepancy between the crude rate ratio and the rate ratios for each of the two age categories is a result of the strong age effect and the fact that the female patients tend to be older than the male patients. It is a good example of confounding by age, in this case biasing the crude rate ratio downward because the male person-time experience is younger than that of the females.

Stratification into age categories allows us to assess the presence of confounding. It also permits us to refine the estimate of the rate ratio by controlling age confounding. Later we will show how to remove confounding for this trigeminal neuralgia example and examples of other types of data by using stratification.

Table 10–2 Mortality Rates Among Patients with Trigeminal Neuralgia by Sex and Age Category[1]

	Age			
	<65 Years		65+ Years	
	Males	Females	Males	Females
Deaths	14	10	76	121
Person-years	1516	1701	949	2245
Mortality rate (cases/1000 person-years)	9.2	5.9	80.1	53.9
Rate ratio	1.57		1.49	

Data from Rothman and Monson.[1]

UNCONFOUNDED EFFECT ESTIMATES AND CONFIDENCE INTERVALS FROM STRATIFIED DATA

How does stratification control confounding? Confounding, as explained in Chapter 7, comes from the mixing of the effect of the confounding variable with the effect of the exposure. If a variable that is a risk factor for the disease is associated with the exposure in the study population, confounding will result. Confounding occurs because the comparison of exposed with unexposed people is also a comparison of those with differing distributions of the confounding factor. In the trigeminal neuralgia example, comparing men with women was also a comparison of younger people (ie, men in the study) with older people (ie, women in the study). Stratification creates subgroups in which the confounding factor either does not vary at all or does not vary much. Stratification by nominal scale variables, such as sex or country of birth, theoretically results in strata in which the variables of sex or country of birth do not vary; in actuality, there may still be some residual variability because some people may be misclassified into the wrong strata. Stratification by a continuously measured variable, such as age, will result in age categories within which age can vary, although over a restricted range. With either kind of variable, nominal scale or continuous, a stratified analysis proceeds under the assumption that within the categories of the stratification variable there is no meaningful variability of the potential confounding factor. If the stratification variable is continuous, such as age, the more categories that are used to form strata, the less variability by age there can be within those categories.

In some stratified analyses, the end result is nothing more than the presentation of the data within each of the strata, with estimates of rates, risks, or effect estimates for each stratum. Often, however, the investigator hopes to summarize the relation between exposure and disease over the strata. The methods that do so compare exposed and unexposed subjects within each stratum and then aggregate the information from these comparisons over all the strata. The two basic approaches to aggregate the information over strata are referred to as *pooling* and *standardization*, representing two different methods for combining the data across the strata.

Pooling

Pooling is one method for obtaining unconfounded estimates of effect across a set of strata. When pooling is used, it comes with an important assumption: that the effect being estimated is constant across the strata. With this assumption, each stratum can be viewed as providing a separate estimate, referred to as a *stratum-specific estimate*, of the overall effect. The principle behind pooling is to take an average of these stratum-specific estimates of effect. The average is taken as a weighted average, which is a method of averaging that assigns more weight to some values than to others. In pooling, the weights are assigned so that the strata that provide the most information, which is to say the strata with the most data get the most weight. This weighting is built directly into the formulas for obtaining the pooled estimate. When the data do not conform to the assumption that the effect is constant across all strata, pooling is not applicable. In that situation, it is still possible to obtain an unconfounded summary estimate of the effect over the strata using *standardization*, which is discussed later.

Cohort Studies with Risk Data or Prevalence Data

Consider risk data; for analytic purposes, prevalence data may be treated the same as risk data. We use the same basic notation as we did for unstratified data, but we add a stratum-identifying subscript, i, which ranges from 1 to the total number of strata. The notation for stratum i in a set of strata of risk data is as follows:

	Exposed	Unexposed	Total
Cases	a_i	b_i	M_{1i}
Noncases	c_i	d_i	M_{0i}
Total at risk	N_{1i}	N_{0i}	T_i

For risk data, we can calculate a pooled estimate of the risk difference or the risk ratio. The pooled risk difference may be estimated from stratified data using Equation 10–1:

$$RD_{MH} = \frac{\sum_i \dfrac{a_i N_{0i} - b_i N_{1i}}{T_i}}{\sum_i \dfrac{N_{1i} N_{0i}}{T_i}} \qquad [10\text{--}1]$$

Σ signifies summation over all values of the stratum indicator i. The subscript "MH" for the pooled risk difference measure refers to Mantel-Haenszel, indicating that the equation is one of a group of equations for pooled estimates that derive from an approach that was originally introduced by Mantel and Haenszel.[2]

The pooled risk ratio from stratified risk or prevalence data can be calculated by Equation 10–2:

$$RR_{MH} = \frac{\sum_i \dfrac{a_i N_{0i}}{T_i}}{\sum_i \dfrac{b_i N_{1i}}{T_i}} \qquad [10\text{--}2]$$

Example: Stratification of Risk Data

The stratification of risk data is illustrated in the example of the University Group Diabetes Program (see Tables 7–7 and 7–8 in Chapter 7). For convenience, the age-specific data are repeated in Table 10–3.

First, we consider the risk difference. From the crude data (see right part of Table 10–3), the risk difference is 4.5%. Contrary to expectations, the tolbutamide group had a greater risk of death than the placebo group, despite the fact

Table 10–3 RISK OF DEATH FOR GROUPS RECEIVING TOLBUTAMIDE OR
PLACEBO IN THE UNIVERSITY GROUP DIABETES PROGRAM IN 1970[3]

	Age					
	<55 Years		55+ Years		Total	
	Tolb.	Placebo	Tolb.	Placebo	Tolb.	Placebo
Deaths	8	5	22	16	30	21
Total at risk	106	120	98	85	204	205
Risk of death	0.076	0.042	0.224	0.188	0.147	0.102
Risk difference	0.034		0.036		0.045	
Risk ratio	1.81		1.19		1.44	

Data from University Group Diabetes Program.[3]

that tolbutamide was thought to prevent complications of diabetes that might lead
to death. Critics of the study believed this finding to be erroneous and looked for
explanations such as confounding that might account for this surprising result. Age
was one of the possible confounding factors. By chance, the tolbutamide group
tended to be slightly older than the placebo group. This age difference is evident
in Table 10–3: 48% (98/204) of the tolbutamide group is at least 55 years old,
whereas only 41% (85/205) of the placebo group is at least 55 years old. Older
people have a greater risk of death, a relation that is also evident in Table 10–3.
Consider the placebo group: The risk of death during the study period was 18.8%
for the older age group but only 4.2% for the younger age group. We therefore
suspect that the greater risk of death in the tolbutamide group is in part due to
confounding by age. We can explore this issue further by obtaining a pooled estimate of the risk difference for tolbutamide compared with placebo after stratifying
by the two age strata in Table 10–3.

We obtain a pooled estimate of the risk difference by applying Equation 10–1:

$$RD_{MH} = \frac{\dfrac{8 \cdot 120 - 5 \cdot 106}{226} + \dfrac{22 \cdot 85 - 16 \cdot 98}{183}}{\dfrac{106 \cdot 120}{226} + \dfrac{98 \cdot 85}{183}} = \frac{1.903 + 1.650}{56.283 + 45.519} = 0.035$$

The result, 3.5%, is smaller than the risk difference in the crude data, 4.5%.
Notice that 3.5% is within the narrow range of the two stratum-specific risk
differences in Table 10–3, 3.4% for age <55 years and 3.6% for age 55+ years.
Mathematically, the pooled estimate is a weighted average of the stratum-specific
values, and it will always be within the range of the stratum-specific estimates
of the effect. The crude estimate of effect, however, is not within this range. We
should regard 3.5% as a more appropriate estimate of the risk difference than the
value of 4.5% from the crude data, because it removes age confounding. The crude
risk difference differs from the unconfounded estimate of risk difference because
the crude estimate reflects a combination of the effect of tolbutamide (which we
estimate to be 3.5% from this analysis) and the confounding effect of age. Because
the tolbutamide group is older on average than the placebo group, the risk difference in the crude data is greater than the unconfounded risk difference. If the

tolbutamide group had been younger than the placebo group, the confounding would have worked in the opposite direction, resulting in a lower risk difference in the crude data than from the pooled analysis after stratification.

RESIDUAL CONFOUNDING

The two age categories for the data in Table 10–3 may not be sufficient to control all of the age confounding in the data. More strata with narrower boundaries usually can control confounding more effectively than fewer strata with broader boundaries. If age strata (or strata by any continuously measured stratification factor) are broad, there may be confounding within them. A stratified analysis controls only between-stratum confounding, not within-stratum confounding. Within-stratum confounding is often referred to as *residual confounding*. The same term is used to describe confounding from factors that are not controlled at all in a study or from factors that are controlled but are measured inaccurately.

To avoid within-stratum residual confounding, it is desirable to carve the data into more strata and to avoid open-ended strata (eg, age 55+) when possible. On the other hand, stratifying too finely may stretch the data unreasonably, producing small frequencies of events within cells and leading to imprecise results. Finding the best number of strata to use in a given analysis often requires balancing the need to control confounding against the need to avoid random error in the estimation and ends up being a compromise.

The unconfounded estimate of the risk difference, 3.5%, is unconfounded only to the extent that stratification into these two broad age categories removes age confounding. It is likely that some residual confounding remains (see box) and that the risk difference that is fully unconfounded by age is smaller than 3.5%.

We can also calculate a pooled estimate of the risk ratio from the data in Table 10–3 using Equation 10–2:

$$RR_{MH} = \frac{\dfrac{8 \cdot 120}{226} + \dfrac{22 \cdot 85}{183}}{\dfrac{5 \cdot 106}{226} + \dfrac{16 \cdot 98}{183}} = \frac{4.248 + 10.219}{2.345 + 8.568} = 1.33$$

This result, like that for the risk difference, is closer to the null value than the crude risk ratio of 1.44, indicating that some age confounding has been removed by the stratification. The pooled estimate is within the range of the stratum-specific estimates, as it must be mathematically. Note, however, that for the risk ratio, the stratum-specific estimates for the data in Table 10–3, 1.81 and 1.19, differ considerably from one another. The wide range between them includes the pooled estimate and the estimate of effect from the crude data. When the stratum-specific estimates of effect are almost identical, as they are for the risk differences in the data in Table 10–3, we have a good idea of what the pooled estimate will be just from inspecting the stratum-specific data. When the stratum-specific estimates vary, it is not clear on inspection what the pooled estimate will be.

As stated earlier, the equations used to obtain pooled estimates are premised on the assumption that the effect is constant across strata. The pooled risk ratio of 1.33 for the previous example is premised on the assumption that there is a single value for the risk ratio that applies to both the young and the old stratum. This assumption seems reasonable for the risk difference calculation, for which the two strata gave almost the same estimate of risk difference, but how can we use this assumption to estimate the risk ratio when the two age strata give such different risk ratio estimates? The assumption does not imply that the estimates of effect will be the same or even almost the same in each stratum. It allows for statistical variation over the strata. It is possible to conduct a statistical evaluation, called a *test of heterogeneity* or a *test of homogeneity*, to determine whether the variation in estimates from one stratum to another is compatible with the assumption that the effect is uniform.[4] In any event, it is helpful to bear in mind that the assumption that the effect is uniform is probably wrong in most situations. It is asking too much to have the effect be absolutely constant over the categories of some stratification factor. It is more realistic to consider the assumption as a fictional convenience, one that facilitates the computation of a pooled estimate. Unless the data demonstrate some clear pattern of variation that undermines the assumption that the effect is uniform over the strata, it is usually reasonable to use a pooled approach, despite the fiction of the assumption. In Table 10–3, the variation of the risk ratio estimates for the two age strata is not striking enough to warrant concern about the assumption that the risk ratio is uniform. If a more formal statistical evaluation of the assumption of uniformity were undertaken for these data (calculating a P value to test the assumption), it would support the view that the assumption of a uniform risk ratio for the data in Table 10–3 is reasonable.

Confidence Intervals for Pooled Estimates

To obtain confidence intervals for the pooled estimates of effect we need variance formulas to combine with the point estimates. Table 10–4 lists variance formulas for the various pooled estimates that we consider in this chapter.

Although the formulas may look complicated, they are easy to apply. Each variance formula corresponds to a particular type of stratified data. First consider the pooled risk difference. For the data in Table 10–3, we calculated an RD_{MH} of 0.035. We can derive the variance for this estimate and a confidence interval by applying the first formula from Table 10–4 to the data in Table 10–3.

$$\mathrm{Var}(RD_{MH}) = \frac{\left(\dfrac{106 \cdot 120}{226}\right)^2 \left(\dfrac{8 \cdot 115}{106^2 \cdot 105} + \dfrac{5 \cdot 98}{120^2 \cdot 119}\right) + \left(\dfrac{98 \cdot 85}{183}\right)^2 \left(\dfrac{22 \cdot 69}{98^2 \cdot 97} + \dfrac{16 \cdot 76}{85^2 \cdot 84}\right)}{\left[\left(\dfrac{106 \cdot 120}{226}\right) + \left(\dfrac{98 \cdot 85}{183}\right)\right]^2}$$

$$= \frac{3.1681 + 7.4879}{10{,}363.7} = 0.001028$$

This gives a standard error of $(0.001028)^{\frac{1}{2}} = 0.0321$ and a 90% confidence interval of $0.035 \pm 1.645 \cdot 0.0321 = 0.035 \pm 0.053 = -0.018$ to 0.088. The

Table 10–4 VARIANCE FORMULAS FOR POOLED ANALYSES

Risk Difference:
$$\mathrm{Var}(RD_{\mathrm{MH}}) = \frac{\sum_i \left(\dfrac{N_{1i}N_{0i}}{T_i}\right)^2 \left[\dfrac{a_i c_i}{N_{1i}^2(N_{1i}-1)} + \dfrac{b_i d_i}{N_{0i}^2(N_{0i}-1)}\right]}{\left(\sum_i \dfrac{N_{1i}N_{0i}}{T_i}\right)^2}$$

Risk Ratio:
$$\mathrm{Var}[\ln(RR_{\mathrm{MH}})] = \frac{\sum_i (M_{1i}N_{1i}N_{0i}/T_i^2 - a_i b_i/T_i)}{\left(\sum_i \dfrac{a_i N_{0i}}{T_i}\right)\left(\sum_i \dfrac{b_i N_{1i}}{T_i}\right)}$$

Incidence Rate Difference:
$$\mathrm{Var}(ID_{\mathrm{MH}}) = \frac{\sum_i (PT_{1i}PT_{0i}/T_i)^2 \left(a_i/PT_{1i}^2 + b_i/PT_{0i}^2\right)}{\left(\sum_i (PT_{1i}PT_{0i}/T_i)\right)^2}$$

Incidence Rate Ratio:
$$\mathrm{Var}[\ln(IR_{\mathrm{MH}})] = \frac{\sum_i M_{1i}PT_{1i}PT_{0i}/T_i^2}{\left(\sum_i \dfrac{a_i PT_{0i}}{T_i}\right)\left(\sum_i \dfrac{b_i PT_{1i}}{T_i}\right)}$$

Odds Ratio:
$$\mathrm{Var}[\ln(OR_{\mathrm{MH}})] = \frac{\sum_i G_i P_i}{2\left(\sum_i G_i\right)^2} + \frac{\sum_i (G_i Q_i + H_i P_i)}{2\left(\sum_i G_i \sum_i H_i\right)} + \frac{\sum_i H_i Q_i}{2\left(\sum_i H_i\right)^2}$$

where

$$G_i = (a_i d_i/T_i) \quad H_i = (b_i c_i/T_i)$$
$$P_i = (a_i + d_i)/T_i \quad Q_i = (b_i + c_i)/T_i$$

confidence interval is broad enough to indicate a fair amount of statistical uncertainty in the finding that tolbutamide is worse than placebo. It is notable, however, that the data are not very compatible with any compelling benefit for tolbutamide.

A confidence interval can be constructed for the risk ratio estimated from the same stratified data. In that case, an investigator would use the second formula in Table 10–4, setting limits on the log scale, as we did in the previous chapter for crude data. The variance for the logarithm of the RR_{MH} can be calculated as

$$\mathrm{Var}[\ln(RR_{\mathrm{MH}})] = \frac{\left(\dfrac{13\cdot106\cdot120}{226^2} - \dfrac{8\cdot5}{226}\right) + \left(\dfrac{38\cdot98\cdot85}{183^2} - \dfrac{22\cdot16}{183}\right)}{\left(\dfrac{8\cdot120}{226} + \dfrac{22\cdot85}{183}\right)\cdot\left(\dfrac{5\cdot106}{226} + \dfrac{16\cdot98}{183}\right)}$$

$$= \frac{3.0605 + 7.5286}{14.466 \cdot 10.913} = \frac{10.5891}{157.88} = 0.0671$$

This result gives a standard error for the logarithm of the RR of $(0.0671)^{1/2} = 0.259$ and a 90% confidence interval of 0.87 to 2.0.

$$RR_L = e^{\ln(1.33) - 1.645 \cdot 0.259} = 0.87$$

$$RR_U = e^{\ln(1.33) + 1.645 \cdot 0.259} = 2.0$$

The interpretation for this result is similar to the interpretation for the confidence interval of the risk difference, which is as expected because the two measures of effect and their respective confidence intervals are alternative ways of expressing the same finding from the same set of data.

As another example, consider again the data in Table 1–2. We can calculate the risk ratio for 20-year risk of death among smokers compared with nonsmokers across the seven age strata using Equation 10–2. This calculation gives an overall Mantel-Haenszel risk ratio of 1.21, with a 90% confidence interval of 1.06 to 1.38. The Mantel-Haenszel risk ratio is different from the crude risk ratio of 0.76, and as discussed in Chapter 1, it points in the opposite direction.

Cohort Studies with Incidence Rate Data

For rate data, we have the following notation for stratum i of a stratified analysis:

	Exposed	Unexposed	Total
Cases	a_i	b_i	M_i
Person-time at risk	PT_{1i}	PT_{0i}	T_i

As we did for risk data, we can calculate a pooled estimate of the rate difference or the rate ratio. The pooled rate difference may be estimated from stratified data using Equations 10–4 and 10–5:

$$ID_{MH} = \frac{\displaystyle\sum_i \frac{a_i PT_{0i} - b_i PT_{1i}}{T_i}}{\displaystyle\sum_i \frac{PT_{1i} PT_{0i}}{T_i}} \qquad [10\text{–}4]$$

$$IR_{MH} = \frac{\displaystyle\sum_i \frac{a_i PT_{0i}}{T_i}}{\displaystyle\sum_i \frac{b_i PT_{1i}}{T_i}} \qquad [10\text{–}5]$$

A pooled estimate of the rate ratio may be calculated as follows. Consider the rate data in Table 10–5. These data come from a study of mortality rates among current users and past users of clozapine, a drug used to treat schizophrenia. Clozapine is thought to affect mortality primarily for current users. The experience of past users, who still have many of the indications for using the drug but who have for various reasons

Table 10–5 MORTALITY RATES FOR CURRENT AND PAST CLOZAPINE USERS,
OVERALL AND BY AGE CATEGORY[5]

| | Age | | | | | |
| | 10–54 Years | | 55–94 Years | | Total | |
	Current	Past	Current	Past	Current	Past
Deaths	196	111	167	157	363	268
Person-years	62,119	15,763	6,085	2,780	68,204	18,543
Rate ($\times 10^5$ yr)	315.5	704.2	2,744	5,647	532.2	1,445
Rate Difference ($\times 10^5$ yr)	−388.7		−2903		−912.8	
Rate Ratio	0.45		0.49		0.37	

Data of Walker et al.[5]

discontinued it, was used as the reference for judging the effect of current use. As for the tolbutamide example, the data are stratified into two broad age categories.

The death rates are much greater for older patients than for younger patients, as expected. Among schizophrenia patients, as for the general population, death rates climb strikingly with age. There is also an association between age and current versus past use of clozapine. Among current users, 9% (6085/68,204) of the person-time is in the older age category, whereas among past users, 15% (2780/18,543) of the person-time is in the older age category. This difference is enough to introduce some confounding, although it is not large enough to produce more than a modest amount. Because the person-time for past use has an older age distribution, the age differences will lead to lower death rates among current users. The crude data do indicate a lower death rate among current users, with a rate difference of −912.8 cases per 100,000 person-years. At least some of this difference is attributable to age confounding. We can obtain an estimate of the mortality rate difference that is unconfounded by age (apart from any residual age confounding within these broad age categories) from Equation 10–4:

$$ID_{MH} = \frac{\dfrac{196 \cdot 15{,}763 - 111 \cdot 62{,}119}{77{,}882} + \dfrac{167 \cdot 2780 - 157 \cdot 6085}{8865}}{\dfrac{62{,}119 \cdot 15{,}763}{77{,}882} + \dfrac{6085 \cdot 2780}{8865}}$$

$$= \frac{-48.864 - 55.396}{12{,}572.633 + 1908.212} = -720.0 \times 10^{-5} \, \text{yr}^{-1}$$

This result is smaller in absolute value than the crude rate difference of −912.8 × 10⁻⁵ person-years, as was predictable from the direction of the difference in the age distributions. The amount of the confounding is modest, despite age being a strong risk factor, because the difference in the age distributions between current and past use is also modest. We cannot say that the remaining difference of −720.0 × 10⁻⁵ person-years is completely unconfounded by age because our age categorization comprises only two broad age categories, but the pooled estimate removes some of the age confounding. Further control of age confounding might move the estimate further in the same direction, but it is unlikely that age confounding could account for the entire effect of current use on mortality.

What is the confidence interval for the pooled estimate? To obtain the interval, we use the third variance equation in Table 10–4:

$$\mathrm{Var}(ID_{MH}) = \frac{\left(\dfrac{62{,}119 \cdot 15{,}763}{77{,}882}\right)^2 \left(\dfrac{196}{62{,}119^2} + \dfrac{111}{15{,}763^2}\right) + \left(\dfrac{6085 \cdot 2780}{8865}\right)^2 \left(\dfrac{167}{6085^2} + \dfrac{157}{2780^2}\right)}{\left(\dfrac{62{,}119 \cdot 15{,}763}{77{,}882} + \dfrac{6085 \cdot 2780}{8865}\right)^2}$$

$$= \frac{78.644 + 90.394}{209694871.6} = 8.061 \times 10^{-7}$$

The square root of the variance gives a standard error of 89.8×10^{-5} person-years, for a 90% confidence interval of $(-720.0 \pm 1.645 \cdot 89.8) \times 10^{-5}$ person-years = -867.7×10^{-5} person-years, -572.3×10^{-5} person-years. The narrow confidence interval is the result of the large numbers of observations in the two strata.

The pooled incidence rate ratio for these same data is calculated from Equation 10–5 as

$$IR_{MH} = \frac{\dfrac{196 \cdot 15{,}763}{77{,}882} + \dfrac{167 \cdot 2780}{8865}}{\dfrac{111 \cdot 62{,}119}{77{,}882} + \dfrac{157 \cdot 6085}{8865}} = \frac{39.67 + 52.37}{88.53 + 107.77} = 0.47$$

This value indicates that after control of confounding by age in these two age categories, current users have about one half the mortality rate of past users. (We have been using the notation of incidence rate in these formulas, but we are actually describing mortality data. This use is legitimate because a mortality rate is an incidence rate of death.)

The 90% confidence interval for this pooled estimate of the mortality rate ratio can be calculated from the fourth variance equation in Table 10–4:

$$\mathrm{Var}[\ln(IR_{MH})] = \frac{\dfrac{307 \cdot 62{,}119 \cdot 15{,}763}{77{,}882^2} + \dfrac{324 \cdot 6085 \cdot 2780}{8865^2}}{\left(\dfrac{196 \cdot 15{,}763}{77{,}882} + \dfrac{167 \cdot 2780}{8865}\right) \cdot \left(\dfrac{111 \cdot 62{,}119}{77{,}882} + \dfrac{157 \cdot 6085}{8865}\right)}$$

$$= \frac{49.56 + 69.74}{92.04 \cdot 196.30} = \frac{119.30}{18067.4} = 0.00660$$

The corresponding standard error is $(0.00660)^{1/2} = 0.081$. The 90% confidence interval for the pooled rate ratio is calculated as

$$IR_L = e^{\ln(0.47) - 1.645 \cdot 0.081} = 0.41$$

$$IR_U = e^{\ln(0.47) + 1.645 \cdot 0.081} = 0.54$$

This confidence interval is narrow, as is that for the rate difference, because there is a large number of deaths in the study. Thus, the study indicates with substantial precision that current users of clozapine had a much lower death rate than past users.

Case-Control Studies

For case-control data, we use the following notation for stratum i of a stratified analysis:

	Exposed	Unexposed	Total
Cases	a_i	b_i	M_{1i}
Controls	c_i	d_i	M_{0i}
Total	N_{1i}	N_{0i}	T_i

The pooled incidence rate ratio is estimated as a pooled odds ratio from Equation 10–6:

$$OR_{MH} = \frac{\sum_i \dfrac{a_i d_i}{T_i}}{\sum_i \dfrac{b_i c_i}{T_i}} \qquad [10\text{--}6]$$

The data in Table 10–6 are from a case-control study of congenital heart disease that examined the relation between spermicide use and Down syndrome among the subset of cases who had both congenital heart disease and Down syndrome. The total congenital heart disease case series comprised more than 300 subjects, but the Down syndrome case series was a small subset of the original series that was of interest with regard to the specific issue of a possible relation with spermicide use.

For the crude data, combining the previous strata into a single table, the odds ratio is 3.50. Applying Equation 10–6 gives us an estimate of the effect of spermicide use unconfounded by age.

$$OR_{MH} = \frac{\dfrac{3 \cdot 1059}{1175} + \dfrac{1 \cdot 86}{95}}{\dfrac{104 \cdot 9}{1175} + \dfrac{5 \cdot 3}{95}} = \frac{2.704 + 0.905}{0.797 + 0.158} = 3.78$$

Table 10.6 INFANTS WITH CONGENITAL HEART DISEASE AND DOWN SYNDROME, AND HEALTHY CONTROLS, BY MATERNAL SPERMICIDE USE BEFORE CONCEPTION AND MATERNAL AGE AT DELIVERY[6]

Maternal Age (years), Spermicide Use

	<35			35+		
	Yes	No	Total	Yes	No	Total
Cases	3	9	12	1	3	4
Controls	104	1,059	1,163	5	86	91
Total	107	1,068	1,175	6	89	95
Odds Ratio	3.39			5.73		

Data from Rothman.[6]

This result is slightly larger than the crude estimate of 3.50, indicating that there was modest confounding by maternal age. We can obtain a confidence interval for the pooled estimate from the last variance formula in Table 10–4:

$$G_1 = 2.704 \qquad G_2 = 0.905$$
$$H_1 = 0.797 \qquad H_2 = 0.158$$
$$P_1 = 0.904 \qquad P_2 = 0.916$$
$$Q_1 = 0.096 \qquad Q_2 = 0.084$$

$$
\begin{aligned}
\mathrm{Var}[\ln(OR_{MH})] = {} & \frac{2.704 \cdot 0.904 + 0.905 \cdot 0.916}{2(2.704 + 0.905)^2} \\
& + \frac{(2.704 \cdot 0.096 + 0.797 \cdot 0.904) + (0.905 \cdot 0.084 + 0.158 \cdot 0.916)}{2(2.704 + 0.905) \cdot (0.797 + 0.158)} \\
& + \frac{0.797 \cdot 0.096 + 0.158 \cdot 0.084}{2(0.797 + 0.158)^2} \\
= {} & 0.126 + 0.174 + 0.049 = 0.349
\end{aligned}
$$

The corresponding standard error is $(0.349)^{\frac{1}{2}} = 0.591$. The 90% confidence interval for the pooled odds ratio is calculated as follows:

$$OR_L = e^{\ln(3.78) - 1.645 \cdot 0.591} = 1.43$$
$$OR_U = e^{\ln(3.78) + 1.645 \cdot 0.591} = 10.0$$

STANDARDIZATION

Standardization is a method of combining category-specific rates into a single summary value by taking a weighted average. The weights used in averaging come from a *standard* population or distribution. The weights define the standard. Suppose an investigator is standardizing a set of age-specific rates to conform to a specific age standard. He or she may decide to use the U.S. population of 2010 as the standard. That choice means that the weights used to average the age-specific rates reflect the age distribution of the U.S. population in the year 2010. Standardization is a process of averaging the rates in two or more categories using a specified set of weights.

Suppose we have a rate of $10/1000 \ yr^{-1}$ for males and a rate of $5/1000 \ yr^{-1}$ for females. We can standardize these sex-specific rates to any standard that we wish. A reasonable standard may be one that weights males and females equally. We would then get a weighted average of the two rates that would equal $7.5/1000 \ yr^{-1}$. Suppose the rates reflected the disease experience of nurses, 95% of whom are female. In that case, we may wish to use as a standard a weight of 5% for males and 95% for females. The standardized rate would then be

$$0.05 \times 10/1000 \ yr^{-1} + 0.95 \times 5/1000 \ yr^{-1} = 5.25/1000 \ yr^{-1}$$

If all categories had similar rates, the choice of weights would not matter much. Suppose that males and females had the same rate, 8.0/1000 yr^{-1}. The standardized rate, after standardizing for sex, would have to be 8.0/1000 yr^{-1}, because the standardization would involve taking a weighted average of two values, both of which were 8.0/1000 yr^{-1}. In this situation, the choice of weights is not important. When rates do vary over categories, however, the choice of weights, which means the choice of a standard, can greatly affect the overall summary result. If the standard couples large weights with categories that have high rates, the standardized rate will be high, whereas if it assigns large weights to categories with low rates, the standardized rate will be low. Some epidemiologists prefer not to derive a summary measure when the value of the summary is so dependent on the choice of weights. Nevertheless, it may be convenient or even necessary to obtain a single summary value, in which case a standardized rate at least provides some information about how the category-specific information was weighted, by disclosing which standard was used.

Although an investigator can standardize a single set of rates, the main reason to standardize is to facilitate comparisons; therefore, there are usually two or more sets of rates that are standardized. To compare rates for exposed and unexposed people, we would standardize both groups to the same standard. The standardized comparison is akin to pooling. Both standardization and pooling involve comparing a weighted average of the stratum-specific results. With pooling, the weights for each stratum are buried within the Mantel-Haenszel equations, and their values are not immediately obvious. The built-in weights reflect the information content of the stratum-specific data. These Mantel-Haenszel weights are large for strata that have more information and small for strata that have less information. Because the weighting reflects the amount of information in each stratum, the result of pooling is an overall estimate that is optimal from the point of view of statistical efficiency. That efficiency translates to a narrower confidence interval for the effect estimate than what would be obtained using a less efficient approach. Standardization also assigns a weight to each stratum and also involves taking a weighted average of the results across the strata. Unlike pooling, however, in standardization, the weights may have nothing to do with the amount of data in each stratum. In pooling, the weights come from the data themselves, whereas in standardization, the weights can come from outside the data. The standard may correspond to a specific population of interest or may be chosen arbitrarily. The study population itself could be chosen as the standard, which will lead to an efficient analysis that will approximate the efficiency of pooling, but the standard is not required to be based on the study data.

Standardization also differs from pooling in that pooling requires the assumption that the effect is the same in all strata (often called the *assumption of uniformity of effect*). This assumption is the premise from which the formulas for pooling are derived. As explained earlier, even when the assumption of uniformity of effect is wrong, pooling may still be reasonable. We do not necessarily expect that the effect is strictly uniform across strata when we make the assumption of uniformity; rather, it is an assumption of convenience. We may be willing to tolerate substantial variation in the effect across strata as a price for the convenience and efficiency of pooling as long as we are comfortable with the idea that the actual relation of the effect to the stratification variable is not strikingly different for different strata. When the effect is strikingly different for different strata, however, we can still use standardization to obtain a summary estimate representing the net effect across strata, because standardization has no requirement that the effect be uniform across strata.

CRUDE RATES AND STANDARDIZED RATES

A crude rate may be thought of as a weighted average of category-specific rates, in which the weights correspond to the actual distribution of the population. Consider age for the purpose of discussion. Every population can be divided into age categories. The age-specific rates in a population can be averaged to get an overall rate. If the averaging uses weights that reflect the amount of the population (or person-time) that actually falls into each age category, the weighted average that results is the crude rate. Algebraically, if each age-specific rate is denoted as A_i/PT_i, where A_i is the number of cases in age category i (i ranging from 1 to K) and PT_i is the number of person-time units in that category, the crude rate is as follows:

$$\frac{PT_1 \dfrac{A_1}{PT_1} + PT_2 \dfrac{A_2}{PT_2} + \cdots + PT_K \dfrac{A_K}{PT_K}}{PT_1 + PT_2 + \cdots + PT_K} = \frac{\sum A_i}{\sum PT_i} = \frac{A}{PT}$$

A is the total number of cases in the population, and PT is the total person-time. The crude rate is a weighted average of the age-specific rates in which the weights are the same as the denominators for the rates: PT_1, PT_2, ..., PT_K. These are the *natural* weights, or *latent* weights, for the population. If we change the weights from the denominator values of the rates to an outside set of weights drawn from a standard, the resulting standardized rate can be viewed as the value that the crude rate would have been if the population age structure were changed from what it actually is to that of the standard, and the same age-specific rates applied. A standardized rate is a hypothetical crude rate that would apply if the age structure were that of the standard instead of what it happens to be.

Although standardization is preferable to pooling when an effect apparently varies across strata, standardization may be desirable even when pooling is a reasonable alternative, simply because standardization uses a defined set of weights to combine results across strata. This characteristic of standardization provides for better comparability of stratified results from one study to another or in comparing different subgroups within a study. Standardization can guarantee that differences in the distribution of the standardized variable cannot account for any differences in the summary measures of the exposure effect. In contrast, with pooling, the weights are different for every summary measure, because they come from the data that are being summarized, and therefore differences between pooled summary measures may be influenced by differences in the stratification variable. We say that pooled measures are internally unconfounded (ie, comparing the exposed with unexposed within the measure) but not externally unconfounded (ie, comparing two different summary measures). Standardized estimates that use the same standard weights are both internally and externally unconfounded.

Consider the data on clozapine use and mortality in Table 10–5. We obtained a pooled estimate of the mortality rate difference, using the Mantel-Haenszel approach, of -720×10^{-5} yr^{-1}. Suppose we chose instead to standardize the rates for age over the two age categories. First we must choose an age standard to use. We might standardize to the age distribution of current clozapine use in the study, because that is a reasonable approximation for the age distribution of those who use the drug. There were a total of 68,204 person-years of current clozapine use, of which 62,119 (91.1%) were in the younger age category. To standardize the death rate for past users to this standard, we take a weighted average of past use as follows:

$$0.911 \times 704.2/100,000 \ \text{yr}^{-1} + 0.089 \times 5647/100,000 \ \text{yr}^{-1}$$
$$= 1144/100,000 \ \text{yr}^{-1}$$

The standardized rate for current users, standardized to the age distribution of current users, is the same as the crude rate for current users, which is 532.2/100,000 yr^{-1}. The *standardized rate difference* is the difference between the standardized rates for current and past users, which is $(532.2 - 1144)/100,000$ yr^{-1} $= -612/100,000$ yr^{-1}, slightly smaller in absolute value than the $-720/100,000$ yr^{-1} that was obtained from the pooled analysis. Analogously, we can obtain the *standardized rate ratio* by dividing the rate among current users by that among past users, giving a result of $532.2/1144 = 0.47$, essentially identical to the result obtained through pooling. The stratum-specific rate ratios did not vary much, so any weighting, whether pooled or standardized, will produce a result close to this value.

Both pooling and standardization can be used to control confounding. Because they are different approaches and can give different results, it is fair to ask why we would want to use one rather than the other. Both involve taking weighted averages of the stratum-specific results. The difference is where the weights come from. In pooling, the data determine the weights, which are derived mathematically to give statistically optimal results. This method gives precise results (ie, relatively narrow confidence intervals), but the weights are statistical constructs that come out of the data and cannot easily be specified. Standardization, unlike pooling, may involve weights that are inefficient if large weights are assigned to strata with little data and vice versa. On the other hand, the weights are explicit. Ideally, the weights used in standardization should be presented along with the results. Making the weights used in standardization explicit facilitates comparisons with other data. Standardization may be less efficient, but it may provide for better comparability. A more detailed discussion of standardization, including appropriate confidence interval equations for standardized results, can be found in Rothman, Greenland and Lash[7] (see pages 265–269 of that text).

In a stratified analysis, another option that is always open is to stratify the data and to present the results without aggregating the stratum-specific information over the strata. Stratification is highly useful even if it does not progress beyond the examination of the stratum-specific findings. This approach to presenting the data is especially attractive when the effect measure of interest appears to change

WHAT IS AN SMR?

When the standardized rate ratio is calculated using the exposed group as the standard, the resulting standardized rate ratio is usually referred to as a *standardized mortality ratio* or *standardized morbidity ratio* (SMR). The standardized rate ratio for clozapine that is calculated using the age distribution of current users as the age standard is an example of an SMR. An SMR can be expressed as the ratio of the total number of deaths in the exposed group, which was 363 in the clozapine example, divided by the number expected in the exposed group if the rates among the unexposed prevailed within each of the age categories. For the 10- to 54-year-old age group, if the rate among past users of 704.2/100,000 yr^{-1} had prevailed among the 62,119 person-years experienced by current users, there would have been 437.4 deaths expected in that age category. Similar calculations give 343.6 deaths expected in the 55- to 94-year-old age category. The figure for total expected deaths is 437.4 + 343.6 = 781.0. The SMR is the ratio of observed to expected deaths, which is 363/781.0 = 0.47. This result is algebraically identical to standardization based on taking a weighted average of the age-specific rates and taking the age distribution of current users as the standard.

The SMR is sometimes claimed to result from a method of standardization called *indirect standardization*, as opposed to *direct standardization*. Direct standardization is what we have been describing as standardization. Indirect standardization is a misnomer. The method is actually the same as direct standardization, but it has one additional feature, which is that the standard is always the exposed group. It is sometimes described differently, but mathematically the calculations are the same as direct or ordinary standardization, with the proviso that the standard is the exposed group.

considerably across the strata. In this situation, a single summary estimate is less attractive an option than in a situation in which the effect measure is almost constant across strata.

CALCULATION OF *P* VALUES FOR STRATIFIED DATA

Earlier, we gave the reasons why estimation is preferable to statistical significance testing. Nevertheless, for completeness, the formulas for calculating *P* values from stratified data are given here. These formulas are straightforward extensions of the formulas presented in Chapter 9 for crude data.

For risk, prevalence, or case-control data, all of which consist of a set of 2 × 2 tables, chi can be calculated as follows:

$$\chi = \frac{\sum_i a_i - \sum_i \frac{N_{1i}M_{1i}}{T_i}}{\sqrt{\sum_i \frac{N_{1i}N_{0i}M_{1i}M_{0i}}{T_i^2(T_i-1)}}}$$

Applying this formula to the case-control data in Table 10–6 gives the following chi statistic:

$$\chi = \frac{(3+1)-\left(\dfrac{12\cdot107}{1175}+\dfrac{4\cdot6}{95}\right)}{\sqrt{\dfrac{107\cdot1068\cdot12\cdot1163}{1175^2\cdot1174}+\dfrac{6\cdot89\cdot4\cdot91}{95^2\cdot94}}} = 2.41$$

This result translates to a P value of 0.016 (see Appendix).

For rate data, the corresponding formula is as follows:

$$\chi = \frac{\displaystyle\sum_i a_i - \sum_i \dfrac{PT_{1i}M_i}{T_i}}{\sqrt{\displaystyle\sum_i M_i \dfrac{PT_{1i}PT_{0i}}{T_i^2}}}$$

Applying this equation to the data in Table 10–5, we obtain the following:

$$\chi = \frac{(196+167)-\left(\dfrac{62,119\cdot307}{77,882}+\dfrac{6085\cdot324}{8865}\right)}{\sqrt{\dfrac{307\cdot62,119\cdot15,763}{77,882^2}+\dfrac{324\cdot6085\cdot2780}{8865^2}}} = -9.55$$

This result is too large in absolute value to be found in the Appendix table, implying an extremely small P value.

MEASURING CONFOUNDING

The control of confounding and the assessment of confounding are closely intertwined. It may seem reasonable to assess how much confounding a given variable produces in a body of data before we control for that confounding. The assessment may indicate, for example, that there is not enough confounding to present a problem, and we may therefore ignore that variable in the analysis. It is possible to predict the amount of confounding from the general characteristics of confounding variables, that is, the associations of a confounder with both exposure and disease. To measure confounding directly, however, requires that we control it: The procedure is to remove the confounding from the data and then see how much has been removed.

An example of the measurement of confounding can be found in Tables 1–1 and 1–2 (see Chapter 1). In Table 1–1, we have a risk of death over a 20-year period of 0.24 among smokers and 0.31 among nonsmokers. The crude risk ratio is 0.24/0.31 = 0.76, indicating a risk among smokers that is 24% lower than that among nonsmokers. As was indicated in Chapter 1 and earlier in this chapter, this apparent protective effect of smoking on the risk of death is confounded by age, which can be seen from the data in Table 1–2. The age confounding can be removed by applying Equation 10–2, which gives a result of 1.21. This value indicates a risk of death among smokers that is 21% greater than that of nonsmokers. The discrepancy between the crude risk ratio of 0.76 and the unconfounded risk ratio of 1.21 is a direct measure of the age confounding. Were these two values equal, there would be no indication of age confounding in the data. To the extent that they differ, it indicates the presence of age confounding. The age confounding is strong enough in this instance to have reversed the apparent effect of smoking, making it appear that smoking is related to a reduced risk of death in the crude data. This biased result occurs because the smokers tend to be younger than the nonsmokers, and the crude comparison between smokers and nonsmokers is to some extent a comparison of younger women with older women, mixing the smoking effect with an age effect that negates it. By stratifying, the age confounding can be removed, revealing the adverse effect of smoking. The direct measure of this confounding effect is the comparison of the pooled estimate of the risk ratio with the crude estimate of the risk ratio.

A common mistake is to use statistical significance tests to evaluate the presence or absence of confounding. This mistaken approach to the evaluation of confounding applies a significance test to the association between a confounder and the exposure or the disease. The amount of confounding, however, is a result of the strength of the two associations between the confounder and both exposure and disease. Confounding does not depend on the statistical significance of these associations, only the magnitude of the associations. Furthermore, a significance test evaluates only one of the two component associations that give rise to confounding. A common situation in which this mistaken approach to evaluating confounding is applied is in the analysis of randomized trials, when baseline characteristics are compared for the randomized groups. Baseline comparisons are useful, but they often are conducted with the sole aim of checking for statistically significant differences in any of the baseline variables as a means of detecting confounding. A better way to evaluate confounding in a trial or any study is to control for the potential confounder and determine the extent to which the unconfounded result differs from the crude, potentially confounded, result.

STRATIFICATION BY TWO OR MORE VARIABLES

For convenience of presentation, the examples in this chapter have used few strata with only one stratification variable. Nevertheless, stratified analysis can be conducted with two or more stratification variables. Suppose that an investigator wished to control confounding by sex and age simultaneously, with five age categories. The combination of age and sex categories will produce 10 strata. All of the methods discussed in this chapter can be applied without any modification to a stratified analysis with two or more stratification variables. The only real difficulty with such analyses is that with several variables to control, the number of strata increases quickly and can stretch the data too far. Controlling five different variables with three categories each in a stratified analysis would require $3 \times 3 \times 3 \times 3 \times 3 = 243$ strata. With so many strata, many of them would contain few observations and would end up contributing little or no information to the data summary. When the numbers within strata become very small, and in particular when zeroes become frequent in the tables, some tables may not contribute any information to the summary measures, and some of the study information is effectively lost. As a result, the analysis as a whole becomes less precise. Consequently, stratified analysis is not a practical method to control for many confounding factors at once. Fortunately, it is rare to have substantial confounding by many variables at once.

STRATIFICATION AFTER MATCHING

When matching is used in study design to control confounding, the matching should be taken into account in the data analysis. As described in Chapter 7, the implications of matching are very different in case-control studies and in cohort studies. In cohort studies, matching on potential confounding factors prevents confounding by creating a balance of risk factors for the outcome in the compared cohort. As a result, the matching can be ignored in the analysis without introducing any bias; matching has done its job in the selection of subjects, which suffices to prevent confounding by the matched factors. Even so, it is worthwhile to take the matching into account in the analysis by stratifying by the matched sets of subjects. Doing so does not remove any confounding, which has already been prevented, but it can lead to narrower confidence intervals than would be obtained if the matching had been ignored.

For case-control studies, unlike cohort studies, matching by one or more factors that are related to exposure will result in selection bias, which must be removed in the data analysis (see Chapter 7). Stratification by the matched sets (each set consisting of a case and its matched controls is an individual stratum) can accomplish this goal. If some matched sets have the same values for all the matching factors, they can be lumped together into one stratum, which may narrow the resulting confidence interval. Usually, epidemiologists employ a specialized regression model rather than stratification to remove the bias introduced by matching in case-control studies. This model is the *conditional logistic* model, which is a version of the logistic regression model that conditions on the sets that comprise a case and all its matched controls (see Chapter 12 for a discussion of logistic models). Conditional logistic models provide the same or almost the same result as stratified analysis, but they have the advantage of allowing the investigator to include in the regression model other confounders that were not matched, something not easily accomplished in a stratified analysis.

IMPORTANCE OF STRATIFICATION

The equations in this chapter may look imposing, but they can be applied readily with a hand calculator, a spreadsheet, or a pencil and paper. Consequently, the methods described to control confounding are widely accessible without heavy reliance on technology. These are not the only methods available to control confounding. In Chapter 12, we discuss multivariate modeling to control confounding. Multivariate modeling requires computer hardware and software but offers the possibility of convenient methods to control confounding not merely for a single variable but simultaneously for a set of variables. The allure of these multivariate methods is almost irresistible. Nevertheless, stratified analysis is preferable and should always be the method of choice to control confounding. This is not to say that multivariate modeling should be ignored; it does have its uses. Stratification, however, is a preferred approach, at least as the initial approach to data analysis. Stratification has several advantages over multivariate analysis:

1. With stratified analysis, the investigator can visualize the distribution of subjects by exposure, disease, and the potential confounder. Strange features in the distributions of the major variables, such as data that have been miscoded during programming, can become immediately apparent. Regression models do not divulge this kind of information as readily.
2. Not only the investigator, but the consumer of the research as well can visualize the distributions. Indeed, from detailed tables of stratified data, a reader can check the calculations or conduct his or her own pooled or standardized analysis.
3. Fewer assumptions are needed for a stratified analysis, reducing the possibility of obtaining a biased result.

It should be standard practice to examine the data by categories of the primary potential confounding factors, that is, to conduct a stratified analysis. A multivariate analysis rarely changes the interpretation produced by a competent stratified analysis. The stratified analysis can keep the researcher and the reader better informed about the nature of the data. Even when it is reasonable to conduct a multivariate analysis, it should be undertaken only after the researcher has conducted a stratified analysis and has a good appreciation for the confounding in the data or lack of it by the main study variables.

QUESTIONS

1. In Table 10–3, the crude value of the risk ratio is 1.44, which is between the values for the risk ratio in the two age strata. Could the crude risk ratio have been outside the range of the stratum-specific values, or must it always fall within the range of the stratum-specific values? Why or why not?

2. The pooled estimate for the risk ratio from Table 10–3 was 1.33, also within the range of the stratum-specific values. Does the pooled estimate always fall within the range of the stratum-specific estimates of the risk ratio? Why or why not?

3. If you were comparing the effect of exposure at several levels and needed to control confounding, would you prefer to compare a pooled estimate of the effect at each level or a standardized estimate of the effect at each level? Why?

4. Prove that an SMR is directly standardized to the distribution of the exposed group; that is, prove that an SMR is the ratio of two standardized rates that are both standardized to the distribution of the exposed group.

5. Suppose that an investigator conducting a randomized trial of an old and a new treatment examines baseline characteristics of the subjects (eg, age, sex, stage of disease) that may be confounding factors and finds that the two groups are different with respect to several characteristics. Why is it unimportant whether these differences are "statistically significant"?

6. Suppose one of the differences in question 5 is statistically significant. A significance test is a test of the null hypothesis, which is a hypothesis that chance alone can account for the observed difference. What is the explanation for baseline differences in a randomized trial? What implication does that explanation have for dealing with these differences?

7. The larger a randomized trial, the smaller the expected confounding. Why? Explain why the size of a study does not affect confounding in nonexperimental studies.

8. Imagine a stratum of a case-control study in which all subjects were unexposed. What is the mathematic contribution of that stratum to the estimate of the pooled odds ratio (see Equation 10–6)? What is the mathematic contribution of that stratum to the variance of the pooled odds ratio (see bottom equation in Table 10–4)?

REFERENCES

1. Rothman KJ, Monson RR. Survival in trigeminal neuralgia. *J Chron Dis.* 1973;26: 303–309.
2. Mantel N, Haenszel WH. Statistical aspects of the analysis of data from retrospective studies of disease. *J Natl Cancer Inst.* 1959;22:719–748.
3. University Group Diabetes Program. A study of the effects of hypoglycemic agents on vascular complications in patients with adult onset diabetes. *Diabetes.* 1970;19(Suppl. 2):747–830.
4. Rothman KJ, Greenland S, Lash TL. *Modern Epidemiology.* 3rd ed. Philadelphia, PA: Lippincott-Raven; 2008: Chapter 15, Introduction to Stratified Analysis, pp 279–280.
5. Walker AM, Lanza LL, Arellano F, Rothman KJ: Mortality in current and former users of clozapine. *Epidemiology* 1997;8:671–677.
6. Rothman KJ: Spermicide use and Down syndrome. *Am J Public Health.* 1982;72:399–401.
7. Rothman KJ, Greenland SL, Lash TL. *Modern Epidemiology.* 3rd ed. Philadelphia, PA: Lippincott-Raven; 2008: Chapter 15, Introduction to Stratified Analysis, pp 265–269.

11

Measuring Interactions

The nature of causal mechanisms is complicated enough that we expect some causes to have an effect only under certain conditions. This principle is illustrated by the observation that even among the heaviest of cigarette smokers, only 1 in 10 will develop lung cancer during their lives. If we accept the proposition that cigarette smoking causes lung cancer, this observation implies that some complementary causes that act together with cigarette smoking to cause lung cancer play their causal role in only 10% of heavy smokers. These complementary causes interact biologically with cigarette smoke. Some form of causal interaction occurs in every case of every disease, so there is good reason for epidemiologists to be interested in interaction. Unfortunately, there is substantial confusion surrounding the evaluation of interaction, much of which stems from the fact that the term is used differently in statistics and in epidemiology.

Knowledge about causal interactions is not just of academic interest; it has important public-health implications. By identifying groups or settings in which interaction occurs, preventive actions can be more effective. Three examples illustrate how knowledge of causal interactions affects public health. First, influenza can lead to serious complications, but those at highest risk for complications are the young, the elderly, and people with heart and lung disorders. These groups can be targeted for influenza vaccination (but also see discussion of influenza vaccine efficacy in Chapter 7). Second, people who do get influenza are sometimes treated with aspirin. A rare but potentially deadly consequence of aspirin therapy is Reyes syndrome, which can also occur without aspirin use but is more likely to occur among youngsters who take aspirin for a viral illness. Rather than deter everyone from using aspirin, which is a useful drug with many indications in adults, epidemiologic knowledge of the interaction between aspirin and age has enabled preventive efforts to focus on discouraging aspirin use only in children. Third, one of the best-known efforts based on a causal interaction is the public-health campaign against drunk driving. Both driving and alcohol consumption are risk factors for injury, but their combination is a much more potent cause of injury than either alone.

EFFECT-MEASURE MODIFICATION

In statistics, the term *interaction* is used to refer to a departure from additivity on the scale used in a statistical model. Because various statistical models use different scales, interaction does not have a consistent, universal meaning; statistical interaction in one model may be different from the interaction in another model based on a transformed scale, even with the same data. The arbitrariness of this concept of interaction has a counterpart in epidemiology in the term *effect-measure modification,* which refers to the common situation in which a measure of effect changes over values of some other variable.

Suppose, for example, that we are measuring the effect of an exposure and that the other variable is age. Consider the age-incidence curves in Figure 11–1. The rate of disease rises linearly with age among those who are unexposed. If it also rose linearly and with the same slope among those who are exposed, as depicted by the other solid line in Figure 11–1, the difference in incidence rate between exposed and unexposed people would be constant with age (ie, the two lines are parallel). In that case, we would say that age does not modify the rate difference measure of effect. Looking at the same two curves, however, we can see that the rate ratio measure of effect does change with age—that is, the ratio of the incidence rate among exposed versus unexposed people is large at younger ages and small at older ages, despite the constant rate difference. The reason that the rate ratio declines with age is the steady rise in rate among the unexposed with age.

Figure 11–1 also illustrates an alternative situation, in which the rate among the exposed increases linearly with age, so that the ratio of the rate in exposed

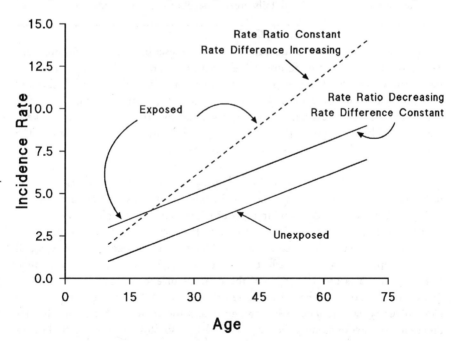

Figure 11–1   Age-incidence curves showing disease incidence increasing linearly with age for unexposed people and two possible linear relations with age for exposed people.

versus unexposed people remains constant with increasing age; this alternative is depicted by the dashed line. In this situation, we would say that because the rate ratio is constant over age, age does not modify the rate ratio effect measure. The rate difference measure, however, does increase with age, as is evident from the increasing distance between the dashed line for exposed and the solid line for unexposed as age increases.

From these examples, it is easy to see that even in the unusual situation in which one of the effect measures is not modified by age, the other is likely to be modified. Therefore, we typically cannot make a blanket statement about the presence or absence of effect-measure modification, because the answer depends on which effect measure is under discussion.

EFFECT MODIFICATION VERSUS EFFECT-MEASURE MODIFICATION

Epidemiologists often use the term *effect modification* to mean what is described here as effect-measure modification. The addition of the word *measure* to the phrase is intended to emphasize the dependence of this phenomenon on the choice of the effect measure and its consequent ambiguity. One cannot speak in general terms about the presence or absence of effect modification, any more than one can speak in general terms about the presence or absence of clouds in the sky, without being more specific as to the details. For clouds in the sky, the details would include the geographic area, the time, and perhaps what is meant by a cloud. In the case of effect-measure modification, the details are in the choice of effect measure.

Consider the hypothetical data in Table 11–1 describing the risk of lung cancer according to two environmental exposures, cigarette smoke and asbestos. What can we say about how exposure to smoking modifies the effect of asbestos? Suppose that we measure the risk difference. Among nonsmokers, the risk difference for the effect of asbestos is $5 - 1 = 4$ cases per 100,000. Among smokers, the risk difference is $50 - 10 = 40$ cases per 100,000, ten times as great. On this basis, we would say that smoking is an effect modifier of the risk difference measuring the effect of asbestos. If we look at the risk ratio measure instead, however, we find that the risk ratio measuring an effect of asbestos is 5 among nonsmokers and also 5 among smokers. In both groups, five times more people with asbestos exposure develop lung cancer compared with people not exposed to asbestos. Therefore, smoking does not modify the risk ratio measure of the asbestos effect. Is smoking an effect-measure modifier of the asbestos effect? It is and it is not, depending on which effect measure we use. This example, like the previous one, illustrates the ambiguity of the concept of effect-measure modification. The example also could be turned around to ask whether asbestos modifies the effect of smoking. The pattern is symmetric, and the answer is the same: the risk difference of the smoking effect is modified by asbestos exposure, but the risk ratio is not.

The ambiguity of the concept of effect-measure modification corresponds directly to arbitrariness in the concept of *statistical interaction*. Some key statistical

Table 11–1 Hypothetical 1-Year
Risk of Lung Cancer According
to Exposure to Cigarette
Smoke and Exposure to
Asbestos (Cases per 100,000)

Smoke Exposure	Asbestos Exposure	
	No	Yes
Nonsmokers	1	5
Smokers	10	50

models used in epidemiology are discussed in Chapter 12. If a statistical model is based on additivity of effects, as an ordinary linear regression model is, the data in Table 11–1 would indicate the presence of statistical interaction, because the separate effects of smoking and asbestos are not additive when both are present. If a statistical model is based on the multiplication of relative effects, as is the case for many popular statistical models used in epidemiologic applications (logistic regression is one example), the data in Table 11–1 would indicate no statistical interaction, because the relative effects of smoking and asbestos are multiplicative. That is, the risk ratio of smoking alone, 10, multiplied by the risk ratio of asbestos alone, 5, gives the risk ratio of 50 for those with both exposures compared with those with neither exposure.

POOLING AND A MULTIPLICATIVE RELATION

A stratified analysis that uses pooling to summarize an effect across strata is based on the assumption that the effect measure is constant over strata. If the effect measure is the risk ratio or the rate ratio, pooling requires the assumption that the ratio is constant over the strata. This amounts to assumption of a multiplicative relation between the exposure and the stratification variable. In Table 11–1, suppose that asbestos is the exposure and the data are stratified by smoking. Within the stratum of nonsmokers, the risk ratio for asbestos is 5/1, or 5. Within the stratum of smokers, the risk ratio for asbestos is 50/10 or 5. Therefore, the risk ratio for asbestos is 5 within each stratum of smoking. The relation is symmetric: if we consider smoking to be the exposure and asbestos the stratification variable, we would find that the risk ratio for smoking is 10 within each stratum of asbestos.

A uniform risk ratio across strata is equivalent to a multiplicative relation between exposure and the stratification variable. As explained in this chapter, a multiplicative relation is evidence of biologic interaction, because multiplicative relations are more than additive. Consequently, pooling over strata to estimate a uniform risk ratio requires us to assume that there is a biologic interaction between the exposure and the stratification variable. This implicit assumption is not necessarily a problem with pooling, but it is a feature of stratified analysis worth keeping in mind.

These examples illustrate the arbitrariness in the terms "effect-measure modification" and "statistical interaction." Both depend on an arbitrary choice of measure or scale. In contrast, *biologic interaction* refers to a mechanistic interaction that either exists or does not exist. It is not a feature that can be turned off or on by the arbitrary choice of an effect measure or a statistical model. Statistical interaction, having an interpretation that is model dependent, cannot correspond to the specific concept of biologic interaction among component causes. For this reason, it is important not to confuse statistical with biologic interaction.[1] Unfortunately, when statistical interaction is discussed, it is usually described as simply "interaction" and is often confused with biologic interaction. Often, the only way to distinguish one from the other is by a careful reading of what is being reported or described. Here, we will use the terms *biologic interaction* and *statistical interaction* to keep these concepts separate.

Biologic interaction between two causes occurs whenever the effect of one is partially or wholly dependent on the presence of the other. For example, being exposed to someone with an active measles infection is a causal risk factor for getting measles, but the effect of the exposure depends on another risk factor, lack of immunity. Someone who has been vaccinated or has already had measles will not experience any effect from being exposed to someone with an active measles infection. The effect is limited to people who lack immunity. Lack of immunity is sometimes referred to as *susceptibility*, a term that in its broadest sense refers to the condition of already having one of two interacting causes and therefore being predisposed to the effect of the other. (Other terms commonly used to describe aspects of biologic interaction include *predisposition, promotion, predisposing factor*, and *cofactor*.)

Another example of biologic interaction is the development of melanoma among those with high levels of exposure to ultraviolet light who also have fair skin. Dark skin protects against the adverse effects of ultraviolet light exposure, whereas those with fair skin experience a much greater increase in risk from ultraviolet light exposure. Many environmental causes of disease interact with genetic predisposing factors. People who carry the predisposing gene constitute a group that has high susceptibility to the environmental factor. For example, people who carry a gene that codes for faulty receptor sites for low-density lipoprotein ("bad cholesterol") have a greater risk for cardiovascular disease from a diet high in saturated fat than do those who do not carry the gene. For these genetically predisposed people, the effect of the dietary exposure to saturated fat interacts with the presence of the gene to cause disease.

A DEFINITION OF BIOLOGIC INTERACTION

How can we derive an unambiguous definition for biologic interaction? We have already described what we mean by interaction between causes in terms of the sufficient/component cause model (ie, coparticipation in a causal mechanism of two or more component causes). Interaction between causes A and B in a given instance corresponds to the occurrence of a case of disease in which A and B both played a causal role. It means that both A and B were part of the causal mechanism for that case, or, in terms of the model, both A and B were parts of the same causal pie. Factors A and B can both be causes of the same disease without any direct interaction, but for that to happen they would have to operate through different mechanisms and would be causes of different cases, rather than acting together as causes of the same case. In other words, suppose that A plays a role in causal mechanisms in which B does not, and vice versa. Under those circumstances, some cases would occur as a result of causal mechanisms involving A, and others would occur from causal mechanisms involving B. In this situation, both factors would act independently as causes of the disease.

With regard to the interaction of factors A and B, there are four possible classes into which all causal mechanisms of the disease fall (Fig. 11–2). The first class (far left pie diagram in Fig. 11–2) comprises those mechanisms in which A and B interact in producing the disease. The piece of the causal pie labeled U refers to the unidentified complementary component causes that also interact with A and B to produce disease. Because U could represent many different combinations of component causes that act in concert with A and B through the same mechanism, we refer to the first pie as a set, or class, of causal mechanisms. Within this class of mechanisms, every specific causal mechanism includes both A and B as component causes. If either A or B were absent in a given person, that person could not get the disease through any mechanism in this class. Cases that occur through these mechanisms would not have occurred if either A or B had not been present. We can therefore say that these cases depend on the joint presence of both A and B.

The second and third diagrams in Figure 11–2 denote classes of causal mechanisms in which either A or B plays a causal role but the other does not. Again, U refers to unidentified complementary component causes other than A or B and could represent various combinations of complementary causes, explaining why each pie is an entire class of causal mechanisms.

The fourth class of mechanisms, often referred to as the *background occurrence*, consists of causal mechanisms that produce disease without either A or B playing any causal role. The solitary U in that pie represents all combinations of causal components that can cause the disease, with the proviso that these combinations include neither A nor B. This background occurrence represents disease mechanisms that are independent of the causal action of A or B.

One way to measure the interaction between A and B would be to measure the risk of developing disease that was caused by mechanisms in which both A and B played a role—in other words, the risk of disease caused by mechanisms in the first class in Figure 11–2. Unfortunately, there is no way to tell, by direct observation alone, which class of causal mechanisms is responsible for an individual

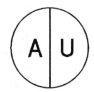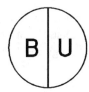

Figure 11–2   Four classes of causal mechanisms involving component causes A and B. U refers to unidentified complementary component causes other than A or B.

case. Even if a person were exposed to both A and B and developed the disease, the disease might have been caused by a causal mechanism in any of the classes in Figure 11–2, and one or both of the exposures to A and B might have been just an incidental characteristic rather than a factor that played a causal role for that case of disease. We can, however, indirectly estimate the risk of becoming a case through mechanisms involving both A and B. We start by measuring the risk among people exposed to both factor A and factor B. Cases of disease among people exposed to both A and B will include cases occurring from all four classes of mechanisms in Figure 11–2. We narrow these down to the first class of mechanisms in Figure 11–2 by subtraction. For simplicity, we assume that all risks are low, and we ignore competing risks.

Let us define R_{AB} as the risk of disease among those with exposure to both A and B. People exposed to both A and B will get disease through all four classes of mechanisms in Figure 11–2. Let us now subtract that component of the total risk for those with exposure to A and B that corresponds to the risk of getting disease from mechanisms that include factor A but not factor B. We can estimate this component by measuring the disease risk among people exposed to A but not to B. We will call this risk R_A. People exposed to A but not B cannot get disease from any causal mechanism that involves B. Therefore, the first and third classes of mechanisms in Figure 11–2 do not occur among these people. They can get disease through mechanisms that involve A but not B and through mechanisms that involve neither A nor B (the background). Therefore, of the original four classes of causal mechanisms, the expression $R_{AB} - R_A$ removes cases stemming from two of those classes and leaves two others: the class of causal mechanisms involving biologic interaction between A and B and the class of causal mechanisms involving factor B without factor A. (For this subtraction of risks to be valid, we have to assume that there was no confounding, which we must always assume when we use the risk or rate in one group to estimate what would happen in another group under counterfactual circumstances.)

Next, to eliminate the class of mechanisms that involve B without A, so that we are left with just the class of mechanisms that include both A and B, we subtract the risk of disease among those with exposure B who lack exposure A. We will designate this risk R_B. This subtraction removes disease mechanisms that involve B without A, but it also subtracts disease mechanisms that involve neither B nor A (the background). Because the background was already subtracted once when we subtracted R_A, if we subtract it a second time with R_B we need to add it back again. We then have the following equation:

$$\text{Interaction Risk} = R_{AB} - R_A - R_B + R_U \qquad [11\text{–}1]$$

Expression 11–1 is a measure that quantifies the risk of disease stemming from causal mechanisms that include both factor A and factor B. Thus, it measures the risk of getting disease through mechanisms in which A and B interact biologically. If this expression is zero, we would say that there is no interaction between A and B, which means that A and B act as causes only in distinct causal mechanisms, rather than acting together in the same mechanism. By setting Equation 11–1 equal to zero, which corresponds to no biologic interaction, we can derive an expression that gives the relation among the risks if A and B are biologically independent:

$$\text{Interaction Risk} = 0 = R_{AB} - R_A - R_B + R_U$$
$$R_{AB} = R_A + R_B - R_U$$
$$(R_{AB} - R_U) = (R_A - R_U) + (R_B - R_U) \qquad [11\text{--}2]$$

Equation 11–2 expresses the relation between the risks under conditions of biologic independence. This equation says that the risk difference between those with joint exposure to A and B and those with exposure to neither A nor B is equal to the sum of the risk differences for the effect of exposure to A in the absence of B and the effect of exposure to B in the absence of A, both compared with the risk among those who lack exposure to both factors (ie, the background risk). In short, the risk differences are additive under independence. (Technically, the converse is not strictly true: although independence implies additivity of risk differences, additivity does not guarantee complete independence between the two causes, because there may be two or more types of biologic interactions that cancel each other and produce, on balance, additivity. Nevertheless, when there is additivity of risk differences, the net effect of the two causes on a population is equivalent to what occurs under biologic independence. For a more detailed discussion, see Chapter 5 in *Modern Epidemiology*.[2])

Because Equation 11–2 involves absolute risks, it appears to be useful only for cohort studies, in which risks can be measured. Is there an analogous expression for case-control studies, from which risk ratios can be estimated but risks and risk differences are not obtainable? To derive an equivalent expression for risk ratios, we need only divide each term in Equation 11–2 by the background risk, R_U:

$$(RR_{AB} - 1) = (RR_A - 1) + (RR_B - 1) \qquad [11\text{--}3]$$

In Equation 11–3, RR_{AB} denotes the risk ratio for those exposed jointly to A and B compared with those exposed to neither factor (for whom the risk is R_U); RR_A denotes the risk ratio for those exposed to A but not B compared with R_U; and RR_B denotes the risk ratio for those exposed to B but not A compared with R_U. All of the risk ratios in Equation 11–3 can be obtained from a case-control study that measures the effect of factors A and B.

PARTITIONING THE RISK AMONG THOSE WITH JOINT EXPOSURE

Equations 11–2 and 11–3 allow us to predict the risk or the risk ratio that would occur under biologic independence for those exposed jointly to two factors. In fact, these equations allow us to partition the observed risk of disease for those with exposure to A and B into four components that correspond to the four classes of causal mechanisms depicted in Figure 11–2.

As an illustration, let us partition the risk in Table 11–1 for people jointly exposed to cigarette smoke and asbestos into its four components. The value of the risk for those with joint exposure is 50 cases per 100,000. From Table 11–1, the risk among those who are nonsmokers and are not exposed to asbestos is 1 per 100,000. This value is the background risk, which is equal to the background component in the partitioning of the risk among those with joint exposure. It means that for every 50 cases of lung cancer occurring among those who were exposed to both smoke and asbestos, an average of 1 of those cases would be expected to have occurred from background causes that involve neither smoking nor asbestos. How many cases would we expect from smoking acting in the absence of asbestos? The risk difference for smokers who are not exposed to asbestos is $10 - 1 = 9$ cases per 100,000. Therefore, among every 50 cases with exposure to both smoking and asbestos, we would expect 9 cases to have occurred from smoking through causal mechanisms that do not involve asbestos. Similarly, from the risk difference for asbestos alone, we would expect 4 of the cases to have occurred from mechanisms involving asbestos but not smoking. These three components add to $1 + 9 + 4 = 14$ cases.

We have so far accounted for 14 cases of every 50 that occur among those with joint exposure. If smoking and asbestos acted independently of one another, we would expect the risk among those with both exposures to be 14 per 100,000. This is the value if there is no biologic interaction. All of the excess above 14 cases in every 50 corresponds to the effect of biologic interaction between smoking and asbestos. This excess is 36 cases out of 50. Therefore, most of the risk among people with both exposures is attributable to biologic interaction between asbestos and smoking. Every 50 cases among those with both exposures can be partitioned into those resulting from the effect of background (1 case), the effect of smoking alone (9 cases), the effect of asbestos alone (4 cases), and the biologic interaction between smoking and asbestos (36 cases). Thus, the data in Table 11–1 show considerable biologic interaction; quantitatively, we can say that 36/50 or 72% of the cases occurring among people with joint exposure are attributable to causal mechanisms in which both factors play a causal role, which is to say that 72% of the cases are attributable to biologic interaction.

As another example, let us consider the risk ratio data in Table 11–2, which reports on the interaction between oral contraceptives and hypertension in the causation of stroke. These data come from a case-control study, but we can use the same approach as we used for the lung cancer data in Table 11–1 to evaluate interaction. The idea, once again, is to partition the effect measure for those with joint exposure into four parts: the background effect, the effects relating to each of the two exposures in the absence of the other (ie, the independent effects of the two risk factors), and the effect attributable to the biologic interaction. The risk ratio for those who are hypertensive and who also use oral contraceptives is 13.6. The background component is 1.0 out of 13.6, because the value of 1.0 for the risk ratio is by definition the value among those with neither exposure. How do we determine the effect of oral contraceptives in the absence of hypertension?

Among those without hypertension, oral contraceptive users had a risk ratio of 3.1, which means that oral contraceptive use increased the risk ratio from 1.0 to 3.1. The difference, 2.1, is the effect of oral contraceptives in the absence of hypertension. Similarly, the effect of hypertension in the absence of oral contraceptive use was $6.9 - 1.0 = 5.9$. That gives us three of the four components of

Oral Contraceptive Use	Hypertension	
	No	Yes
Nonusers	1.0	6.9
Users	3.1	13.6

Data from Collaborative Group for the Study
of Stroke in Young Women.[3]

the 13.6 cases: 1.0 for the background, 2.1 for oral contraceptives alone, and 5.9 for hypertension alone. The remainder, 4.6 cases, represents the part of the risk ratio that is attributable to the biologic interaction between oral contraceptive use and hypertension in the causation of stroke. We can describe the amount of biologic interaction by estimating the proportion of stroke cases, among women with hypertension who also use oral contraceptives, that is attributable to the biologic interaction of these two causes. This proportion is 4.6/13.6 = 34%. The proportion would be zero if the two causes were biologically independent; the fact that about one third of all cases result from biologic interaction between the two causes indicates that the interaction is considerable.

The data in Table 11–2 provide an interesting contrast between the evaluation of biologic interaction and that of statistical interaction. A purely statistical approach to these case-control data would ordinarily fit a multiplicative model to the data, because such models are typically used for the analysis of case-control data (see Chapter 12). Using such a model, we would find that there is a statistical interaction in the data in Table 11–2, but it goes in the opposite direction to the biologic interaction that we have just described. A multiplicative model would predict a value of the risk ratio for women who use oral contraceptives and are hypertensive by multiplying the product of the individual risk ratios for each risk factor alone. The predicted risk ratio for joint exposure in this case would be 3.1 × 6.9 = 21.4, whereas the observed risk ratio for the group with joint exposure was 13.6. Therefore, evaluation of statistical interaction based on a multiplicative model indicates that those with joint exposure exhibit a smaller effect than would be predicted from the separate effects of the two causes. This conclusion is strikingly different from the interpretation that emerges from an evaluation of biologic interaction, as previously shown.

The evaluation of statistical interaction means only that the effect in those with joint exposure is less than multiplicative; it has no biologic implication. The data in this example demonstrate how misleading it can be to examine statistical interaction when the interest is in the biologic interaction between two causes. Use of multiplicative models as the baseline from which to measure (statistical) interaction will lead to an estimate of interaction that is smaller than an evaluation based on departures from additivity of risk differences. In the worst-case scenario, such as in this example of stroke, the two approaches can be so different that they point in opposite directions.

Assessing Biologic Interaction with Preventive Factors

The approach to measuring biologic interaction described in this chapter involves partitioning the cases that have simultaneous exposure to two factors into four subsets, according to the types of causal mechanisms involved. The method assumes that both factors are causes, rather than preventives. If both factors are preventives, or if one is a cause and the other is a preventive, the assessment can be more complicated. It is possible to avoid the complication of preventive factors, however, if one chooses the high-risk category of both factors to be the "exposed" category for that factor, making the group with the lowest risk, considering the combination of the two risk factors, the referent category for comparisons.[4] This technique changes a preventive factor into a causal factor by considering lack of the preventive to be the cause. For example, suppose that a vaccine prevents disease. We could say that being unvaccinated is a cause of disease. Similarly, if regular exercise reduces the risk of cardiovascular disease, we could just as well say that the absence of regular exercise increases the risk. By defining the exposure category so that each factor is viewed as a cause of disease, rather than a preventive, one can avoid the problem of dealing with preventive factors or a combination of causes and preventives in assessing biologic interaction.

Why is it that biologic interaction should be evaluated as departures from additivity of effect? Perhaps the easiest way to understand the connection between additivity and biologic independence is to reflect on the derivation of Equation 11–2, which establishes additivity as the definition of biologic independence. This derivation depends on the concept that we can partition the cases occurring among those with joint exposure to two factors into the four causal subsets depicted in Figure 11–2. Partitioning of a set of objects implies classifying them into subsets that are mutually exclusive and collectively exhaustive, and this is the case for the subsets in Figure 11–2. This partitioning process would not make much sense if one were to invoke scale transformations first. For example, you can partition a collection of colored marbles into subsets by color or by size, but it makes less sense to consider partitioning the logarithm of the number of marbles into equivalent subsets. Multiplicative models typically involve logarithmic transformations of the original scale for which partitioning into the four biologically distinct causal subsets is sensible. It is because the partitioning into subsets can be easily understood only on the original scale in which the cases are enumerated that the definition of biologic interaction is linked logically to that original scale. Because of this linkage, biologic independence is inherently linked to the additivity of risk differences. A more thorough discussion of this topic is given in Chapter 5 of *Modern Epidemiology*.[2]

Although multivariable modeling is not discussed until the next chapter, it is worth noting here that most of the multivariable models in common use for epidemiologic data employ logarithmic transformations. As a result, attempting to evaluate interaction from these models using the conventional statistical

INDEPENDENCE IS NOT A MODEL

Some writers have pointed out that under certain circumstances we should expect to see variables that have a multiplicative relation, and under other circumstances we should expect to see an additive relation. They have used this observation to argue in favor of flexibility for choosing different types of models in epidemiologic analysis. The argument is flawed, however, if it is used to suggest that we should be flexible about which model to use as a starting point for measuring interaction. The main problem is confusion between the goal of modeling, which is to find a succinct mathematical expression to explain the patterns in the data, and the goal of measuring biologic interaction, which requires that we know the reference point from which we are measuring the interaction. The reference point for measuring biologic interaction is additivity of risk differences, as has been shown in this chapter. Taking this reference point as the definition of biological independence is not the same thing as applying an additive model; in fact, it is not modeling at all.

It may be that two causes have a multiplicative relation, as they do in Table 11–1. Nevertheless, even then, the amount of biologic interaction in the data is measured by taking the excess over additivity of effects. Doing so does not amount to the application of an additive model, or of any model, but rather the application of a specific definition of biologic independence. It is important to avoid confusion between modeling, on the one hand, and defining the relation specified by biologic independence, on the other hand. We can be flexible in modeling, but there is less room for arbitrariness when defining biologic independence. In short, evaluating interaction is not the same as choosing a statistical model.

approaches (ie, inclusion of "product terms" in the model) amounts to the evaluation of departures from a multiplicative model rather than departures from additivity. Therefore, statistical evaluation of interaction using these models will not yield an appropriate assessment of biologic interaction. It is possible, however, to use multivariable models to assess biologic interaction appropriately; in fact, it is straightforward. The method for doing so is given in the next chapter.

QUESTIONS

1. Explain why the mere observation that not every cigarette smoker gets lung cancer implies that cigarette smoking interacts with other factors in causing lung cancer.

2. From the data in Table 11–2, estimate the proportion of stroke cases among hypertensive women who use oral contraceptives that is attributable to the causal role of oral contraceptives.

3. In an analysis of the effect of oral contraceptives on stroke based on the data in Table 11–2, suppose that you were interested in the oral-contraceptive effect and wished only to control for possible confounding by hypertension using stratification. What would be the stratum-specific risk ratio estimates for oral contraceptive use for the two strata of hypertension? In an ordinary stratified analysis, why is there a separate referent category in each stratum?

4. Show that if there is an excess over a multiplicative effect among those with joint exposure to two causes, there will also be an excess over an additive effect.

5. The investigators of the study described in Table 11–2 claimed that women who faced increased risk from one risk factor ought to avoid additional risk from another risk factor, regardless of whether the two factors interacted in the causation of the disease. Does this suggestion make sense? What would it imply about seat belt use for women who take oral contraceptives?

6. List reasons why the study of biologic interaction is more difficult than the study of the effects of single factors.

REFERENCES

1. Ahlbom A, Alfredsson L. Interaction: a word with two meanings creates confusion. *Eur J Epidemiol.* 2005;20:563–564.
2. Rothman KJ, Greenland S, Lash TL. *Modern Epidemiology.* 3rd ed. Philadelphia, PA: Lippincott Williams & Wilkins; 2008:Chapter 5, Concepts of Interaction.
3. Collaborative Group for the Study of Stroke in Young Women. Oral contraceptives and stroke in young women. *JAMA.* 1975;231:718–722.
4. Knol MJ, Vanderweele TJ, Groenwold RH, Klungel OH, Rovers MM, Grobbee DE. Estimating measures of interaction on an additive scale for preventive exposures. *Eur J Epidemiol.* 2011;26:433–438.

12

Using Regression Models in Epidemiologic Analysis

The straight line depicted in Figure 12–1 is an example of a simple mathematical model. It is a model because we use the mathematical equation for the straight line that is fitted to the data as a way of describing the relation between the two variables in the graph, in this case cigarette smoking and laryngeal cancer mortality. Models in epidemiology are used for various purposes, the two primary ones being to make predictions and to control for confounding. Prediction models are used to estimate risk (or other epidemiologic measures) based on information from risk predictors. For example, an equation can be used to estimate a person's risk of heart attack during a 10-year period based on information about the person's age, sex, family history, blood pressure, smoking history, weight, height, exercise habits, and medical history. Values for each of these predictors could be inserted into an equation that predicts the risk of heart attack from the combination of risk factors. The model must have terms in it for all the risk factors listed.

In contrast to the goal of risk prediction for specific people, much of epidemiologic research is aimed at learning about the causal role of specific factors for disease. In causal research, regression models are used to evaluate the causal role of one or more factors while simultaneously controlling for possible confounding effects of other factors. Because this use of multivariable regression models differs from the use of models to obtain estimates of risk for people, there are different considerations that apply to the construction of multivariable models for causal research. Unfortunately, many courses in statistics do not distinguish between the use of regression models for prediction of individual risk and the use of such models for causal inference.

The data in Figure 12–1 illustrate an almost perfect linear relation between the number of cigarettes smoked per day and the age-standardized mortality rate of laryngeal cancer. Seldom do epidemiologic data conform to such a striking linear pattern. The line drawn through the data points is a *regression line*, meaning that

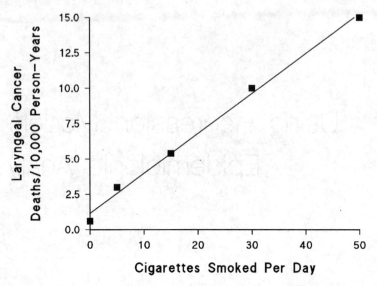

Figure 12–1   Age-standardized mortality from laryngeal cancer according to number of cigarettes smoked daily, derived from data of Kahn.[1] (Adapted from Rothman et al[2] with permission of the *American Journal of Epidemiology*.)

it estimates average values for the variable on the vertical scale (Y) according to values of the variable on the horizontal scale (X). In this case, it is a *simple regression* because it can be described as a single straight line in the following form:

$$\hat{Y} = a_0 + a_1 X$$

$\hat{Y}$ (often called "Y-hat") is the estimated value of Y for any given value of X; a_0 is the intercept, or the value of $\hat{Y}$ when X is zero; and a_1 is the coefficient of X, which describes the slope of the line, or the number of units of change in $\hat{Y}$ for every unit change in X. In the figure, $\hat{Y}$ is the age-standardized mortality rate from laryngeal cancer, and X is the number of cigarettes smoked daily.

The equation for the regression line in Figure 12–1 is $\hat{Y} = 1.15 + 0.282X$. These values refer to deaths per 10,000 person-years. The intercept, 1.15, represents the number of deaths per 10,000 person-years that are estimated to occur in the absence of cigarette smoking. There is also a direct observation for the rate at the zero level of smoking, which is 0.6 deaths per 10,000 person-years. The regression line estimates a slightly larger value, 1.15, than the value that was observed; this estimate is based not just on the zero level for smoking but on all five data points. The regression line slope, 0.282, indicates that the number of deaths per 10,000 person-years is estimated to increase by 0.282 for every additional cigarette smoked daily.

Assuming that confounding and other biases have been properly addressed, the slope value of 0.282 quantifies the effect of cigarette smoking on death from laryngeal cancer. The regression line also allows us to estimate mortality rate ratios at different smoking levels. For example, from the regression line, we can estimate the mortality rate among those who smoke 50 cigarettes daily (equivalent to 2.5 packs/day) to be 15.2 deaths per 10,000 person-years. Compared with the estimated rate among nonsmokers of 1.15 deaths per 10,000 person-years, the estimated rate ratio for smoking 2.5 packs daily is 15.2/1.15 = 13.3. Put in these terms, we can readily see that the regression coefficient indicates a strong effect of smoking on laryngeal cancer mortality.

THE GENERAL LINEAR MODEL

Models that incorporate terms for more than one factor at a time can be used as an alternative to stratification to achieve control of confounding. These models succeed in controlling confounding because when several risk factors are included, the effect of each is unconfounded by the others. Let us consider an extension of the simple linear model in Figure 12–1 to a third variable.

$$\hat{Y} = a_0 + a_1 X_1 + a_2 X_2 \qquad [12\text{--}1]$$

Equation 12–1, like the one for Figure 12–1, has the same outcome variable, $\hat{Y}$ (also known as the *dependent* variable), but there are now two predictor variables, X_1 and X_2, which are referred to as *independent* variables. Suppose that Y is the mortality rate from laryngeal cancer, as in Figure 12–1, and that X_1, as before, is the number of cigarettes smoked daily. The new variable, X_2, might be the number of grams of alcohol consumed daily (alcohol is also a risk factor for laryngeal cancer). With two independent variables and one dependent variable, the data points must now be visualized as being located within a three-dimensional space: two dimensions for the two independent variables and one dimension for the dependent variable. Imagine a room in which the edge of the floor against one wall is the axis for X_1 and the edge where the adjacent wall meets the floor is the axis for X_2. The line from floor to ceiling where these two adjacent walls meet would be the Y axis. Equation 12–1 is a straight line through the three-dimensional space of this room.

What is the advantage of adding the term X_2 to the model? Ordinarily, because cigarette smoking and alcohol consumption are correlated, we might expect that cigarette smoking and alcohol drinking would be mutually confounding risk factors for laryngeal cancer. A stratified analysis could remove that confounding, but the confounding can also be removed by fitting Equation 12–1 to the data. In a model such as Equation 12–1 with terms for two predictive factors, smoking (X_1) and alcohol (X_2), the coefficients for these terms, a_1 and a_2 respectively, provide estimates of the effects of cigarette smoking and alcohol drinking that are mutually unconfounded. Mathematically, there is no limit to the number of terms that could be included as independent variables in a model, although limitations of the data provide a practical limit. The general form of Equation 12–1 is referred to as the *general linear model*.

TRANSFORMING THE GENERAL LINEAR MODEL

The dependent variable in a regression model is not constrained mathematically to any specific range of values. In actual epidemiologic applications, however, the dependent variable might be constrained in various ways. For example, the dependent variable might be FEV_1 (forced expiratory volume in 1 second), a measure of lung function that cannot be negative. As another example, the dependent variable might be the occurrence of disease, which is measured as either *no* or *yes* and is usually assigned a value of 0 or 1. This dichotomy is a highly constrained variable, because only two values are observable, and the estimates would theoretically be constrained to be within the range [0,1]. It is common when using constrained outcome variables to use a transformation to avoid getting impossible values for the dependent variable. For example, the straight line in Figure 12–1 has an intercept of 1.15 deaths per 10,000 person-years. With only slightly different data points, however, it would have been possible to have the line cross the Y-axis at a value less than 0, implying a negative mortality rate for nonsmokers. A negative mortality rate is impossible, but mathematically there is nothing in the fitting of a straight line that confines the line to positive territory.

How could we fit a model for rate data that avoids the possibility of the dependent variable taking negative values? We can transform the data to confine the line to positive territory. One way to achieve that is to fit the straight line to the logarithm of the mortality rate rather than to the mortality rate itself:

$$\ln(\hat{Y}) = a_0 + a_1 X_1 + a_2 X_2 \qquad [12\text{–}2]$$

where $\ln(\hat{Y})$ is the natural logarithm of $\hat{Y}$. In Equation 12–2, the left side can range from minus infinity to plus infinity, as can the right side, but $\hat{Y}$ itself must always be positive because one cannot take the logarithm of a negative number. This equation can be solved for $\hat{Y}$ by taking the antilogarithm of both sides, giving

$$\hat{Y} = e^{a_0 + a_1 X_1 + a_2 X_2} \qquad [12\text{–}3]$$

Equation 12–3 allows only positive values for $\hat{Y}$. On the other hand, to achieve this nicely, we no longer have a simple linear model but an exponential model instead.

Having an exponential model has some implications for the interpretation of the coefficients. Consider again the simple linear model in Figure 12–1. The slope, 0.282, is a measure of the absolute amount of increase in the death rate from laryngeal cancer with each additional cigarette smoked per day. If a similar model were applied to an exposure that was measured on a dichotomous scale, with the "unexposed" condition assigned a value of 0 and the "exposed" condition assigned a value of 1, the coefficient a_1 would correspond to the rate difference between the exposed and unexposed states, which can be determined by subtracting the equation given that a person is unexposed (when $X = 0$) from the equation given that a person is exposed (when $X = 1$).

$$\text{exposed } (X = 1): \quad \hat{Y}_e = a_0 + a_1 X = a_0 + a_1$$

$$\text{unexposed } (X = 0): \quad \hat{Y}_u = a_0 + a_1 X = a_0$$

$$\text{exposed-unexposed:} \quad \hat{Y}_e - \hat{Y}_u = a_1$$

Thus, without any transformation, a_1 can be interpreted as an estimate of the rate difference between exposed and unexposed persons. If, however, we use the logarithmic transformation that is shown in Equations 12–2 and 12–3, we find that the coefficient a_1 in that model is not interpretable as a rate difference:

$$\text{exposed:} \quad \ln(\hat{Y}_e) = a_0 + a_1 X = a_0 + a_1$$

$$\text{unexposed:} \quad \ln(\hat{Y}_u) = a_0 + a_1 X = a_0$$

$$\text{difference:} \quad \ln(\hat{Y}_e) - \ln(\hat{Y}_u) = a_1$$

$$\text{ratio:} \quad \frac{\hat{Y}_e}{\hat{Y}_u} = e^{a_1}$$

Rather, the antilogarithm of the coefficient (which is what you get when you raise the constant e to the power of the coefficient) is the rate ratio of exposed to unexposed persons. Thus, the transformation that provides for the good behavior of the predictions from the model with respect to avoiding negative rate estimates also has an implication for the interpretation of the coefficient. Without the transformation, the coefficient estimates rate differences; with the transformation, the coefficient estimates rate ratios (after exponentiating).

THE LOGISTIC TRANSFORMATION

Suppose that we had data for which the dependent variable was a risk measure. Whereas rates are never negative but can go as high as infinity, risks are mathematically confined to the narrower range, $[0,1]$. For any straight line with nonzero slope, Y ranges from minus infinity to plus infinity rather than from 0 to 1. Consequently, a straight line model without transformation could lead to individual predicted risk values that are either negative or greater than 1. There is a commonly used transformation, however, the *logistic transformation*, that will confine the predicted risk values to the proper range.

It is easier to understand the logistic transformation if we think of it as two transformations. The first converts the risk measure, R, to a transformed measure that ranges from zero to infinity instead of $[0,1]$. This transformation is accomplished by using $R/(1-R)$ in place of R. For values of R near 0, the quantity $R/(1-R)$ will be little different from R, but as R approaches 1, the denominator of the transformed value approaches 0 and the ratio $R/(1-R)$ approaches infinity. Thus, this transformation raises the upper end of the range from 1 to infinity. The quantity $R/(1-R)$ is called the *risk-odds* (any proportion divided by its complement is an odds). The second transformation converts the risk-odds to a measure that ranges all the way from minus infinity to plus infinity. That transformation is the same as the one used previously for incidence rates: one simply takes the logarithm of the risk-odds. The resulting measure, after both transformations, is $\ln[R/(1-R)]$, a quantity that is called a "logit." The two-step transformation is known as the logistic transformation.

The logistic model is one in which the logit is the dependent variable of a straight-line equation:

$$\ln\left[\frac{R}{1-R}\right] = a_0 + a_1 X \qquad [12\text{-}4]$$

Equation 12–4 shows only a single independent variable, but, just as in other linear models, it is possible to add additional independent variables to the model, making it a "multiple logistic" model. What is the interpretation of the coefficient a_1 in this model? For an X that is dichotomous (ie, $X = 1$ for exposed and $X = 0$ for unexposed), the coefficient a_1 is the ratio of logits for exposed relative to unexposed. This ratio is equal to the logarithm of the risk-odds ratio:

$$\ln\left[\frac{R_1}{1-R_1}\right] - \ln\left[\frac{R_0}{1-R_0}\right] = \ln\left[\frac{\dfrac{R_1}{1-R_1}}{\dfrac{R_0}{1-R_0}}\right] = \ln\left[\frac{R_1(1-R_0)}{R_0(1-R_1)}\right] = a_1 \qquad [12\text{-}5]$$

This result means that, in the logistic model, the antilogarithm of the coefficient of a dichotomous exposure term estimates the odds ratio of risks.

$$\frac{R_1(1-R_0)}{R_0(1-R_1)} = e^{a_1}$$

As a consequence of this interpretation for the logistic coefficient, the logistic model has become a popular tool for the analysis of case-control studies, in which the odds ratio is the primary statistic of interest.

CHOICES AMONG MODELS

From a mathematical perspective, the advantages of these transformations are tied to the mathematical behavior of the measures, ensuring that individual estimates from the models conform to the allowed range. From a practical standpoint, however, the transformations dictate what type of measure the coefficients in the model will estimate. If one has risk data and wishes to estimate risk difference, the logistic model will not conveniently provide it will provide odds ratios. If one is using a model to obtain risk estimates for people, it may be important to avoid getting estimates of risk that are negative or greater than 100%, because these are invalid estimates. On the other hand, if the model is being used primarily to assess an overall effect of the exposure from the coefficient in the fitted model, there may be less concern about whether all the individual estimates stay within their allowable ranges and more interest in which effect measure the model can provide. In many epidemiologic applications, it is the choice among effect measures that dictates the type of model the investigator ought to use.

Consider the data in Table 12–1, which describe the risk of acquiring a hypothetical disease over a 5-year period according to the subject's age at the start of the period. Twenty subjects were followed for 5 years, and each either did or did

Table 12–1 RISK
OF DEVELOPING A
HYPOTHETICAL DISEASE
DURING A 5-YEAR PERIOD
FOR 20 SUBJECTS

Subject No.	Age	Disease
1	18	0
2	21	0
3	22	0
4	25	0
5	26	0
6	28	0
7	33	0
8	34	0
9	35	0
10	37	0
11	42	1
12	47	1
13	55	0
14	56	1
15	58	0
16	61	1
17	65	1
18	68	1
19	75	1
20	77	1

not develop the disease. These data are plotted as a scatterplot in Figure 12–2. In a scatterplot with a binary outcome variable that takes values of either 0 or 1, all the observations fall either at 0 or at 1 on the vertical axis. Figure 12–2 also shows the linear regression line through the 20 data points and its equation. The intercept of the regression line is the estimated value of the risk for those with age 0. The value of the intercept is −0.49, an impossible value for a risk. In fact, the line estimates a negative risk for all ages less than 24 years and a risk greater than 100% for all ages greater than 74 years.

One can avoid the inadmissible risk estimates from the regression line in Figure 12–2 by fitting a logistic model instead of a straight line. The logistic model for the same data from Table 12–1 is illustrated in Figure 12–3. Its sigmoid shape is characteristic of the logistic curve. This shape keeps the curve within the range [0,1] for any age, preventing the impossible estimates that come from the linear model in Figure 12–2.

It might appear from a comparison of these two figures that the logistic model is always preferable for risk data, because it cannot result in estimates of risk that are inadmissible (ie, either less than zero or greater than one). This example is presented, however, to make the point that the logistic model is not always preferable. The age coefficient in the straight-line equation in Figure 12–2 is interpretable as a risk difference for each year of age: it indicates that the risk increases by an estimated 2% for each year of age. It is true that the fitted straight

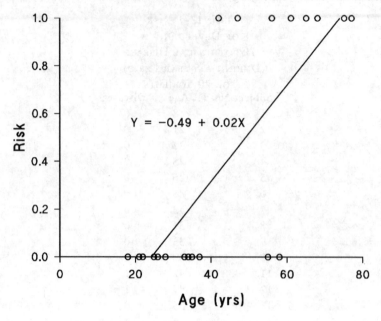

Figure 12–2   Scatterplot of risk data from Table 12–1 and a linear regression line fitted to the data.

line is not expected to fit the data well outside the central region of the graph. Nevertheless, for this central region in the middle of the age span, the straight line provides a simple and useful way of estimating the risk difference for each year of age. In contrast, the logistic model in Figure 12–3 does not permit direct estimation of a risk difference. Instead, it allows estimation of an odds ratio associated with a 1-year increase in age, from the antilogarithm of the logistic coefficient: $e^{0.144} = 1.15$, which is the risk-odds ratio for each 1-year increase in age. Although there is nothing fundamentally wrong with estimating the odds ratio, the straight-line model may be preferable if one wishes to estimate a risk difference. As mentioned earlier, the logistic model is particularly appropriate for the analysis of case-control studies because the odds ratio can be obtained from it, and the odds ratio is the statistic of central interest for estimating rate ratios in case-control studies.

CONTROL OF CONFOUNDING WITH REGRESSION MODELS

One of the principal advantages of multivariable regression models for epidemiologic analysis is the ease with which several confounding variables can be controlled simultaneously. In a multivariable regression model, the inclusion of several variables results in a model in which each term is unconfounded by the other terms in the model. This approach makes it easy and efficient to control confounding by several variables at once, something that might be difficult to achieve through a stratified analysis.

For example, as described in Chapter 10, suppose that you were conducting an analysis with five confounding variables, each of which had three categories.

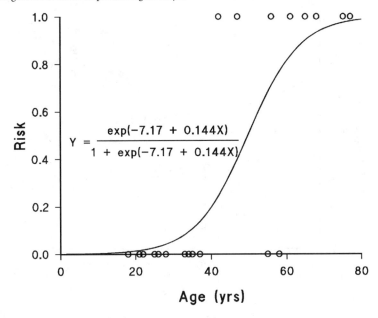

Figure 12-3 Scatterplot of risk data from Table 12-1 and a logistic regression line fitted to the data.

To control for these variables in a stratified analysis, you would need to create three strata for the first variable, then divide each of those three strata into three more substrata for the second variable, giving nine strata, and so on until there are $3 \times 3 \times 3 \times 3 \times 3 = 243$ strata. If any of the variables required more than three categories, or if there were more than five variables to control, the number of strata would rise accordingly. With such a large number of strata required for a stratified analysis to control several variables, the data could easily become uninformative because there are too few subjects within each stratum to give useful estimates. Multivariable regression modeling solves this problem by allowing a much more efficient way to control for several variables simultaneously. Everything has its price, however, and so it is for multivariable regression analysis. The price is that the results from the regression model are readily susceptible to bias if the model is not a good fit to the data.

To illustrate the problem, consider the hypothetical data in Figure 12-4, with data points for exposed and unexposed people by age and by some unspecified but continuous outcome measure. These data show an unfortunate situation in which there is no overlap in the age distributions between the exposed population and unexposed population. If a stratified analysis were undertaken to control for age, there would be little or no overlap in any age category between exposed and unexposed groups, and the stratified analysis would produce no estimate of effect. In essence, a stratified analysis attempting to control for age would give the result that there is no information in the data.

In contrast, in a multiple regression with both age and exposure terms, the model will essentially fit two parallel straight lines through the data, one relating age to the outcome for unexposed people and the other relating age to the outcome for exposed people. If the dichotomous exposure term is coded 0 or 1, at

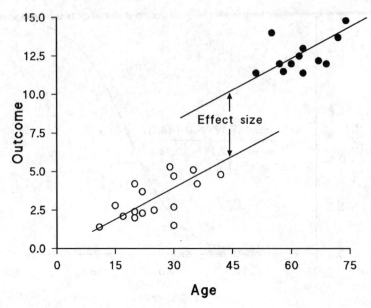

Figure 12–4   Hypothetical example of a multivariable linear regression of outcome data involving a dichotomous exposure variable (exposed = *solid circles*, unexposed = *open circles*) and age.

any age the difference in the outcome between exposed and unexposed is equal to the coefficient for the exposure, which measures the exposure effect:

$$\text{Outcome} = a_0 + a_1 \cdot \text{Exposure} + a_2 \cdot \text{Age}$$

Thus the regression model produces a statistically stable estimate from the nonoverlapping sets of data points. Basically, the model extrapolates the age relation for the unexposed and exposed persons and estimates the effect from the extrapolated lines, as indicated in Figure 12–4. This estimation process is much more efficient than a stratified analysis, which for these data would not produce any effect estimate at all.

But what if the actual relation between age and the outcome were as pictured in Figure 12–5? If age has the curvilinear relation pictured there, there is no effect of exposure on the outcome, and the effect estimated from the model depicted in Figure 12–4 would be incorrect. The apparent effect in Figure 12–4 is simply a bias introduced by the model and its inappropriate extrapolation beyond the observations. Because we cannot know whether the model in Figure 12–4 is appropriate or whether the relation is actually like the pattern depicted in Figure 12–5, the lack of results from a stratified analysis of these data begins to look good compared with the regression analysis, which might produce an incorrect result. Saying nothing is better than saying something incorrect.

Stratified analysis has other advantages over regression analysis. With stratified analysis, both the investigator and the reader (if the stratified data are presented) are aware of the distribution of the data by the key study variables. When examining the output from a multiple regression analysis, on the other hand, the reader

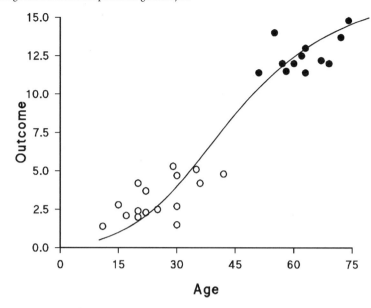

Figure 12–5   A possible age-outcome curve for the data in Figure 12–4 (exposed = *solid circles*, unexposed = *open circles*).

is typically in the dark, and the researcher may not be much better off than the reader. For this reason, a multivariable regression analysis should be used only as a supplement to a stratified analysis, rather than as the primary analytic tool. Unfortunately, many researchers tend to leap into regression modeling without arming themselves first with the knowledge that would come from a stratified analysis. Typically, the reader is also deprived and is presented with no more than the coefficients from the regression model. This approach has the lure of seeming sophisticated, but it is a mistake to plunge into regression modeling until one has viewed the distribution of the data and analyzed them according to the methods presented in Chapter 10.

PREDICTING RISK FOR A PERSON

Much of the advice on how to construct a regression model is crafted for models aimed at making individual predictions regarding the outcome of interest. For example, Murabito et al[3] published a logistic model that provided 4-year risk estimates for intermittent claudication (the symptomatic expression of atherosclerosis in the lower extremities). The model is given in Table 12–2.

To obtain individual risk estimates from this model, one would multiply the coefficients for each variable in the table by the values for a given person for each variable, which gives the logit for a given person. Because the exponentiated logit equals the risk-odds, $exp(\text{logit}) = [R/(1{-}R)]$, the logit can be converted to a risk estimate by taking into account the relation between risk and risk-odds:

$$\text{Odds} = \frac{\text{Risk}}{1-\text{Risk}} \quad \text{or} \quad \text{Risk} = \frac{\text{Odds}}{1+\text{Odds}}$$

Table 12–2 LOGISTIC MODEL TO OBTAIN ESTIMATES
OF 4-YEAR RISK FOR INTERMITTENT CLAUDICATION

Variable	Coefficient
Intercept	−8.915
Male sex	0.503
Age	0.037
Blood pressure	
Normal	0.000
High-normal	0.262
Stage 1 hypertension	0.407
Stage 2+ hypertension	0.798
Diabetes	0.950
Cigarettes/day	0.031
Cholesterol (mg/dL)	0.005
Coronary heart disease	0.994

Thus, the risk can be estimated as $R = exp(\text{logit})/[1 + exp(\text{logit})]$. For example, suppose we wish to estimate the 4-year risk of intermittent claudication for a 70-year-old nonsmoking man who has normal blood pressure, diabetes, coronary heart disease, and a cholesterol level of 250 mg/dL. The logit would be $−8.915 + 1 \cdot 0.503 + 70 \cdot 0.037 + 0 \cdot 0.000 + 1 \cdot 0.950 + 0 \cdot 0.031 + 250 \cdot 0.005 + 1 \cdot 0.994 = −2.628$, and the risk estimate over the next 4 years for intermittent claudication to develop would be $exp(−2.628)/[1 + exp(−2.628)] = 6.7\%$. If the man had stage 2 hypertension instead of normal blood pressure, the logit would be $−1.830$ and the risk estimate would be 13.8%.

In a model such as the one in Table 12–2, the purpose of including each individual term in the model is to improve the estimate of risk. To produce a useful risk estimate, it does not matter whether any of the predictor terms is causally related to the outcome. In the model in Table 12–2, some of the predictors cannot be viewed as causes: age is an example of a noncausal predictor, as is heart disease, which presumably does not cause intermittent claudication, although the two diseases may have causes in common. Nevertheless, despite not being causes of intermittent claudication, both age and the presence of coronary heart disease are good predictors of the risk of developing intermittent claudication; therefore, it makes sense to include them in the prediction model. Other predictors, such as cigarette smoking, hypertension, and diabetes, may be causes of intermittent claudication.

STRATEGY FOR CONSTRUCTING REGRESSION MODELS FOR EPIDEMIOLOGIC ANALYSIS

Although a detailed discussion of the strategy for constructing multivariable regression models for epidemiologic analysis goes beyond the scope of this book, I outline here some basic principles for the use of these models in causal research.

CENTERING OF VARIABLES IN REGRESSION MODELS

The intercept in a regression model is the predicted outcome when all independent predictors equal 0. In a model with one predictor, the intercept is the predicted value when that predictor equals 0. But how can we interpret the intercept when 0 is not a meaningful value for the predictor? For example, suppose we fit a regression that predicts mortality rate according to body mass index (BMI), which is defined as weight in kilograms divided by the square of height in meters. The intercept would correspond to the predicted mortality rate for people with a BMI of 0, which is impossible. In such situations, it is useful to "center" the predictor variable around some central value, such as a BMI of 22 kg/m^2. Centering is accomplished simply by subtracting 22 from each BMI value, so that the new BMI variable is the difference above or below a BMI of 22 kg/m^2. With the centered variable, the intercept corresponds to the mortality rate predicted when BMI is 22 kg/m^2, rather than 0, which is much more interpretable. Centering does not affect the basic interrelationships of the study variables, but it does make it easier to interpret the coefficients, especially when there are product terms in the model that would further complicate the interpretations.

DO A STRATIFIED ANALYSIS FIRST

The first step should always be a stratified analysis. The main contribution of a multivariable regression analysis to causal research is to enable the simultaneous control of several confounding factors. In accomplishing this goal, multivariable modeling ought to be thought of as a supplement to stratified analysis, to be used in situations in which there are too many confounders to be handled comfortably in a stratified analysis. Even is those circumstances, it is common that most of the confounding stems from one or two variables and a multivariable regression model will give essentially the same result as a properly conducted stratified analysis.

DETERMINE WHICH CONFOUNDERS TO INCLUDE IN THE MODEL

Start with a set of predictors of the outcome based on the strength of their relation to the outcome, as indicated from analyses of each factor separately or from a preliminary model in which all potential confounders are included. Then, build a model by introducing predictor variables one at a time. After each term is introduced, examine the amount of change in the coefficient of the exposure term. If the exposure coefficient changes considerably (most investigators look for a 10% change), then the variable just added to the model is a confounder (provided that it also meets the conditions for a confounder described in Chapter 7); if not, it is not an important confounder. To judge the confounding effect in this way, it is essential for the exposure to be included in the model as a single term. For example, if the exposure is cigarette smoking, one might enter a single term that quantifies the amount of cigarette smoking rather than several terms for levels of cigarette smoking. It is likewise important to avoid any product terms that

STEPWISE MODELS IN EPIDEMIOLOGIC ANALYSIS

Stepwise construction of regression models is accomplished by an algorithm that automatically selects which terms to include in the final model. The algorithm typically selects terms based on the level of statistical significance of the coefficient for each term. Stepwise modeling makes much more sense for the construction of a prediction model than for a causal model. As discussed in Chapter 8, statistical testing does not allow us to grasp either the strength of a relation or the precision of an estimate in isolation; it mixes the two. Using statistical significance levels to determine which potential confounders to include in a model is a bad idea, whether it is part of an automatic stepwise algorithm or not, for several reasons. First, the amount of confounding depends on two associations—the relation between the potential confounder and the exposure, and the relation between the potential confounder and the outcome. The coefficient that is tested for significance in a stepwise algorithm evaluates only the latter relation; it ignores the relation between the potential confounder and the exposure. Therefore, this method can result in the inclusion of variables that are not confounding. It can also omit variables that are confounding but for which the relation with the outcome is not "statistically significant."

involve cigarette smoking (or whatever the exposure variable is) at this stage of the analysis.

ESTIMATE THE SHAPE OF THE EXPOSURE-DISEASE RELATION

If the exposure is a simple dichotomy, one can estimate the exposure effect directly from the coefficient of the exposure term after the confounders have been entered into the model. If, however, the exposure is a continuous variable, such as the number of cigarettes smoked daily, the exposure term needs to be redefined after the confounders are entered into the model. The reason for redefining the exposure term is that the single exposure term that was in the model for the purpose of evaluating confounding will not reveal the shape of the exposure-disease relation for a continuous exposure variable. If the model involves a logarithmic transformation, as do most of the models commonly used in epidemiologic analysis, a single term for a continuous exposure variable will be mathematically constrained to take the shape dictated by the model. In a logistic model, the exposure coefficient is the logarithm of the odds ratio for a unit change in the exposure variable. If the exposure is the number of cigarettes smoked daily, the coefficient of a single term that corresponds to the number of cigarettes smoked daily would be the logarithm of the odds ratio for each single cigarette smoked. Because there is only a single term, the model dictates that the effect of each cigarette multiplies the odds ratio by a constant amount. The result is an exponential dose-response curve between exposure and disease (Fig. 12–6).

This exponential shape will be fit to the data regardless of the actual shape of the relation between exposure and disease, as long as the exposure variable is continuous and confined to a single term in a model that uses a logarithmic

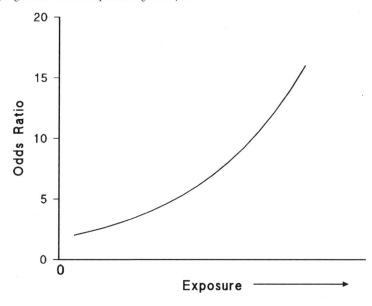

Figure 12–6 Shape of a positive dose-response relation between exposure and disease from a logistic model with a single continuous exposure term.

transformation. In linear models, a linear relation, rather than an exponential relation, will be guaranteed. The problem is that the actual relation set by nature may be nothing like the shape of the relation posed by the model. Indeed, few dose-response relations in nature look like the curve in Figure 12–6.

To avoid this difficulty of having the model dictate the shape of the dose-response relation, the investigator can allow the data, rather than the model, to determine the shape. To accomplish this goal, the investigator must redefine the exposure term in the model. One popular approach is *factoring* the exposure. Factoring here refers to categorizing the exposure into ranges and then creating a separate term for each subrange of exposure, except for one category that becomes by default the reference value. For example, cigarette smoking could be categorized as zero cigarettes per day, 1 to 9 per day, 10 to 19 per day, and so on. The model would have a term for each cigarette-smoking category except 0, which is the reference category. The variable corresponding to each term would be dichotomous, simply revealing in which category a given person fell. Each smoker would have a value of 1 for the smoking category that applied and a value of 0 for every other category; a nonsmoker would have a 0 for all smoking categories. The resulting set of coefficients in the fitted model indicate a separately estimated effect for each level of smoking, determined by the data and not by the mathematics of the model.

Another approach for estimating the shape of the dose-response trend is to use curve-smoothing methods, such as *spline regression*, which allow a different fitted curve to apply in different ranges of the exposure variable.

The important point in evaluating dose-response relations is to avoid letting the model determine the shape of the relation between exposure and disease. Whether one uses factoring, splines, or other smoothing methods, it is desirable to allow the data, not the model, to define the shape of the dose-response curve.

EVALUATE INTERACTION

To evaluate interaction appropriately, the investigator should redefine the two exposures in question by considering them jointly as a single composite exposure variable and entering combinations of the exposures into the model as a factored set of terms. For two dichotomous exposures, A and B, the composite variable would have four categories: exposed to neither, exposed to A but not B, exposed to B but not A, and exposed to both. Each person will fall into only one category of the joint exposure to the two variables. Using *exposed to neither* as the reference category, the model will provide estimates of relative effect for each of the other three categories, enabling the investigator to partition the risk or risk ratio among those with joint exposure to two agents into the four categories described in Chapter 11.[4,5] If one or both of the variables is a preventive rather than a cause, then it should be redefined so that the referent category is the lower risk category of the variable.[6] For more discussion related to the evaluation of interaction, see Chapter 11.

OVERFITTING OF REGRESSION MODELS AND SUMMARY CONFOUNDER SCORES

The great advantage of regression models for epidemiologic analysis is the ability to control simultaneously for several confounding variables. Very often, there is little confounding from most of the potential confounders in a body of data, apart from one or two that exhibit moderate or strong confounding. When it is not necessary to control for more than one or two variables, it is often advisable to present the results of a stratified analysis as the primary findings. With several confounders that all contribute at least moderate amounts of confounding, however, some multivariable regression approach is preferred. In extreme cases, there may be a large number of variables that all contribute substantial confounding, and in some of these situations, it may not be feasible to fit a regression model. For example, in a cohort study with a small number of outcomes, the sparsity of outcomes may pose a problem. One rule of thumb that is commonly cited is that there should be at least 10 or 15 observations for every term in a regression model. With fewer observations than that, the fitted model may be *overfitted*, which means that the model will be too heavily influenced by random error in the data.[7,8]

In most epidemiologic studies, "observations" are equivalent to people, but in many studies, it is not the total number of people that serves as the limiting factor but the number of people with the study outcome. Suppose that you conducted a cohort study in 10,000,000 people aimed at learning about the causes of acute liver failure. This is a large cohort, but because acute liver failure is rare, in 1 year you might observe only 70 cases. This small number of cases is the limiting number for determining how many terms could be included in a regression model without overfitting. With 70 cases, the maximum that the model can reasonably accommodate will be about 7 to 10 terms. The number of variables may be less than the number of terms. For example, if a variable such as age is categorized into 10-year age categories, age alone may require several terms in the model, one for each category apart from the referent category. Therefore, the number of variables that can be accommodated may be quite limited if overfitting is to be avoided.

One way to avoid overfitting is to use a *confounder summary score* to control for confounding. There are two types of confounder summary scores. One is a *disease risk score*. To obtain a disease risk score, a regression model is fitted that predicts disease risk for every person in a study based on the information from confounding factors. Then the actual risk estimates are calculated for each person, and these estimates of risk are added to the data as a new variable. This new variable in theory summarizes the confounding information from all the disease risk predictors that were used to obtain it. In the final stage of the analysis, the investigator only needs to control for one variable, the disease risk score. This control can be accomplished by a stratified analysis, matching, or a regression model that contains no more than the disease risk score along with the exposure variable.[9]

Use of a disease risk score as a confounder summary would not overcome the problem of overfitting if the regression model used to fit the disease risk score contained many confounders and just a handful of people with the outcome, as in the example of acute liver failure. In these situations, another type of confounder summary score may be used. It is an exposure summary score, usually referred to as a *propensity score*. Suppose that the aim of the acute liver failure study is to examine the relation between administration of antibiotics and the development of acute liver failure. To get a summary exposure score, one could fit a regression model that predicts whether each person would receive an antibiotic. Overfitting that model is less of a problem than overfitting a model that predicts risk of acute liver failure: although few people get acute liver failure, many people use antibiotics. From the regression model that predicts antibiotic exposure, one would calculate a propensity score for each person in the study and treat that score as a summary confounder. Then, in the final analysis, the investigator would need to control for only a single variable, the propensity score, which effectively will control for all the component variables used to estimate the propensity score. Because exposures typically are not as rare as many disease outcomes, propensity scores can often be used to control for a large number of confounding factors in a regression model without the difficulty of overfitting the model.

Using a summary confounding score amounts to more work than fitting the typical multivariable regression model, and despite the greater effort it does not always appear to result in substantially better control of confounding.[10] Nevertheless, the use of summary confounder scores, especially propensity scores, is increasing. One reason, as just described, is the ability to control for numerous confounders when there are few outcome events in the data. Another value in using a confounder summary score is the ability to examine the range of confounder scores for all subjects and to exclude outlier subjects who are outside the range common to both exposed and unexposed subjects (a procedure called *trimming*). Suppose one looked at the age distribution of exposed and unexposed subjects and discovered that exposed subjects tend to be older, with the oldest exposed subjects having ages well above those of the oldest unexposed subjects. On the other end of the age distribution, there may be unexposed subjects younger than any exposed subjects. It would be good practice to restrict the age distributions of exposed and unexposed subjects to the range common to both. Doing so would reduce residual confounding by age. The same approach could be used with a confounder summary score, likewise reducing residual confounding (Fig. 12–7). The advantage of trimming the distributions based on a summary confounder score is that one needs to

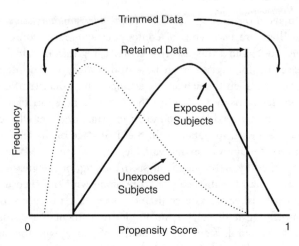

Figure 12–7 Trimming of subjects outside the range of propensity scores that is common to both exposed and unexposed subjects.

trim for only that one variable. Trimming for age may reduce residual confounding by age, but it does not affect residual confounding by other variables. Trimming for several variables may control residual confounding at the price of losing much of the data. Trimming the data once according to a summary confounder score reduces residual confounding much more effectively than trimming by a single variable, and it conserves data by making the trimming process efficient.[11]

There is an important caution to keep in mind when selecting variables for propensity score models. When regression modeling is taught, students are often told that the aim is to put into the model the best predictors of the outcome. That may be true for regression models that are used to make individual predictions. When the purpose of the model is to control confounding, however, as it is in propensity score models, putting in the best predictors of the outcome may be undesirable. Very strong predictors of exposure may or may not be confounders, depending on their relation to the disease. If a strong predictor of exposure is unrelated to the disease, including it in a propensity score regression model will not accomplish any control of confounding. Including such a variable will, however, lead to separation of the exposed and unexposed distributions, as depicted in Figure 12–7, resulting in loss of data that are useful for direct comparison and ultimately resulting in wider confidence intervals. Therefore, it is important to avoid including strong predictors of exposure in a propensity score regression model unless they are also confounders, which means that they are also predictors of disease and that they are not in the causal pathway between exposure and disease.

EXAMPLE OF USING PROPENSITY SCORES: ARE DRUG-ELUTING STENTS BETTER THAN BARE-METAL STENTS?

In pharmacoepidemiology, the use of propensity scores to model the probability of treatment as a summary confounder score has become a dominant method for the control of confounding. This method was employed by Mauri et al[13] in a 2008

VARIABLE MATCHING RATIOS, CONFOUNDING, AND TRIMMING

Suppose you were conducting a cohort study of treated (exposed) and untreated (unexposed) patients in which there was expected to be substantial confounding by indication. Accordingly, you have decided to compute a propensity score for each subject to control for confounding. One option in the data analysis is to match an untreated patient to every treated patient, ending up with two cohorts that are matched by their propensity scores. All of the variables that went into the propensity score model should be adequately controlled in the comparison between the treated cohort and the individually matched untreated cohort. In fact, one can usually demonstrate that the compared cohorts show a balance for all the risk factors that went into the propensity score model, even if they were severely unbalanced before the matching process.[12] Such a demonstration can persuade skeptics that a propensity score model can indeed control effectively for many confounding variables simultaneously. Another advantage of matching is that it automatically achieves the trimming illustrated in Figure 12–7.

Matching one untreated subject to each treated subject comes at a cost, however. Many subjects may have propensity scores that put them in the range to be matched, but simply do not get matched. They are omitted from the analysis, resulting in a loss of information and leading to a wider confidence interval. These subjects could be retained in the study if either a stratified analysis or a regression model were used to analyze the data. Alternatively, the matching could be expanded so that instead of matching only one unexposed person with each exposed person, all unexposed persons who have approximately the same propensity score as the exposed person would be included. Including as many subjects as possible that match on propensity score produces a variable matching ratio rather than a fixed ratio of untreated patients for every treated patient. A variable matching ratio simply means that the ratio of untreated to treated subjects varies across matched sets. A drawback to a variable matching ratio is that one cannot display a simple table that shows the desired balance between all treated and untreated subjects for each of the variables that goes into the propensity score. Such overall balance will result only if the matching ratio is fixed, yielding the same number of unexposed people for each exposed person. A table that demonstrates balance is a useful way to persuade skeptics that use of the propensity score has successfully controlled for all its component variables that could be confounding, but this persuasive demonstration is not possible when the matching ratio varies across matched sets.

Rather than exclude subjects from the study who could have been included simply to obtain a table showing a balance of potential confounders, one might consider using a two-step process: first, select matched pairs (ie, using a fixed matching ratio of 1) to produce a table that shows balance for the individual variables in the propensity score model; second, add back into the data those subjects who could have been matched but were excluded to keep the matching ratio to a value of 1. The first step shows that the propensity score achieves balance between the cohorts, because it uses a fixed matching ratio. The second step expands the comparison group by allowing a variable matching ratio, which avoids the loss of information from those who would have been omitted from the matched-pair analysis.

The above discussion of a cohort study does not apply to a case-control study. For case-control studies, matching on any variable related to exposure induces a selection bias that must be controlled in the analysis (see Chapter 7). Showing balance between cases and controls is no reassurance that the bias has been removed. The different behavior of matching in cohort and case-control studies derives from the fact that the matching in cohort studies is between exposed and unexposed subjects, whereas in case-control studies it is between subjects who have disease (the cases) and those at risk for disease (the controls)—an entirely different phenomenon.

study on the comparative safety of two different kinds of stents. Stents are tubular wire cages used to keep arteries patent after narrowed vessels have been widened by angioplasty. The authors identified adults undergoing stenting at Massachusetts hospitals for acute myocardial infarction during an 18-month period. They then measured the risk of death over the 2 years following insertion of the stent, comparing the risk for patients receiving bare-metal stents and those receiving drug-eluting stents. The latter stents are coated with medication to prevent scar tissue formation within the artery walls. Some previous studies, but not all, had indicated that patients with drug-eluting stents had a greater risk of eventual cardiac complications and death than patients receiving bare-metal stents.

The study by Mauri et al.[13] showed some differences in the characteristics of patients receiving the two kinds of stents. These differences were consistent with the explanation that a greater proportion of those receiving bare-metal stents were treated under emergency conditions. It is possible that drug-eluting stents were more widely used in big referral centers, whereas patients with an immediate cardiac crisis were more likely to be treated at local hospitals that were more likely to use bare-metal stents. Of course, this difference in prognosis would bias the study results unless it could be controlled adequately in the analysis. To attempt to control for these confounding differences, the authors calculated the propensity for each patient to receive a drug-eluting stent rather than a bare-metal stent, and then they matched patients receiving one kind of stent to patients receiving the other kind according to their propensity score.

No analytic method is perfect in controlling for confounding, because of unmeasured confounders or imperfect measurement of identified confounders. Mauri et al.[13] proposed an ingenious way to gauge the effectiveness of control of confounding in their study. The risk of death after a myocardial infarction is highest during the first few days and then declines gradually over time. Based on the mechanism of action, drug elution from a stent is thought to have no effect during the first days after placement of the stent. Therefore, the researchers compared the risk of death among patients receiving the two types of stents during the 2 days following insertion of the stent, a period in which the type of stent should make no difference. If the propensity score model were effective in controlling for confounding, then one would expect to see the same risk of death over the 2 days following insertion for patients receiving drug-eluting versus bare-metal stents. In fact, however, the 2-day risk for those receiving a bare-metal stent was almost double the 2-day risk for those receiving a drug-eluting stent: 1.2% versus 0.7%. This difference indicates that matching on the propensity score did not balance the risk factors that predict death between the two groups of patients.

Unfortunately, Mauri et al. incorrectly focused on the lack of statistical significance of the difference in 2-day risk of death between the two study cohorts. The P value was 0.06, but using statistical significance to assess a difference is a poor approach to interpreting the data, as explained in Chapter 8. In this situation, the authors' mistake was even more profound, because the question at hand was not whether the difference between the cohorts might have been compatible with chance. Rather, the question was the size of the imbalance in risk factors and how much it biased the final results of the study. The authors claimed that their study showed a lower risk of death over 2 years for patients receiving drug-eluting stents. After control of confounding, they found that the 2-year risk of death was 10.7% among patients receiving a drug-eluting stent and 12.8% (20% greater) among those receiving a bare-metal stent. These conclusions, however, ignored the analysis that demonstrated residual confounding, which indicated almost double the risk for short-term death among the bare-metal stent group. If the confounding that was evident during the mortality experience of the first 2 days stemmed from risk factors that persisted over the next 2 years, then we would expect that, from confounding alone, the risk over 2 years would be almost twice as high for patients receiving bare-metal stents as for those receiving drug-eluting stents. Because the risk of death for patients receiving bare-metal stents was in fact much less than twice as high (only 20% higher), one can conclude that these data indicate that it was actually much safer to receive a bare-metal stent, a conclusion opposite to that drawn by the authors.

One problem in this interesting case study was the authors' focus on the P value instead of the magnitude of the risk imbalance that they reported. Another problem surfaced in later published correspondence,[14,15] when the authors suggested that the differences in 2-day risks were unimportant for another reason. They dismissed the greater risk of death over the first 2 days for patients getting bare-metal stents because the risk difference for death over 2 days was 0.5%, small in relation to the difference of 2.1% in the other direction seen over 2 years. The value of a risk, however, is cumulative over the time period for which the risk is measured (see Chapter 4). The risks and the corresponding risk differences for the first 2 days are necessarily smaller than the risks that accumulate over 2 years. Suppose that the patients receiving bare-metal stents had a greater risk over 2 days because they were older than those receiving drug-eluting stents. The age difference would continue to contribute to the risk difference between the two cohorts over the next 2 years, with the cumulative effect being roughly proportional to the period of time. Differences in propensity score would likely work similarly.

To adjust the study findings for the discrepancy seen in the 2-day risk, one would need to project the difference in risk over 2 days to the full 2 years, which requires using the proportionality of the risks as an adjustment factor. Over 2 days, those getting bare-metal stents had a risk that was 73% higher than the risk for those getting drug-eluting stents. Over 2 years, the risk observed in the bare-metal stent group was 20% higher than in the drug-eluting stent group. If the confounding alone would have led to a risk that was 73% higher, it seems that these data indicate that getting the bare-metal stent was considerably safer than getting the drug-eluting stent. After using the ratio of risks over the first 2 days to adjust the risk ratio at 2 years, one can then convert that 2-year risk ratio to a risk difference with some simple assumptions that we will not elaborate here. Using such methods, one can infer that based on the study of Mauri et al.[13] the bare-metal stent patients had an *absolute* risk of death that was actually 4.4% lower over 2 years than that of the drug-eluting stent patients, rather than the 2.1% greater risk the authors reported.

SUMMARY

Regression models are extremely useful in epidemiologic analysis, both for predicting disease risk and for controlling confounding, especially when there are several important confounders that must be controlled simultaneously. Many advanced techniques, which are beyond the scope of this text, rely on different types of regression models in various ways. Nevertheless, there is a case to be made that epidemiologists have demonstrated an overreliance on regression models. As suggested earlier in this chapter, in almost all situations a stratified analysis should be undertaken as a first approach to analyzing the data in an epidemiologic study. If there are several important confounders, it may not be possible for all of them to be controlled simultaneously, but it is rare that there are more than one or two substantial confounders. Even when there are, a stratified analysis can be conducted that will measure and control confounding for each variable singly, a process that informs the multivariable regressions done subsequently. Furthermore, it may be feasible to control for two or three confounders with simple stratification and to get a good estimate of the exposure effect from the tables used for this analysis.

A great strength of a stratified analysis is that the data are revealed for all to peruse. To capitalize on that advantage, when stratified analyses are presented, the researcher should include more than just the summary results. The tables with the stratified data should also be presented. In this way, readers will have access to the key data from which unconfounded effect estimates can be calculated, and this approach keeps everyone well informed about the data. Presenting these tables will lead to fewer mistakes.

Another strength of stratified analysis is that for cohort studies it lends itself more readily than regression models to presentation of exposure-specific rates or risks. For example, one can use standardization to obtain exposure-specific rates of disease from a cohort. From those standardized rates, it is easy to calculate standardized rate differences and rate ratios. In contrast, most regression models are limited to one effect measure and do not offer estimation of exposure-specific rates or risks. Thus, although epidemiologists are taught that an advantage of cohort studies is the ability to measure absolute rates or risks rather than just relative measures, many cohort studies are analyzed and reported using regression models that provide estimates solely of ratio measures, with no information on difference measures or actual rates or risks. This approach negates one of the important advantages of cohort studies. Using stratified analysis as the primary analysis will avert this problem.

In many cases, there will be enough recorded information on variables that have confounding effects so that fitting a regression model will ultimately be useful, after a thorough stratified analysis. The results from the regression model in most situations should be well anticipated by a preliminary stratified analysis. The regression results should be presented in the published work or final report only to the extent that they represent an important refinement of the findings. Rather than being the first analysis and often the only analysis presented, regression models should ordinarily reinforce what has already been shown.

QUESTIONS

1. In a multivariable regression model with a nominal scale variable that has three categories, how many indicator terms would need to be included? In general, for a variable with n categories, what is the expression for the number of terms that would need to be included in the model?

2. The analysis depicted in Figure 12–4 is more efficient than a stratified analysis but also more biased. Why is it more biased?

3. Why is an exponential curve, such as the one in Figure 12–6, not a reasonable model for the shape of a dose-response trend? What would be the biologic implication of a dose-response curve that had the shape of the curve in Figure 12–6?

4. If the age term is removed from the model shown in Table 12–2, what would happen to the coefficients for blood pressure? Why?

5. In a regression model with a continuous exposure variable, why is it desirable to have a single exposure term in the model when evaluating confounding?

6. If we have a continuous exposure variable and use a single exposure term to evaluate confounding, the shape of the dose-response curve for that term will be implied by the model. That imposition can be avoided by factoring the exposure into several terms defined by categories of the exposure. The use of several exposure terms, however, will make it difficult to evaluate confounding. How can we evaluate confounding and also avoid the model-imposed restrictions on the shape of the dose-response curve?

REFERENCES

1. Kahn HA. The Dorn study of smoking and mortality among U.S. Veterans: report on eight and one-half years of observation. National Cancer Institute Monograph 19. US DHEW, Public Health Service, 1966.

2. Rothman KJ, Cann CI, Flanders D, Fried MP. Epidemiology of laryngeal cancer. *Epidemiol Rev.* 1980;2:195–209.

3. Murabito JM, D'Agostino RB, Sibershatz H, Wilson PWF. Intermittent claudication: a risk profile from the Framingham Heart Study. *Circulation.* 1997;96:44–49.

4. Rothman KJ. *Modern Epidemiology.* 1st ed. Boston: Little, Brown; 1986.

5. Assman SF, Hosmer DW, Lemeshow S, Mundt KA. Confidence intervals for measures of interaction. *Epidemiology.* 1996;7:286–290.

6. Knol MJ, Vanderweele TJ, Groenwold RH, Klungel OH, Rovers MM, Grobbee DE. Estimating measures of interaction on an additive scale for preventive exposures. *Eur J Epidemiol.* 2011;26:433–438.

7. Babyak MA. What you see may not be what you get: a brief, nontechnical introduction to overfitting in regression-type models. *Psychosom Med.* 2004;66:411–421.

8. Green SB. How many subjects does it take to do a regression analysis? *Multivar Behav Res.* 1991;26:499–510.

9. Miettinen OS. Stratification by a multivariate confounder score. *Am J Epidemiol.* 1976;104:609–620.

10. Stürmer T, Joshi M, Glynn RJ, Avorn J, Rothman KJ, Schneeweiss S. A review of the application of propensity score methods yielded increasing use, advantages in specific settings, but not substantially different estimates compared with conventional multivariable methods. *J Clin Epidemiol.* 2006;59:437–447.

11. Stürmer T, Rothman KJ, Avorn J, Glynn RJ. Treatment effects in the presence of unmeasured confounding: dealing with observations in the tails of the propensity score distribution—a simulation study. *Am J Epidemiol.* 2010;172:843–854.

12. Seeger JD, Williams PL, Walker AM. An application of propensity score matching using claims data. *Pharmacoepidemiol Drug Saf.* 2005;14:465–476.

13. Mauri L, Silbaugh TS, Garg P, et al. Drug-eluting or bare-metal stents for acute myocardial infarction. *N Engl J Med.* 2008;359:1330–1342.

14. Rothman KJ. Drug-eluting versus bare-metal stents in acute myocardial infarction. *N Engl J Med.* 2009;360:301.

15. Mauri L, Normand S-LT. Drug-eluting versus bare-metal stents in acute myocardial infarction. *N Engl J Med.* 2009;360:301–302.

13

Epidemiology in Clinical Settings

Clinical epidemiology focuses the application of epidemiologic principles on questions that relate to diagnosis, prognosis, and therapy. It also encompasses screening and other aspects of preventive medicine at both the population and the individual level. Therapeutic thinking has been greatly affected by advances in pharmacoepidemiology, an area that has extended the reach of epidemiologic research from the study of drug benefits to that of adverse effects and has led to the burgeoning fields of *outcomes research* and *comparative effectiveness*. Outcomes research marries epidemiologic methods with clinical decision theory to determine which therapeutic approaches are the most cost-effective, whereas comparative effectiveness aims to evaluate the effect of different interventions against one another in a variety of settings.

DIAGNOSIS

Assigning a diagnosis is both crucial and subtle. To a large extent, the process of diagnosis may appear to involve intuition, conviction, and guesswork, processes that are opaque to quantification and analysis. Nevertheless, formal approaches to understanding and refining the steps in assigning a diagnosis have helped to clarify the thinking and solidify the foundation for diagnostic decision making. The basis for formulating a diagnosis comprises the data from signs, symptoms, and diagnostic test results that distinguish those with a specific disease from those who do not have that disease.

The Gold Standard

Diagnosis cannot be a perfect process. Rarely does any sign or symptom, or any combination of them, distinguish completely between those with and those without a disease. Often a diagnosis is considered established when a specific combination of signs and symptoms that has been posed as the criterion for disease is present. A diagnosis meeting this standard may be "definitive" but only in a circular sense, that is, by definition. Another way that a definitive diagnosis can be reached is by expert judgment, often by consensus; but once again this approach makes a diagnosis definitive only by definition. No approach is perfect, and two different approaches to the same disease will not necessarily lead to the same classification for every patient. Nevertheless, even if it is arbitrary, we need to have some definition of disease to use as a "gold standard" by which to judge the findings from individual signs and symptoms or screening tests.

Sensitivity and Specificity

For years, the diagnosis of tuberculosis (TB) has rested on detection of the *Mycobacterium tuberculosis* organism from smears of acid-fast bacilli and from culture, but this method requires 10,000 bacteria/mL and does not distinguish among various mycobacteria. Catanzaro et al.[1] investigated how well an acid-fast smear predicted the diagnosis of clinical TB among patients who were suspected to have active pulmonary TB solely on the basis of clinical judgment. The diagnosis of TB was established by an expert panel of three judges, who used culture information and clinical information according to specific guidelines to classify patients into those who had and those who did not have TB. The distribution by diagnosis and by outcome of the acid-fast smear results is given in Table 13–1.

A total of 338 patients with suspected active pulmonary TB were studied. Of these, 72 (21%) were diagnosed as having it. Among these 72 TB patients, 43 (60%) had a positive smear. This proportion is known as the *sensitivity* of the smear. The sensitivity of a test, sign, or symptom is defined as the proportion of people with the disease who also have a positive result for the test, sign, or symptom. If everyone who has the disease has a given sign or symptom, the sensitivity of that sign or symptom is 100%. It is easy to find signs or symptoms that have high sensitivities. For example, in diagnosing headache, we might note that all patients have heads, making the sensitivity of having a head 100%. Having a head would have a low *specificity*, however. The specificity of a test, sign, or symptom is the proportion of people among those who do not have the disease

Table 13–1 DISTRIBUTION OF PATIENTS WITH SUSPECTED ACTIVE PULMONARY TUBERCULOSIS, BY DIAGNOSIS AND BY RESULTS OF ACID-FAST BACILLUS SMEAR TESTING

	Tuberculosis		
Smear	Present	Absent	Total
Positive	43	22	65
Negative	29	244	273
Total	72	266	338

$$\text{Sensitivity of smear} = \frac{43}{72} = 60\% \quad \text{Predictive Value Positive of smear} = \frac{43}{65} = 66\%$$

$$\text{Specificity of smear} = \frac{244}{266} = 92\% \quad \text{Predictive Value Negative of smear} = \frac{244}{273} = 89\%$$

who have a negative test, sign, or symptom. The specificity of the acid-fast smear test, based on the data in Table 13–1, was 244/266 (92%). The specificity of having a head in diagnosing a headache would be zero, because everyone has a head. The most useful tests, signs, or symptoms for diagnosing a disease are those with both high sensitivity and high specificity. A test with 100% sensitivity and 100% specificity would be positive for everyone with disease and negative for everyone without disease. Almost all tests, however, fall short of providing perfect separation of those with and without disease.

Tests, signs, and symptoms can be used in combination to improve either the sensitivity or the specificity. Suppose test A had a sensitivity of 80% and a specificity of 90% by itself, and test B also had a sensitivity of 80% and a specificity of 90%. If we used the two tests in combination to indicate disease, we might postulate that a positive result on both tests would be required to indicate the presence of disease. If the tests results were independent of each other, then $0.8 \times 0.8 = 0.64$ of all patients with disease would test positive on both, making the sensitivity of the combination 64%, worse than the sensitivity of either test alone. On the other hand, the specificity would improve, because those who are negative for the combination of tests would include all those who tested negative on either test. In this example, 90% of those without disease would test negative on the first test, and among the 10% who did not, 90% would test negative on the second test, making the specificity of the combination $0.9 + (0.1 \times 0.9) = 99\%$. Therefore, requiring a positive result from two tests increases the specificity but decreases the sensitivity.

The reverse occurs if a positive result on either test is taken to indicate the presence of disease. For the example given, 80% of those with disease would test positive on the first test, and of the remaining 20%, 80% would test positive on the second test, making the sensitivity $0.8 + (0.2 \times 0.8) = 96\%$. The price paid to obtain a higher sensitivity is a lower specificity, which would be the proportion of those without disease who test negative on both tests, $0.9 \times 0.9 = 81\%$.

This discussion assumes that the test results are independent, which is rarely the case. Nevertheless, the principle always applies that combinations of tests, signs, and symptoms can be used to increase either the sensitivity or the specificity—one at the cost of the other—depending on how a positive outcome for the combination of tests is defined. This principle is used to detect cervical cancer by a Papanicolaou smear, which has a high sensitivity but a lower specificity. As a result, a Pap smear will detect almost all cervical cancers but has a high proportion of false-positive results. By requiring a sequence of positive Pap smears before taking further diagnostic action, however, it is possible to improve the specificity of the smear (ie, reduce the false-positive results) without compromising by much the already high sensitivity. In recent years there has been improvement on the approach of repeated smears: now, a single cervical smear can be simultaneously tested for the DNA of human papilloma virus, another risk factor for cervical cancer, to improve the sensitivity of a single screen rather than having to rely on repeated Pap testing.[2]

Predictive Value

Sensitivity and specificity describe the characteristics of a test, sign, or symptom in correctly classifying those who have or do not have a disease. *Predictive value* is a measure of the usefulness of a test, sign, or symptom in classifying people with disease. It can be calculated from the same basic data from which we calculate sensitivity and specificity. Consider the TB example in Table 13-1. We can use these data to calculate the predictive value of a positive smear. Among the 65 people with a positive smear, 43 had TB. Therefore, a positive smear correctly indicated the presence of TB in 43/65 (66%) of people who were tested. This proportion is referred to as the *predictive value positive*, or the predictive value of a positive test, usually abbreviated as PV+. We can also measure the predictive value negative, or the predictive value of a negative test, which is abbreviated PV−. In the same data, of the 273 who had a negative smear, 244 did not have TB, making the predictive value negative of the smear 244/273 (89%).

Sensitivity and specificity should theoretically be constant properties of a test, regardless of the population that is being tested, but in practice they can vary with the mix of patients. In contrast, predictive value varies even theoretically from one population to another, because it is highly dependent on the prevalence of disease in the population being tested. We can illustrate the dependence of predictive value on the prevalence of disease by examining what would result if we added to the population described in Table 13-1 500 people who did not have TB. The effect is similar to the change one would find in moving from a clinic serving a population in which TB was common to a clinic serving a population in which TB was less common. The augmented data are displayed in Table 13-2.

Let us assume that the sensitivity and specificity of the test remain the same. We still have 72 people with TB, of whom 43 have a positive smear. We now have 766 people without TB, which includes the original 266 plus 500 additional people who do not have TB. We have assumed that the specificity of the test remains the same, 92%, which means that 703 of the 766 patients without TB will have a negative smear. The PV+ and PV− are considerably different in this second population, however. The PV+ is 43/106 = 41%, much less than the PV+ of 66% for the population in Table 13-1. As the prevalence of disease decreases, the predictive value of a positive test will decrease as well. At the same time, the PV− has changed from 89% in the original data to 703/732 = 96% in the augmented data. As the prevalence of the disease decreases, the PV+ decreases but the PV− increases.

Table 13-2 Results from Table 13-1 Augmented with Data from 500 Additional People Without Tuberculosis

Smear	Tuberculosis Present	Tuberculosis Absent	Total
Positive	43	63	106
Negative	29	703	732
Total	72	766	838

$$\text{Sensitivity of smear} = \frac{43}{72} = 60\% \quad \text{Predictive Value Positive of smear} = \frac{43}{106} = 41\%$$

$$\text{Specificity of smear} = \frac{703}{766} = 92\% \quad \text{Predictive Value Negative of smear} = \frac{703}{732} = 96\%$$

These changes in predictive value with changes in prevalence should not be too surprising. If we tested a population in which no one had disease, there would still be some false-positive test results. The predictive value of a positive test in such a population would be zero, because no one in that population actually had the disease. On the other hand, the predictive value of a negative test would be perfect (100%). Taking the other extreme, if everyone in a population had the disease, then the PV+ would be 100% and the PV− would be zero. Changes in predictive value with prevalence of disease have implications for the use of diagnostic and screening tests. Tests that have reasonably good PV+ in a clinic population of patients presenting with symptoms may have little PV+ in an asymptomatic population being screened for disease. For this reason, it may not make sense to convert diagnostic tests into screening tests that would be applied to populations with a low prevalence of disease.

Screening

The premise of screening for disease is that for many diseases early detection improves the prognosis. Otherwise, there would be no point to screening, because it is expensive both in monetary terms and in terms of the burden it places on the screened population. To be suitable for screening, a disease must be detectable during a preclinical phase by some test, and early treatment must convey a benefit over later treatment (ie, the treatment that would occur after the disease comes to attention without screening).[3] Furthermore, the benefit that early treatment conveys should outweigh the overall costs of the screening. These costs are more than just the expense of administering the screening test to a healthy population. Screening will result in some false-positive tests, saddling those who have the false result with the mistaken prospect of facing a disease that they do not have. Furthermore, a false-positive test usually leads to further tests and sometimes even to treatments that are unnecessary and risky. Another cost comes from false-negative results, which provide false reassurance about the absence of disease. Even for those whom the screening test labels correctly with disease, there is a psychological cost that comes from being labeled earlier in the natural history of the process than would have occurred without screening. Weighing against this cost is the useful reassurance for those who do not have the disease that comes from having tested negative.

For screening to succeed, the disease being screened for should have a reasonably long preclinical phase so that the prevalence of people in this preclinical phase is high. If the preclinical phase is short and people who develop the disease promptly pass through it into a clinical phase, there is little point to screening. In such a situation, the low prevalence of the preclinical phase of the disease in the population will produce a low PV+ for the screening test.

LEAD-TIME BIAS
Because screening advances the date of diagnosis for a disease, it can be difficult to measure its effect. Suppose the disease is cancer. The success of treating cancer is usually measured by the survival time after diagnosis or the time to recurrence. If early treatment is advantageous, one would expect it to result in longer survival

time or longer time until recurrence. After screening, however, survival time and time to recurrence will increase even if the screening and earlier treatment do no good. The reason is that the time of diagnosis is moved ahead by screening, so that the diagnosis is registered earlier in the natural history of the disease process than it would have been without screening. The difference in time between the date of diagnosis with screening and the date of diagnosis without screening is called the *lead time*. Lead time should not be counted as part of the survival time after disease diagnosis, because it does not represent any real benefit. If it is counted, it will erroneously inflate the survival time, a problem known as *lead-time bias*. Lead time can be estimated by comparing the course of disease among a screened population with the course of disease among a similar population that has not been screened.

PROGNOSTIC SELECTION BIAS

In addition to lead-time bias, another difficulty in evaluating the success of a screening effort is bias that comes from self-selection of subjects who decide to be screened. This bias is called *prognostic selection bias*. Because screening programs are voluntary, those who volunteer to get screened will differ in many ways from those who refuse to be screened. Volunteers are likely to be more interested in their health, to be more eager to take actions that improve their health, and to have a more favorable clinical course even in the absence of a benefit from screening. One way to avoid this bias, as well as lead-time bias and the effect of length-biased sampling (see next section), is to evaluate the screening test or program in a randomized trial. In nonexperimental studies, however, these biases are important issues that must be taken into account to obtain a valid assessment of screening efficacy.

LENGTH-BIASED SAMPLING

Another difficulty in measuring the effect of screening comes from *length-biased sampling*, which results from natural variability in the progression rate of disease. To simplify the issue, suppose that breast cancer comes in two types, fast-progressing and slow-progressing. Those with fast-progressing breast cancer have the worse prognosis; their disease goes quickly through the preclinical phase into a clinical phase and spreads rapidly, leading to an early demise for many patients. Slow-progressing breast cancer is more benign, taking many more months or years to progress through the preclinical phase into a clinical phase that also is characterized by slow progression. Women with slow-progressing breast cancer have a better prognosis, even without treatment, although they are also more likely to benefit from treatment.

Let us assume that an equal number of cases of slow-progressing and fast-progressing breast cancer occur in a population. Despite the equal incidence, the prevalence of slow-progressing cases would be greater, because prevalence reflects duration as well as incidence. Thus, more individuals with slow-progressing breast cancer will be in the preclinical phase of disease, because each case takes longer to pass through that stage of the disease process. A screening program, therefore, would tend to identify more slow-progressing cases than fast-progressing cases. Even if early identification and treatment of breast cancer had no effect on the disease, cases identified in a screening program would tend to have a better prognosis than the average of all cases because of length-biased sampling: the screening tends to favor identification of slow-progressing cases, which have a better prognosis.

PROGNOSIS

Prognosis is a qualitative or quantitative prediction of the outcome of an illness. A full description of the prognosis involves not merely the duration of the illness and the timing of recovery or progression but also the nature of the illness as it progresses along its clinical course. Epidemiologic evaluation of prognosis focuses specifically on the measurement in epidemiologic terms of serious sequelae or recovery. The most serious sequela is death, and much of epidemiologic prognostication focuses on the occurrence of death among newly diagnosed or treated patients.

The simplest epidemiologic measure of prognosis is the *case-fatality rate*. Despite the name, this measure is an incidence proportion rather than a true rate. It is the proportion of people with newly diagnosed disease who die from the disease. Strictly speaking, the case-fatality rate should be measured over a fixed and stated time period, such as 3 months or 12 months. Traditionally, however, the measure has been used to describe the clinical course of acute infectious illnesses that progress toward recovery or death within a short time. The time period implicit in the measure is the period of active infection and its aftermath and is often left unspecified. For example, we might describe typhoid fever as having a case-fatality rate of 0.01, paralytic poliomyelitis as having a case-fatality rate of 0.05, and Ebola disease as having a case-fatality rate of 0.75, with each disease having its own characteristic time period during which the patient either dies or recovers.[4] Eventually, of course, all the patients with any disease will die from one cause or another. The presumption of the case-fatality rate is that essentially all of the deaths that occur promptly after disease onset are a consequence of the disease.

For diseases with a long clinical course, it becomes more important to specify the time period over which the case-fatality rate is measured. When it is measured over longer periods, the term case-fatality rate is often not even used. Instead, we use terms such as *5-year survival rate* to refer to the proportion of patients surviving for 5 years after diagnosis. This is simply the complement of the proportion who die during the same period. Beyond a simple incidence proportion or survival proportion, we can derive a survival curve, which gives the survival probability according to time since diagnosis. The survival curve conveys information about the survival proportion for all time periods up to the limit of what has been observed, thus providing greater information than any single survival proportion. (A common method for obtaining a survival curve is the *Kaplan-Meier product-limit method*, which is a variant of the life-table approach described in Chapter 4. The Kaplan-Meier method recalculates the proportion of survivors at the time of each death in a cohort.[5])

The complement and close cousin to the survival curve is the curve that expresses the cumulative proportion of patients who reach a specific end point. Figure 13–1 exemplifies a pair of such cumulative incidence curves. They

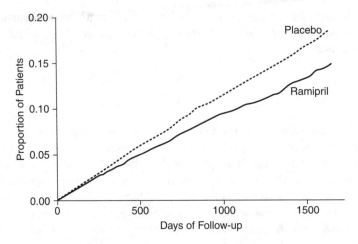

Figure 13-1   Cumulative proportion of patients experiencing a myocardial infarction, stroke, or death from cardiovascular causes, by treatment group. (Adapted with permission from Heart Outcomes Prevention Evaluation Study Investigators. Effects of an angiotensin-converting enzyme inhibitor, ramipril, on cardiovascular events in high-risk patients. *N Engl J Med.* 2000;342:145–153, copyright © 2000, Massachusetts Medical Society. All rights reserved.)

describe the results of a randomized trial that compared the effect of ramipril, an angiotensin-converting enzyme inhibitor, with placebo in preventing the occurrence of myocardial infarction, stroke, or death in patients with certain cardiovascular risk factors.[6] In this example, the curves show the cumulative proportion who experienced any of the end points over a 5-year follow-up period.

THERAPY

It has been said that it was not until the early 20th century that the average patient visiting the average physician was likely to benefit from the encounter. The course of illness today is often greatly affected by the choice of treatment options. The large clinical research enterprise that evaluates new therapies is heavily dependent on epidemiology. In fact, a large part of clinical research is clinical epidemiology.

Clinical Trials

The randomized clinical trial is the epidemiologic centerpiece of clinical epidemiology. Although the clinical trial is but one type of epidemiologic experiment (the others are field trials and community intervention trials), it is by far the most common. (See Chapter 5 for a discussion of the types of epidemiologic experiments.) A full discussion of clinical trials merits a separate textbook; here, I will only touch on some highlights that bear on the interpretation of trial results.

The central advantage of trials over nonexperimental studies is their ability to control confounding effectively. A particularly knotty problem in therapeutics is the problem of *confounding by indication*. When nonexperimental studies are conducted to compare the outcomes of different treatments, confounding by indication can present an insuperable problem. Confounding by indication is a bias that stems from inherent differences in prognosis between patients given different therapies. For example, suppose a new antibiotic shows promise in treating resistant strains of meningitis-causing bacteria but has common adverse effects and is costly. It is likely that the new treatment will be reserved for patients who face the greatest risk of a fatal outcome. Even if the drug is highly effective, the mortality rate among those who receive it could be greater than that among those receiving the standard drugs, because those who get the new drug are at the highest risk. A valid evaluation of the new drug can be achieved only if the prognostic differences can be adjusted or otherwise controlled in the epidemiologic comparison. Nonexperimental studies can deal with such confounding by indication if there is sufficiently good information on measured risk factors for the disease complication that the therapy aims to prevent. Nevertheless, the best efforts to control confounding by indication often fail to remove all of the bias. This problem is the primary motivation to conduct experiments that compare therapies. With the random assignment that is possible in a clinical trial, prognostic factors can be balanced between groups receiving different therapies.

Blinding and Use of Placebos

Blinding refers to hiding information about treatment assignment from the key participants in a trial. The concern is that knowledge of the treatment assignment will influence the evaluation of the outcome. This concern relates most directly to the person or persons who are supposed to make judgments or decisions regarding the outcome. For example, if the outcome is hospitalization for an exacerbation of the disease, the physician who makes the determination about hospitalization might be influenced by knowledge about which treatment was assigned to a given patient. This concern is amplified if the physician has a strong view about the merits of the new therapy. If the physician does not know which treatment the patient has received, then the evaluation should be free of this source of potential bias.

Blinding is not always necessary. If the only outcome of interest is death, there is little reason to be concerned about biased classification of the outcome, because judgment is not an important factor in determining whether someone is dead. In other instances, blinding may be infeasible. If the treatment is an elaborate intervention, such as major surgery, it may be neither possible nor ethical to provide a sham procedure that would allow blinding.

Some trials are described as *double-blind*. This term implies that the evaluator assessing the patient for the possible outcome does not know the treatment assignment, and the patient also does not know the treatment assignment. The person who administers the treatment may also be kept unaware of which treatment is being assigned, in which case the study might be described as *triple-blind*. In all of these situations, the goal is to keep the information about treatment assignment a secret so that the evaluation of the outcome will not be affected.

One method that is often used to facilitate blinding is *placebo* treatment for the comparison group. A placebo (from the Latin, "I shall please") is intended to have no biologic effect outside the offer of treatment itself. Placebo pills typically contain sugar or other essentially inert ingredients. Such pills can be manufactured to be indistinguishable from the new therapy being offered. Other types of placebo treatment involve sham procedures. For example, in a trial of acupuncture, the placebo treatment could involve the application of acupuncture needles at points that are, according to acupuncture theory, not correct. Placebo treatments need to be adapted to the particular experiment in which they are used.

Although a placebo treatment facilitates blinding, that is not the primary reason it is used. It has long been known that even if a treatment has no effect, offering that treatment may have a salubrious effect. An offer of treatment is an offer of hope, and it may bring the expectation of treatment success. Expectations are thought to have a powerful influence on outcome. If so, a new treatment may have an effect that comes only through the lifting of patient expectations. According to some scientists, "The history of medical treatment until recently is largely the history of the placebo effect."[7] The use of a placebo comparison in a trial is intended to distinguish treatments that have only a placebo effect from those that have a greater therapeutic effect. The placebo effect itself is highly variable, depending on the nature of the outcome and the nature of the treatment.

ETHICS OF PLACEBO USE IN RANDOMIZED TRIALS

Only decades ago, it was common for physicians to prescribe placebos so that patients could benefit from improved expectations. Today such practice is rare, and many would consider it unethical. Placebo use continues in randomized trials, however, where the biggest concern is also an ethical one. According to the 1964 Declaration of Helsinki of the World Medical Association,[8] the interests of patients must come before the interests of science and society. Furthermore, every patient in a trial should be assured of getting the equivalent of the best available treatment, even those assigned to the comparison group. Therefore, it is unethical to use a placebo in any trial if there is already an accepted treatment for the condition under study. Instead, an investigator must test a new therapy against the existing standard, to see if it beats the current best treatment.

According to the principles embodied in the Declaration of Helsinki, no researcher should deny a patient the best available treatment solely for the purpose of learning whether a new treatment is better than placebo. Identifying new treatments that are better than placebo but worse than the current best treatment is of less interest than identifying new treatments that are better than the best existing treatment. As medicine progresses, there should be fewer and fewer conditions for which a placebo-controlled study is ethical, because standard therapies that are better than placebo will exist for more and more conditions. Unfortunately, the use of placebos in trials has achieved paradigm status in the minds of many researchers and even official agencies.[9] The paradigm should certainly include a comparison, but not necessarily a placebo comparison.[8,9]

THREATS TO VALIDITY IN TRIALS

Despite the strengths of randomized trials, there are several issues that can lead to biases in assessment. As mentioned, blinding is intended to reduce some of these biases, by reducing opportunities for subjective evaluations to be influenced by knowledge of treatment. Some other sources of bias in trials are incomplete follow-up, intent-to-treat analysis, and confounding imbalances that stem from random assignment.

Incomplete Follow-up

Randomized trials are susceptible to many of the same biases that afflict other types of cohort studies. One source of bias is differential follow-up of the treatment groups. The ideal situation regarding follow-up is for there to be no subjects lost to follow-up, which prevents any bias from this source. In most trials, however, some subjects are not followed to the intended study end point. Reasons for incomplete follow-up are the same ones that occur in other cohort studies, which include subjects moving from the study area, withdrawing their consent to participate in the study, or dying from a disease that is not one of the study end points. If some study subjects are lost to follow-up for any of these reasons, the count of events will be underestimated compared with what it would have been had there been no losses to follow-up.

To deal with this potential source of bias, investigators may analyze the data under the assumption that the experience of those who were lost to follow-up is similar to that of those who remained in the study. This assumption, however, is not always reasonable. For example, subjects with worsening symptoms may be more inclined to drop out of the study than those with a better prognosis. In that case, the risk of the outcome in each treatment group would be underestimated if it were based on the experience of those with complete follow-up. Alternatively, those with the worst prognosis may be less likely to drop out of a study if they believe that they will receive better care by remaining in it. In that case, the study will overestimate the risks of the study outcome, because those dropping out are at lower risk than those remaining in the study. If follow-up is incomplete and is related to both the study intervention and the study outcome, the result is differential loss to follow-up between study groups, a type of selection bias. Differential loss to follow-up can lead to study results that are biased in either direction.

Intent-to-Treat Analysis

As described in Chapter 5, an intent-to-treat analysis is often employed in randomized trials. In this type of analysis, the random assignment at the outset of the trial determines the treatment group in which a subject will be included for the analysis, regardless of whether the subject adhered to that treatment assignment. Therefore, patients who get assigned to a new therapy but for various reasons decide to discontinue it, or never to begin taking it, will still be considered as part of that treatment group for the analysis. This approach maintains the benefits of random assignment for the comparison of a new treatment against an older treatment, but at the cost of misclassification of actual treatment. Those who "cross over" from their assigned treatment to the other treatment group, for example, will be analyzed with their assigned treatment, ignoring the crossover. As a result, the analysis using the intent-to-treat principle incorporates some misclassification of actual exposure. To the extent that the misclassification is independent of the study outcome, the misclassification will be nondifferential and will lead to underestimation of the effect of actual treatment.

Underestimation of the actual treatment effect is often considered acceptable, because it implies that a successful treatment is even better than the value estimated with the intent-to-treat approach. Nevertheless, as mentioned in Chapter 5, adverse effects of a treatment will also be underestimated by this method. This underestimation of risks is a serious drawback to using an intent-to-treat analysis for trials evaluating the safety of a treatment. In such trials, an analysis that classifies subjects according to their actual treatment may be preferred. Because an analysis based on actual treatment would not have all the benefits of a randomized comparison, the usual array of epidemiologic methods would have to be employed to assess and control confounding in the data analysis.

Confounding Imbalances

Baseline risk factors are prognostic factors for the outcome that are measured at the time of random assignment. If randomization succeeds in achieving its goal, the frequency of the outcome will be similar in the various treatment groups created by randomization, apart from the effect of the intervention, because the overall risk for the outcome is balanced between groups. Although there is no direct way to measure whether such a balance in overall prognosis for the treatment groups has been achieved, it is possible to measure the distribution of individual prognostic factors in the compared groups to see how well balanced they are. Any imbalance in a baseline risk factor represents confounding, because a confounding factor is a risk factor that is associated with exposure. To say that a risk factor is imbalanced means that it is not distributed equally in the compared treatment groups and therefore is associated with the assigned treatment.

Randomization is intended to prevent confounding. The outcome of a random process, however, is predictable only if aggregated over many repetitions. In a specific case or in a particular trial, unlikely distributions can result from the randomization. In the University Group Diabetes Program,[10] the group that was randomly assigned to receive tolbutamide was older on average than the group randomly assigned to receive placebo. As a result, there was confounding by age in the evaluation of the tolbutamide effect. This age confounding was illustrated in Chapter 7: the crude difference in mortality proportion between tolbutamide and placebo, ignoring the age imbalance, was 0.045 (Table 7–7), whereas, after stratification into two age strata (Table 7–8), the tolbutamide effect was estimated as 0.035.

Distributions are rarely identical, so how can we tell when the imbalance in a baseline risk factor is severe enough to warrant treating the variable as a confounding factor? If a factor that is severely imbalanced has only a small effect on the outcome, there will be little confounding even with the large imbalance. On the other hand, even a modest imbalance in a strong risk factor for the outcome might lead to worrisome confounding. Therefore, the amount of imbalance in the risk factor is not, by itself, a good guide to the amount of confounding that the baseline imbalance introduces. The best way to assess the confounding is to use the same approach that epidemiologists use in other situations, which is basically the method that was used to compare the effects for tolbutamide estimated in Tables 7–7 and 7–8. Comparison of the crude estimate of effect, which is obtained without control of confounding, with an unconfounded estimate reveals how much confounding is removed when the variable is treated as a confounder (see Chapter 10). It may seem cumbersome that one has to control the confounding to measure how much there is, but no evaluation of the imbalance in the baseline risk factor alone can reveal the amount of confounding, which depends on the interplay between that imbalance and the relation of the risk factor to the outcome.

A common mistake in conducting and reporting clinical trials is to use statistical significance testing to assess imbalances in baseline risk factors. Chapter 8 explains the problems with statistical significance testing in general and suggests that it be avoided. Table 8–3 from that chapter displays the results from a prominently published clinical trial that was misinterpreted because the authors relied on statistical significance for their inference. Use of statistical significance testing for interpretation of the results of a study is undesirable, but it is even less desirable to use statistical significance testing to assess baseline differences in a trial.

Aside from the usual problems with statistical significance testing that are described in Chapter 8, its use in the assessment of baseline imbalances introduces further problems. Perhaps the most obvious problem is that an imbalance in baseline risk factors by itself does not reflect the amount of confounding, as explained earlier. A second problem is that the amount of confounding is the result of the strength of the associations between the baseline risk factor and the two main study variables, treatment (exposure) and outcome (disease). In contrast, the result of a statistical significance test depends not just on the strength of the association being tested but also on the size of the study: for a given strength of association, more data results in a smaller P value. Thus, a given amount of confounding in a large study might yield a statistically significant difference in a baseline risk factor, whereas the same amount of confounding in a small study might not. For these reasons, it does not make much sense to use statistical significance testing to evaluate confounding. Instead, one should simply compare the crude effect estimate with the estimate after controlling for the possible confounder and assess the difference between the two results.

If an imbalance of baseline risk factors is serious enough to induce worrisome confounding into the effect estimate of a trial, how should it be handled? One school of thought holds that any imbalance should be ignored, because the intent of a randomized trial is to compare the experience of the randomized groups, period. According to this theory, one simply hopes that randomization will control successfully for all possible confounding factors, and then one relies on conducting a crude analysis without any control of confounding, no matter what happens after the randomization. The motivation for this view is that if the researcher does control for confounding, problems can be introduced into the analysis that can nullify the benefits of random assignment.

It is true that in an ideal setting randomization will prevent confounding. But if randomization has failed to prevent confounding, the options that the investigator faces are either to rely on a biased comparison of the crude data or to conduct an analysis that controls for the confounding that has been identified. Given the expense and effort of a trial, it makes little sense to ignore confounding that has been identified and thereby risk having the results of the study ignored because critics claim that the study is biased. It makes much more sense to attempt to control for any confounding that has been identified. Critics may still claim that

AN UNREJECTABLE NULL HYPOTHESIS

There is yet another reason why the use of statistical significance testing to evaluate baseline imbalances in a clinical trial makes no sense. If such a statistical test is applied, one might ask what null hypothesis it tests. The answer must be that the null hypothesis is that any observed imbalance is just the result of chance. If a statistically significant result is observed, those who focus on significance testing might take that to mean that the null hypothesis is rejected. In the case of baseline imbalances in a randomized trial, that would mean rejecting the hypothesis that chance produced the imbalances. But we cannot reject that hypothesis! Apart from the possibility of chicanery or incompetence, we know that chance did in fact produce the imbalance: the imbalance is the result of a randomized allocation. Random assignment can produce unusual results, but we already know in a trial that the imbalances that do occur are due to chance. Therefore it makes no sense to test the null hypothesis. Actually, it makes no difference whether the imbalance was caused by chance or not. What matters is that the imbalance exists, and what is important to know is how much confounding it causes. Statistical significance testing cannot reveal that, but the straightforward application of epidemiologic rules for assessment of confounding can.

the randomization has "failed" (although it has not really failed). Nevertheless, the hope that random assignment will prevent confounding has already been defeated if confounding has been identified in the data. The question is how to proceed now that randomization has not prevented confounding.

Some might argue that if an identified confounder is controlled, that process itself can introduce confounding by some other, possibly unidentified factor. Although that is possible, there is no basis to assume that control of a known bias will introduce an unknown bias. Instead, it is more reasonable to control all identified confounders and treat the analysis like any other epidemiologic study.[11,12]

Example: The Alzheimer's Disease Cooperative Study of Selegiline and a-Tocopherol

The question of how to deal with baseline differences arose in a trial[13] of selegiline and a-tocopherol, two treatments intended to slow progression of Alzheimer's disease. The trial followed a factorial design; that is, participants were assigned to groups so that every combination of treatments was studied. In this study with two treatments, there were four groups: one group received only a-tocopherol, one received only selegiline, one received both a-tocopherol and selegiline, and one received a placebo. The mean score on the Mini-Mental State Examination (MMSE) at the start of the trial for the patients randomly assigned to receive a-tocopherol alone was 11.3 on a scale from 0 to 30, whereas the placebo group had a mean score of 13.3 (higher scores indicate better cognitive function). Thus, the random assignment resulted in lower cognitive function at baseline in the group assigned to a-tocopherol compared with the placebo group.

At first the investigators disregarded this difference, and they found that the *a*-tocopherol group had a risk ratio of 0.7 with respect to the occurrence of at least one of several primary end points, including death, institutionalization, and onset of severe dementia. Thus the estimate of the crude effect of *a*-tocopherol indicated a substantial benefit. Adjustment for the baseline difference in MMSE score would be expected to increase the estimated benefit even further, because the *a*-tocopherol group had more signs of dementia to begin with, and this was indeed the case: the estimated rate ratio after adjusting for baseline differences was 0.47, representing an even greater benefit.

These findings were challenged by a correspondent,[14] who claimed that the adjusted results were biased. The critic did not offer a clear rationale for the supposed bias, nor did he discuss its magnitude or direction. When a critic suggests that a result is biased, it is incumbent on that person to quantify the effect of the bias. In this case, the critic implied that the adjusted results should be ignored and that the results from the crude analysis should be used for interpretation. Recall that even the crude effect, with no adjustment for the baseline difference, showed a worthwhile benefit, with a rate ratio of 0.70, indicating a 30% reduction in the occurrence of the primary end-point events. Nevertheless, the critic stated that "no true effect of treatment has been proved," suggesting that *a*-tocopherol had no effect at all. This conclusion was apparently based not on the effect estimate, which showed a 30% reduction in occurrence of the adverse end points, but rather on a lack of statistical significance. This misinterpretation of the findings was aided by the authors of the original report, who themselves placed great emphasis on statistical significance. They also assessed the baseline differences in terms of their statistical significance rather than the amount of confounding that they produced.

In this example, which estimate of effect should be relied on as the best estimate of the effect of *a*-tocopherol on Alzheimer's disease? The crude estimate for the rate ratio is 0.70, and the adjusted estimate is 0.47, but we know that the crude estimate is biased because of baseline differences in the MMSE score. It does not matter what the P value is for these baseline differences, nor exactly how they arose; what matters is the amount of confounding that they introduce. Contrary to what the correspondent asserted, the estimate of the *a*-tocopherol effect after adjustment for those baseline differences contains less bias, not more bias, than the crude estimate of the effect. With adjustment, the estimated benefit of *a*-tocopherol in slowing the progression of Alzheimer's disease is striking. In this example, distrust for an analysis that removed confounding and reliance on statistical significance testing for interpretation wrongly called into question a striking benefit.

Pharmacoepidemiology

Drug epidemiology, also known as *pharmacoepidemiology*, is an active area of epidemiologic research that focuses on the effectiveness and safety of therapeutic drugs and devices. Although randomized trials are, strictly speaking, under the umbrella of pharmacoepidemiology, this discipline is commonly thought to comprise nonexperimental research on drugs and devices. Safety studies are often nonexperimental, because adverse effects are typically much less common than the intended effects of drugs, and the randomized trials that are conducted to evaluate the efficacy of new drugs are seldom large enough to provide an adequate assessment of drug safety. Consequently, most of the epidemiologic information on drug safety comes from studies that are conducted after a drug is marketed.

This research activity is usually referred to as *postmarketing surveillance*. Much of it is not surveillance in the traditional sense; instead, it is based on discrete studies aimed at evaluating specific hypotheses. In the United States, however, the Food and Drug Administration (FDA) encourages the voluntary reporting of suspected adverse drug effects. These *spontaneous reports* are challenging to interpret. First, only a small, but unknown, proportion of suspected adverse drug effects are reported spontaneously; presumably, unexpected deaths, liver or kidney failure, and other serious events are more likely to be reported than skin rashes, but even so it is widely believed that only a small fraction of serious events are reported spontaneously. Second, it is difficult to know whether the number of spontaneously reported exposed cases, who represent only one cell in a 2 × 2 table of exposure versus disease, represent an actual excess of exposed cases or just the number that chance would predict.

Case reports such as those submitted to the FDA as part of their surveillance effort are presumed to represent cases that are attributed to a given drug exposure; that is, the reporting process requires the reporter to make an inference about whether a specific drug exposure caused the adverse event. Although this type of inference is encouraged in clinical practice, it runs counter to the thinking that prevails in an epidemiologic study. As discussed in Chapter 3, it is not possible to infer logically whether a specific factor was the cause of an observed event. We can only theorize about the causal connection and test our theories with data.

Epidemiologists typically collect data from many people before making inferences about a causal connection, and we usually do not apply the inference to any specific person. If a person receives a drug and promptly dies of anaphylactic shock, a causal inference about the connection between the drug and the death may appear strong; but many inferences for individual events are tenuous, based more on conviction than anything else. The danger of thinking in terms of causal inferences in regard to individuals is that if this approach is applied to epidemiologic data, it defeats the validity of the epidemiologic process. If case inclusion in any epidemiologic evaluation takes into account information on exposure, it is apt to lead to biases. Instead, disease should be defined on the basis of criteria that have nothing to do with exposure, and the inferences in an epidemiologic study should relate to the general causal theory rather than what happened to any single person.

One way in which this problem can get out of hand is if a disease is defined in terms of an exposure. Once that occurs, a valid epidemiologic evaluation may be impossible. Consider the example of "analgesic nephropathy." This "disease" refers to kidney failure that is supposedly induced by the effect of analgesic drugs, based on the theory that analgesic drugs cause kidney failure in some people. Although there may be no reason to doubt the theory, if it is applied by defining cases of analgesic nephropathy to be kidney failure in people who have taken analgesics for a specified time, it will be impossible to evaluate epidemiologically the relation of analgesics to kidney failure. A valid evaluation would require that kidney failure be defined and diagnosed on the basis of disease-related criteria alone, with information about analgesic use excluded from the disease definition and diagnosis. Even if the disease is not called analgesic nephropathy, as long as the information on analgesic use is taken into account in making the diagnosis, an epidemiologic evaluation of the relation between analgesics and kidney failure will be biased.

WHEN THE DISEASE DEFINITION INCLUDES AN EXPOSURE

It is not only in the epidemiologic study of drugs that one encounters disease definitions that refer to exposures. If a clear understanding of a causal relation exists, it is a natural tendency to refine the definition of disease to reflect this insight. On the other hand, if the "insight" is only a presumption that a researcher would like to study, it is essential to apply disease definitions that are independent of the exposure. The following is a list of some examples of diseases defined on the basis of an exposure. (Most infectious diseases, such as syphilis, malaria, and influenza, could also be included.)

- Analgesic nephropathy
- Asbestosis
- Berylliosis
- Food poisoning
- Frostbite
- Heatstroke
- Hypervitaminosis D
- Iron-deficiency anemia
- Motion sickness
- Protein-calorie malnutrition
- Radiation sickness
- Silicosis
- Smoker's cough
- Strep throat
- Tennis elbow
- Tuberculosis

Much of the work in pharmacoepidemiology today is conducted using health databases, which allow investigators to design studies from computerized files that include information on drug prescriptions, demographic factors, and health data from medical records or from claims that deal with reimbursement. The Boston Collaborative Drug Surveillance Program was a pioneering effort in pharmacoepidemiology, starting with hospital-based interviews of inpatients using nurse monitors.[15] As the medical world gradually became more computerized, this work and that of other pharmacoepidemiologists evolved to use data that were already entered into computers as part of the record-keeping system, such as in some private prepaid health plans in the United States and in governmental plans such as that of the province of Saskatchewan in Canada. Pharmacoepidemiology is now an active field of research that has established itself as a separate specialty area with its own textbooks.[16,17]

HEALTH OUTCOMES RESEARCH

Health outcomes research and the related field of pharmacoeconomics are comparatively new research areas with lofty goals. Randomized trials and other medical research studies typically focus on a primary end point, such as survival or disease recurrence. Therapeutic evaluations based on narrowly defined end points have been subject to the criticism that they do not adequately take into account the overall quality of life that patients face based on the combination of therapeutic outcomes and unintended effects that a given treatment produces. Furthermore, classic therapeutic research typically does not take into account the economic costs of different therapeutic options. The economic costs are borne either directly by the patient or insurers or indirectly by the government and thus by society as a whole. In either case, there is strong motivation to find therapies that offer desirable results for patients at costs that are attractive to patients or society relative to the therapeutic alternatives. These are the goals that health outcomes research and pharmacoeconomics address, using methods such as meta-analysis, cost-effectiveness analysis, decision analysis, and sensitivity analysis in addition to more traditional epidemiologic methods. The interested reader should consult the text by Petitti[18] for a comprehensive overview.

QUESTIONS

1. Predictive value depends on disease prevalence, but sensitivity and specificity do not. What might cause the sensitivity and specificity of a test to vary from one population to another?

2. Suppose that you wished to conduct a prospective cohort study to evaluate the benefits of prostate-specific antigen testing as a screening tool for prostate cancer. What outcome would most interest you? What biases would affect the study results? Would these biases also affect the results of a randomized trial?

3. Because everyone eventually dies, why would we not say that the case-fatality rate among patients with any disease is 100%?

4. Under what conditions might one find that the baseline difference in a variable in a clinical trial is "statistically significant" but, nevertheless, not confounding? Under what conditions might we find that the baseline difference is not "statistically significant" but, nevertheless, is confounding?

5. The Alzheimer's disease cooperative trial manifested confounding by MMSE score. If the trial were repeated, would you expect that this same risk factor would be confounding again?

6. Equipoise is a state of genuine uncertainty as to which of two treatments is better. Ethicists consider equipoise to be an ethical requirement for

conducting a randomized therapeutic trial: if the researcher is already of the view that one treatment is better than the other, it would be unethical for that researcher to assign patients to the treatment that he or she believes is inferior. Under what conditions can equipoise be achieved in a placebo-controlled trial?

REFERENCES

1. Catanzaro A, Perry S, Clarridge JE, et al. The role of clinical suspicion in evaluating a new diagnostic test for active tuberculosis: results of a multicenter prospective trial. *JAMA*. 2000;283:639–645.

2. Manos MM, Kinney WK, Hurley LB, et al. Identifying women with cervical neoplasia: using human papillomavirus DNA testing for equivocal Papanicolaou results. *JAMA*. 1999;281:1605–1610.

3. Cole P, Morrison AS. Basic issues in population screening for cancer. *J Natl Cancer Inst*. 1980;64:1263–1272.

4. Chin JE, ed. *Control of Communicable Diseases Manual*. 17th ed. Washington, DC: American Public Health Association; 2000.

5. Rothman KJ, Greenland S, Lash TL. *Modern Epidemiology*. 3rd ed. Philadelphia: Lippincott Williams & Wilkins; 2008:42–43.

6. Heart Outcomes Prevention Evaluation Study Investigators. Effects of an angiotensin-converting-enzyme inhibitor, ramipril, on cardiovascular events in high-risk patients. *N Engl J Med*. 2000;342:145–153.

7. Shapiro AK, Shapiro E. The placebo: is it much ado about nothing? In: Harrington A, ed. *The Placebo Effect: An Interdisciplinary Exploration*. Cambridge, MA: Harvard University Press; 1997:19.

8. World Medical Association. *Declaration of Helsinki*. http://www.wma.net/en/30publications/10policies/b3/. Accessed October 21, 2011.

9. Rothman KJ, Michels KB. The continuing unethical use of placebo controls. *N Engl J Med*. 1994;331:394–398.

10. University Group Diabetes Program. A study of the effects of hypoglycemic agents on vascular complications in patients with adult onset diabetes. *Diabetes*. 1970;19(suppl 2):747–830.

11. Rothman KJ. Epidemiologic methods in clinical trials. *Cancer*. 1977;39:1771–1775.

12. Friedman LM, Furberg CD, DeMets DL. *Fundamentals of Clinical Trials*. 3rd ed. St. Louis, MO: Mosby; 1996:297–302.

13. Sano M, Ernesto C, Thomas RG, et al. A controlled trial of selegiline, alpha-tocopherol, or both as treatment for Alzheimer's disease. *N Engl J Med*. 1997;336:1216–1222.

14. Pincus MM. Alpha-tocopherol and Alzheimer's disease [Letter to the editor]. *N Engl J Med*. 1997;337–572.

15. Allen MD, Greenblatt DJ. Role of nurse and pharmacist monitors in the Boston Collaborative Drug Surveillance Program. *Drug Intell Clin Pharm*. 1975;9:648–654.

16. Hartzema AG, Porta MS, Tilson HH. *Pharmacoepidemiology: An Introduction*. Cincinnati, OH: Harvey Whitney Books; 1998.

17. Strom BL. *Pharmacoepidemiology*. New York: John Wiley & Sons; 2000.

18. Petitti DB. *Meta-analysis, Decision Analysis and Cost-effectiveness Analysis*. New York: Oxford University Press; 2000.

Appendix P VALUES CORRESPONDING TO VALUES OF THE STANDARD NORMAL DISTRIBUTION (χ OR Z) RANGING FROM 0.00 TO 3.99

χ Value in Hundredths

χ Value in Tenths	0.00	0.01	0.02	0.03	0.04	0.05	0.06	0.07	0.08	0.09
0.0	1.000000	0.992021	0.984043	0.976067	0.968093	0.960122	0.952156	0.944194	0.936237	0.928287
0.1	0.920344	0.912409	0.904483	0.896566	0.888660	0.880765	0.872881	0.865010	0.857152	0.849309
0.2	0.841480	0.833668	0.825871	0.818092	0.810330	0.802587	0.794864	0.787160	0.779477	0.771816
0.3	0.764177	0.756561	0.748968	0.741400	0.733856	0.726339	0.718847	0.711382	0.703945	0.696536
0.4	0.689156	0.681806	0.674485	0.667196	0.659937	0.652710	0.645516	0.638355	0.631227	0.624134
0.5	0.617075	0.610051	0.603063	0.596112	0.589197	0.582319	0.575479	0.568678	0.561914	0.555190
0.6	0.548506	0.541862	0.535258	0.528694	0.522172	0.515692	0.509254	0.502858	0.496504	0.490194
0.7	0.483927	0.477704	0.471525	0.465390	0.459300	0.453254	0.447254	0.441300	0.435391	0.429528
0.8	0.423711	0.417940	0.412216	0.406539	0.400908	0.395325	0.389789	0.384300	0.378859	0.373466
0.9	0.368120	0.362822	0.357572	0.352371	0.347217	0.342112	0.337055	0.332046	0.327086	0.322174
1.0	0.317310	0.312495	0.307728	0.303010	0.298340	0.293718	0.289144	0.284619	0.280142	0.275713
1.1	0.271332	0.266999	0.262714	0.258476	0.254286	0.250144	0.246048	0.242001	0.238000	0.234046
1.2	0.230139	0.226279	0.222465	0.218697	0.214975	0.211299	0.207669	0.204084	0.200545	0.197050
1.3	0.193601	0.190196	0.186835	0.183518	0.180245	0.177016	0.173830	0.170687	0.167586	0.164528
1.4	0.161513	0.158539	0.155607	0.152717	0.149867	0.147058	0.144290	0.141561	0.138873	0.136224
1.5	0.133614	0.131043	0.128511	0.126016	0.123560	0.121141	0.118760	0.116415	0.114106	0.111834
1.6	0.109598	0.107398	0.105232	0.103101	0.101005	0.098943	0.096914	0.094919	0.092957	0.091028
1.7	0.089131	0.087266	0.085432	0.083630	0.081859	0.080118	0.078407	0.076727	0.075076	0.073454
1.8	0.071860	0.070295	0.068759	0.067250	0.065768	0.064313	0.062885	0.061483	0.060108	0.058758
1.9	0.057433	0.056133	0.054858	0.053606	0.052379	0.051176	0.049995	0.048838	0.047703	0.046591
2.0	0.045500	0.044431	0.043383	0.042356	0.041350	0.040364	0.039398	0.038452	0.037525	0.036617
2.1	0.035728	0.034858	0.034006	0.033171	0.032354	0.031555	0.030772	0.030006	0.029257	0.028524
2.2	0.027806	0.027105	0.026418	0.025747	0.025090	0.024449	0.023821	0.023207	0.022607	0.022021

2.3	0.021448	0.020888	0.020340	0.019806	0.019283	0.018773	0.018274	0.017788	0.017312	0.016848
2.4	0.016395	0.015952	0.015520	0.015098	0.014687	0.014285	0.013893	0.013511	0.013138	0.012774
2.5	0.012419	0.012073	0.011735	0.011406	0.011085	0.010772	0.010467	0.010170	0.009880	0.009597
2.6	0.009322	0.009054	0.008793	0.008538	0.008290	0.008049	0.007814	0.007585	0.007362	0.007145
2.7	0.006934	0.006728	0.006528	0.006333	0.006144	0.005959	0.005780	0.005605	0.005436	0.005270
2.8	0.005110	0.004954	0.004802	0.004654	0.004511	0.004372	0.004236	0.004104	0.003976	0.003852
2.9	0.003731	0.003614	0.003500	0.003389	0.003282	0.003177	0.003076	0.002978	0.002882	0.002789
3.0	0.002699	0.002612	0.002527	0.002445	0.002365	0.002288	0.002213	0.002140	0.002070	0.002001
3.1	0.001935	0.001870	0.001808	0.001748	0.001689	0.001632	0.001577	0.001524	0.001472	0.001422
3.2	0.001374	0.001327	0.001282	0.001238	0.001195	0.001154	0.001114	0.001075	0.001038	0.001002
3.3	0.000966	0.000933	0.000900	0.000868	0.000837	0.000808	0.000779	0.000751	0.000724	0.000698
3.4	0.000674	0.000649	0.000626	0.000603	0.000581	0.000560	0.000540	0.000520	0.000501	0.000483
3.5	0.000465	0.000448	0.000431	0.000415	0.000400	0.000385	0.000370	0.000357	0.000343	0.000330
3.6	0.000318	0.000306	0.000294	0.000283	0.000272	0.000262	0.000252	0.000242	0.000233	0.000224
3.7	0.000215	0.000207	0.000199	0.000191	0.000184	0.000176	0.000170	0.000163	0.000156	0.000150
3.8	0.000144	0.000139	0.000133	0.000128	0.000123	0.000118	0.000113	0.000108	0.000104	0.000100
3.9	0.000096	0.000092	0.000088	0.000084	0.000081	0.000078	0.000074	0.000072	0.000068	0.000066